A Physiotherapist's Guide to Understanding and Managing ME/CFS

A Physiotherapist's Guide to
UNDERSTANDING
and MANAGING
ME/CFS

Karen Leslie, Michelle Bull,
Nicola Clague-Baker,
Natalie Hilliard

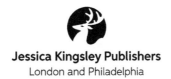

Jessica Kingsley Publishers
London and Philadelphia

First published in Great Britain in 2023 by Jessica Kingsley Publishers
An imprint of John Murray Press

2

A CIP catalogue record for this title is available from the
British Library and the Library of Congress

ISBN 978 1 83997 143 3
eISBN 978 1 83997 144 0

Printed and bound by CPI Group (UK) Ltd, Croydon, CR0 4YY

Jessica Kingsley Publishers' policy is to use papers that are natural, renewable and recyclable products and made from wood grown in sustainable forests. The logging and manufacturing processes are expected to conform to the environmental regulations of the country of origin.

Jessica Kingsley Publishers
Carmelite House
50 Victoria Embankment
London EC4Y 0DZ

www.jkp.com

John Murray Press
Part of Hodder & Stoughton Limited
An Hachette UK Company

Acknowledgements

The authors are grateful to have received commentary and feedback from selected specialists prior to publication, and extend their deepest thanks to:

Dr Charles Shepherd, MB BS, Medical Adviser, the ME Association
Dr Todd E Davenport, PT, DPT, MPH, OCS, Scientific Advisor to
    the Workwell Foundation and Professor in the Department of
    Physical Therapy, University of the Pacific, California
Andrew Kewley

They would also like to thank Ben Howell for his input in collating the appendix of medications.

The specific experiences of a group of people with ME/CFS have been used to create case studies and illustrate the clinical information in each chapter, and the authors thank these people for providing their stories and lending us their valuable voices.

The publication of this book will provide vital education to physiotherapists across the world, and we are extremely grateful to Claire Wilson from Jessica Kingsley Publishers for the opportunity and her support in the process.

Finally, the authors would like to extend special thanks to people living with ME/CFS, who continue to support, inspire and inform us. Their generosity to use their time and energy to contribute to our research and share their knowledge and experiences has been invaluable to the work of Physios for ME and the production of this book.

Contents

Section 3: Physiotherapy Assessment and Management of ME/CFS

Section 4: Case Studies

About this Book

Purpose of this book

Myalgic encephalomyelitis (ME) or chronic fatigue syndrome (CFS) is a debilitating condition that causes a profound intolerance to exertion and significant disability.

The aim of this book is to educate physiotherapists about ME/CFS so they can provide safe and appropriate care. A key priority is to reduce the risk of physiotherapy interventions inadvertently causing adverse effects to a person with ME/CFS.

The book also aims to empower physiotherapists to utilize their skillset to improve the quality of care for people with ME/CFS so that people with ME/CFS can feel confident in seeking physiotherapy advice and support.

Who is this book for?

This book is for all physiotherapists regardless of their speciality, because ME/CFS can involve dysfunction across multiple systems including neurological, musculoskeletal, cardiovascular, endocrine, gastrointestinal and immune. The nature and severity of symptoms can differ considerably between each individual.

The hallmark feature of ME/CFS is post exertional malaise (PEM) where exertion causes additional symptoms and/or an exacerbation of current symptoms. Exertion may be physical, cognitive, sensory or emotional. Physiotherapy interventions and interactions can be a trigger for PEM, which is why all physiotherapists should have an awareness of ME/CFS and how they can adapt their practice to avoid causing PEM, irrespective of the reason for the intervention.

A physiotherapist may see someone with ME/CFS in any setting, whether it is to directly address symptoms caused by ME/CFS, or for a completely unrelated matter. This book is particularly relevant for physiotherapists who work in:

- ME/CFS specialist centres
- Long Covid clinics
- fatigue services
- musculoskeletal services
- neurological rehabilitation
- acute services
- community services
- paediatrics
- rheumatology
- pain services
- orthopaedics
- palliative care
- respiratory care
- cardiology.

It is important to recognize that any type of physiotherapy intervention or interaction may inadvertently cause a worsening of symptoms for a person with ME/CFS.

How to use this book

This book is not a treatment manual for ME/CFS. Any management plan for a person with ME/CFS should be individualized, monitored and regularly evaluated.

This book can be read in order or used as a reference guide. The first section provides information on ME/CFS in general, a brief overview of common co-morbidities, and chapters on specific presentations in people with severe and very severe ME/CFS, children and young people, and acute post viral conditions including discussion of COVID-19 and Long Covid.

The second section takes key symptoms of ME/CFS and explores them in more detail, including a discussion of the current evidence base for management options and treatment. Every symptom may not be experienced by every person with ME/CFS, so this section may provide a helpful reference point for symptoms as and when a physiotherapist may encounter them.

The third section discusses general management principles for physiotherapists, with an overview of assessment and outcome measures, and more in-depth exploration of energy management, heart rate monitoring and exercise.

The final section of this book presents practical examples of different personal experiences of ME/CFS, which demonstrate how the information provided must be individualized when applied to practice.

Limitations of this book

Some underlying physiology of ME/CFS requires a level of understanding of biochemistry and immunology that is beyond the standards required for most physiotherapy practice. Where necessary, information has been simplified or condensed to provide the most relevance for direct application to clinical practice. A physiotherapist with specialist knowledge or interest in these areas may wish to explore the source papers for a more in-depth understanding.

Wherever possible the information in this book is solely based on current evidence, with appropriate critical appraisal to further analysis and understanding. While the authors have made every effort to create a balanced reference guide we acknowledge that there are several limitations of this book in relation to the evidence base:

- There are many areas in which the evidence base is lacking or of poor quality. Such limited research means there are still many 'unknowns' about physiological processes and appropriate management, including physiotherapy. More high quality research in all areas is urgently needed.
- The authors conducted a thorough search of the literature, critically appraised the identified evidence and sought external review to ensure a balanced and comprehensive presentation of the evidence base. However, it is acknowledged that there is always a risk of bias in study selection and level of appraisal.
- The evidence base will continue to evolve up to and beyond the publication of this book, so physiotherapists are encouraged to continue their professional development by conducting literature searches to find the most recent research relevant to the area they are addressing.
- Many areas of physiotherapy management and adaptations

to practice have not yet been explored in research, therefore the authors have had to utilize their own clinical experience, alongside years of collecting feedback from people with ME/CFS. Physiotherapists are responsible for their own clinical practice and must use their own clinical reasoning skills when applying anything to practice. It is important to recognize that management of a person with ME/CFS should be individualized, monitored and regularly evaluated.

Finally, what is reported in research does not always capture or represent the lived experience of a person with ME/CFS. In order to address this problem each chapter will include personal commentary from people with ME/CFS. Their stories give relevance to the objective clinical information and act as a reminder that behind the complex physiology and diverse systemic dysfunction there are individual people experiencing devastating repercussions from this condition.

The lived experience of ME/CFS

This book uses comments and experiences of different people living with ME/CFS throughout each chapter to give relevance to the clinical information provided. Each person is then presented at the end of the book with assessment and management notes written from the treating physiotherapist's perspective to demonstrate how the information in this book can be applied to clinical practice.

While names and identifying information have been changed, they are all real people living with ME/CFS.

Kim, aged 56

Kim has had varying degrees of ME/CFS for over thirty years. The severity of her symptoms have fluctuated between mild and moderate, but became severe following COVID-19 infection.

Oliver, aged 14

Oliver has had ME/CFS since he was 12 years old. He never fully recovered from a viral infection, then suffered a major relapse after playing football and is now unable to attend school.

Mo, aged 37

Mo has been struggling with severe fatigue, cognitive dysfunction and widespread pain since infection with COVID-19 over a year ago.

Ana, aged 53

Ana has had severe or very severe ME/CFS for over twenty years. She experiences regular relapses that leave her completely bedbound and requiring continuous care for all aspects of daily living.

Faith, aged 42

Faith has had ME/CFS for ten years following a viral infection, with symptoms that fluctuate between moderate and severe. Faith has to balance her energy management with the demands of family life.

About the authors

This book has been written by four physiotherapists based in the United Kingdom, who formed the advocacy and education group 'Physios for ME' in 2019. Collectively the team has over 80 years of physiotherapy experience and has worked with people with ME/CFS and acute post viral illnesses both clinically and on a personal level.

The team has experience and qualifications in physiotherapy, sport and exercise science, physical activity, research, teaching, journalism and media communications. Their drive is to improve physiotherapy practice for people with ME/CFS and identify the benefits that this profession has to offer through high quality research.

This book has been written by:

Karen Leslie, BSc(hons) Physiotherapy, BA(hons) Journalism Studies, Chartered Physiotherapist, Co-Founder of Physios for ME

Dr Michelle Bull, DHRes, MSc, GradDipPhys, Chartered Physiotherapist, Co-Founder of Physios for ME

Dr Nicola Clague-Baker, PhD, MPhil, BA(hons) Sports Studies, GradDipPhys, PgCAPHE, SFHEA, Chartered Physiotherapist, Co-Founder of Physios for ME

Natalie Hilliard, BSc(hons) Physiotherapy, BSc(hons) Sports Science, Chartered Physiotherapist, Co-Founder of Physios for ME

SECTION 1

UNDERSTANDING ME/CFS

CHAPTER 1

What Is ME/CFS?

PURPOSE OF THIS CHAPTER

Myalgic encephalomyelitis (ME), or chronic fatigue syndrome (CFS), is a chronic multi-system disease (1) that is serious, systemic and profoundly affects quality of life (2). ME/CFS can have a greater impact on function and quality of life than other chronic health conditions such as heart disease, osteoarthritis, rheumatoid arthritis, diabetes and cancer (3). ME/CFS may inhibit a person from being able to work or attend school, to carry out activities of daily living independently or to leave the house, with some people left completely bedbound. Yet there remains contradiction and uncertainty on the diagnosis and management of the disease across all medical professions including physiotherapy (4).

This chapter will give a general overview of ME/CFS, including the currently known aetiology of ME/CFS, characteristics of key symptoms, diagnostic difficulties and consideration for physiotherapy management.

History of nomenclature

'ME' stands for 'myalgic encephalomyelitis', a term first introduced in 1956 (5) to describe a newly identified condition with symptoms of fatigue and muscle pains that often persisted for years with frequent relapses. 'Myalgic' refers to the typical muscle symptoms and 'encephalomyelitis' describes inflammation of the brain and spinal cord (4). As encephalomyelitis is not a confirmed pathological process in all people with ME/CFS, it has also been proposed to adopt 'encephalopathy' to signify a significant disorder of brain function (4).

An alternative name of 'chronic fatigue syndrome' (CFS) was

introduced in 1988 (6) to initially describe ongoing fatigue symptoms following the Epstein–Barr virus, but then expanded to describe chronic fatigue symptoms akin to those with ME. 'Chronic fatigue syndrome' does not attempt to attribute symptoms to a specific cause, but the term has been strongly criticized for distilling a wide range of complex symptoms and multi-system dysfunction into the generic problem of 'fatigue' (4). This leads to an issue in which 'chronic fatigue syndrome' is often conflated in research and clinical practice with the symptom of 'chronic fatigue', which can be linked to a wide variety of unrelated diseases and conditions. More discussion of fatigue can be found in chapter 7 and issues around diagnostic criteria are detailed later in this chapter.

The term 'post viral fatigue syndrome' (PVFS) was used from the 1980s to describe symptoms arising directly from viral infection (7) and can be applied to issues following an acute infection (4). Post viral fatigue syndrome is discussed in more detail in chapter 5. As ME/CFS can be attributed to causes beyond viral infection, the term 'post viral fatigue syndrome' does not relate to every person.

Another term was developed in 2015 (2), 'systemic exertion intolerance disease' (SEID), which emphasized the intolerance to exertion that is a hallmark feature of the disease. However, the term has also been criticized for failing to capture the role of the immune system and central nervous system dysfunction, and the diagnostic criteria proposed for SEID were not exclusive enough to solely identify ME/CFS from other conditions such as major depressive disorders and other medical illnesses (8).

The debate on an accurate name for this condition is ongoing (4) as more evidence demonstrating the pathophysiology emerges. While some researchers have suggested that ME and CFS are two distinct clinical entities with partial overlaps (9), for simplicity the term 'ME/CFS' will be adopted in this book to reflect the terminology currently used by the National Institute for Health and Care Excellence (NICE) in the United Kingdom (10) and the Centers for Disease Control and Prevention (CDC) in the United States (11), as well as being the most common terminology used in the evidence base.

Due to the variety of nomenclature used to describe this condition, when searching for evidence it is necessary to use all terms to ensure the search fully captures the evidence base.

What is the cause of ME/CFS?

No cause of ME/CFS has so far been identified (4). A primary factor in the lack of clarity around the condition is the limited amount of high quality research. A review of research funding in the United States found that ME/CFS is the most underfunded condition in relation to the size of disease burden (12). Of note is that ME/CFS is more prevalent in women (see 'Who develops ME/CFS' in this chapter) and when conditions primarily affect one sex, funding patterns for research have been found to favour males (13).

Based on current research, one explanation for the development of ME/CFS is that a person may have a predisposition to developing the disease, they are exposed to a triggering event, and ME/CFS is a result of perpetuating pathophysiological processes (4).

Predisposition

As most triggering events such as exposure to an infection are experienced by the general population without the development of ME/CFS, it is presumed that there must be a particular predisposition for a person to develop the condition (4), although there have so far been no identified overarching factors.

Genetic studies have found supporting evidence for a heritable contribution to the predisposition of ME/CFS, with risks of developing the disease increasing in first, second and third degree relatives (14). Increased frequency of specific genetic variants has also been found in relation to immune, hormone and metabolic systems (15). However, studies have so far failed to show consistently significant associations between genetics and the risk of developing ME/CFS (16).

Other factors that may suggest predisposition were found in a prospective epidemiological study of university students in the United States of America. Those with pre-existing gastrointestinal symptoms such as stomach pain, bloating and irritable bowel, as well as abnormally lower levels of certain immune markers, were 80% more likely to develop ME/CFS after a mononucleosis infection (17).

No single genetic characteristic has yet been found that can be attributed to every case of ME/CFS, but this area of research continues to be explored. For example, the world's largest genetic ME/CFS study, 'Decode ME', launched in the United Kingdom in 2021 and aims to collect DNA samples from 20,000 people with ME/CFS so that genetic causes can be explored further (18).

Triggering event

One of the most common triggering events for ME/CFS is infection; however no single infection has been implicated, suggesting the underlying cause may be the immune response as opposed to a particular infectious agent. The type of infection can be viral, bacterial or parasitic (19). For example, infections of Epstein–Barr and enterovirus were reported as triggers in 77% of 873 people with ME/CFS in a 2010 study in Norway (20). The potential for cases of ME/CFS in mass-infectious events such as viral pandemics is discussed in chapter 5.

While infection is the most commonly reported cause of ME/CFS, other triggering events have been identified including (21) (22) (23) (24):

- exposure to toxins, chemical substances or pesticides
- early life immune threats such as developmental immunotoxicity
- vaccinations
- exposure to other significant stressors of the nervous system.

However, diagnostic disparities within research continue to make it difficult to draw any definite conclusions regarding triggering events.

Perpetuating physiological processes

There are many emerging theories that attempt to explain the ongoing processes that are occurring as part of ME/CFS, based on abnormalities that have been found in the central and autonomic nervous system, the metabolic system and the immune system (25). Each theory can only partially explain the whole experience of ME/CFS, and it is possible that there is overlap. Theories include:

- repeated exposure from a stressor such as infection or chemicals leading to prolonged stimulation and hypersensitivity of the nervous system (26)
- a neuroimmune model in which chronic immune activation leads to chronic activation of immune-inflammatory pathways, causing mitochondrial damage and oxidative stress (27)
- dysfunction of the hypothalamic-pituitary-adrenal (HPA) axis, a system designed to maintain homeostasis in response to stressful stimuli (28)
- persistent presence of pathogens interfering with metabolism, gene expression and immunity (29).

Who develops ME/CFS?

Prevalence of ME/CFS is difficult to determine due to the variance in diagnostic criteria (30). Estimates range from 0.42% of the population in 1999 (31) to 0.89% in an international systematic review from 2020 (30), which equates to 8 in every 1000 people.

ME/CFS is more likely to affect women, with estimates of 3:1 in relation to men (1). Sex chromosomes and endocrine function appear to have a significant influence over onset of ME/CFS (32) and sex-based differences have been found in the expression of microRNA in relation to exercise challenge in people with ME/CFS (33).

There appears to be a peak of onset between the ages of 11 to 19 years and 33 to 39 years (1) (34). The specific considerations in relation to ME/CFS in children is discussed further in chapter 4.

ME/CFS in the older population is a cohort that is under-represented in research. One study compared people with ME/CFS over the age of 50 with people aged from 16 to 29 years old and found that the older adults experienced greater levels of fatigue and autonomic dysfunction, potentially due to the physiological effects of aging (35). Contradictory research has found that older adults may have better mental health functioning and less severe autonomic, immune and neuroendocrine symptoms (36). However, neither of these studies used diagnostic criteria that requires the hallmark symptom of ME/CFS, post exertional malaise (PEM), to be essential for diagnosis. Given that fatigue is already a common complaint in older age groups (37), an exclusive diagnostic criteria is essential for any future research to be able to investigate the presence of ME/CFS in older adults.

ME/CFS has been reported globally and across all ethnicities (4). While some black and minority ethnic communities have been shown to have a higher prevalence of ME/CFS in comparison to white communities (38) (39) these groups are also less likely to receive a formal diagnosis, which suggests there may be barriers to diagnosis such as a lack of awareness, religious beliefs, language and the potential racial bias of health professionals (40). However, many studies lack specificity on diagnosis leading to the issues discussed in the diagnosis section of this chapter.

Symptoms of ME/CFS

ME/CFS causes a substantial impairment in function, with symptoms occurring across multiple systems including neurological, musculoskeletal, cardiovascular, endocrine, gastrointestinal and immune (41) (1). Further key symptoms of ME/CFS are explored in individual chapters of this book.

The hallmark feature of ME/CFS is the occurrence of additional symptoms or an exacerbation of current symptoms due to physical, cognitive, sensory or emotional exertion (1). This feature is referred to across various diagnostic criteria as 'post exertional malaise' (PEM), 'post exertional neuroimmune exhaustion' (PENE) or 'post exertional symptom exacerbation' (PESE) (42). For simplicity, the term PEM will be adopted in this book. PEM is a priority for physiotherapists to understand because most physiotherapeutic interventions, such as exercise, are likely to be a trigger and therefore could cause an exacerbation of symptoms. Understanding how to identify, manage and avoid PEM is essential for a physiotherapist working with any person who has ME/CFS, and this is discussed in detail in chapter 6.

Other symptoms identified by various diagnostic criteria of ME/CFS include: fatigue that is unexplained, persistent and significantly impacts on daily life; pain; unrefreshing sleep; cognitive dysfunction; autonomic nervous system dysfunction; and orthostatic intolerance (1) (41). The range of diverse symptoms associated with ME/CFS can be seen through the various diagnostic criteria discussed in this chapter.

Co-morbidities

There are many co-morbidities of ME/CFS, which are discussed in more depth in chapter 2. These include:

- endometriosis
- fibromyalgia
- hypermobility syndromes
- irritable bowel syndrome
- mast cell activation syndrome (MCAS)
- migraines
- postural orthostatic tachycardia syndrome (POTS)
- spinal cord and brain stem co-morbidities
- temporomandibular disorders (TMDs).

Diagnosis

There are currently no widely accepted diagnostic tests or biomarkers for ME/CFS (43) and over twenty different diagnostic criteria are used in research and clinical practice (44), with no agreement on which should be universally used (4). This makes accurate diagnosis very difficult. The wide range of symptoms can also be commonly found in many other conditions so it is important that a person has had a thorough medical review to rule out differential diagnoses. A list of conditions that commonly feature chronic fatigue as a symptom can be found in chapter 7.

As Table 1.1 demonstrates, each set of diagnostic criteria varies in terms of which symptoms are essential for diagnosis. The inconsistency in which they categorize or prioritize symptoms makes comparison between criteria very difficult. It is not the role of a physiotherapist to formally diagnose ME/CFS; however, it is helpful to understand the issues around diagnosis in order to competently appraise the evidence base.

Criticism of diagnostic criteria includes the over-reliance on a subjective history for diagnosis, and the limited acknowledgement of potential subgroups of the condition (43). A lack of consistency in diagnostic criteria used in research means many research findings are difficult to compare and lack reliability (43). 'Fatigue' is a symptom found in a wide array of diseases (see chapter 7) so some diagnostic criteria may incorrectly include people with unspecified 'chronic fatigue' with the risk then of generalizing the results of studies (44).

One symptom described as cardinal and a key diagnostic feature is PEM (4) (41). This symptom is discussed in chapter 6. When diagnostic criteria do not include PEM as essential, there is a risk that people who do not have ME/CFS will be included in data (49). For example, a study measured the sleep patterns of people diagnosed with 'chronic fatigue syndrome' using the Fukuda Criteria, which does not include PEM as essential. Of the 343 people assessed, 30.3% were found to have a primary sleep disorder that could explain their diagnosis (50). Another study (51) looked at the volume of the hippocampus and compared people diagnosed using the Fukuda Criteria and the ICC criteria, which does include PEM, and found significant differences between the two groups, noting that stricter criteria are essential when investigating the pathophysiology of ME/CFS.

Table 1.1 Diagnostic criteria for ME/CFS

Symptom	Institute of Medicine (IOM) / National Academy of Medicine (NAM) Criteria (2015) (45)	International Consensus Criteria (2011) (41)	Canadian Clinical Criteria (2003) (46)	CDC (Fukuda) Criteria (1994) (47)	Oxford Criteria (1991) (48)
Timeframe of symptoms	At least six months	Acute phase: less than six months Chronic phase: more than six months	At least six months in adults At least three months in children	At least six months	At least six months
Post exertional malaise / Post exertional neuroimmune exhaustion	Essential Profound, of new or definite onset, not the result of ongoing exertion and not substantially relieved by rest	Essential	Essential	Not essential Grouped in 'four or more' symptoms required	Not included
Fatigue	Essential	Essential	Essential Significant degree of new onset, unexplained, persistent, or recurrent physical and mental fatigue that substantially reduces activity level	Essential Fatigue is not due to ongoing exertion or other medical conditions, and significantly interferes with daily activities and work	Essential Disabling and affects physical and mental functioning

Sleep dysfunction	Essential	Not essential Section B: '1 from at least 3 of 4 categories'	Essential	Not essential Grouped in 'four or more' symptoms required	Not essential 'May be present'
Pain	Not essential Muscle pain Pain in joints without swelling or redness Headaches	Not essential Section B: '1 from at least 3 of 4 categories'	Essential Muscles and/or joints, widespread	Not essential Grouped in 'four or more' symptoms required Pain in joints Headaches	Not essential 'May be present'
Cognitive impairments	Not essential, but must be present if no orthostatic intolerance Impaired thinking, memory, executive function, and information processing Attention deficit and impaired psychomotor functions	Not essential Section B: '1 from at least 3 of 4 categories' Impaired processing Impaired short-term memory	Not essential Must have two or more, grouped with neurological: confusion, impaired concentration, impaired short-term memory, disorientation, information processing, categorizing and word retrieval	Not essential Included in 'four or more' symptoms required Impaired short-term memory Impaired concentration	Not included

cont.

Symptom	Institute of Medicine (IOM) / National Academy of Medicine (NAM) Criteria (2015) (45)	International Consensus Criteria (2011) (41)	Canadian Clinical Criteria (2003) (46)	CDC (Fukuda) Criteria (1994) (47)	Oxford Criteria (1991) (48)
Neurological impairments	Not essential Visual disturbances Sensitivity to light and sound	Not essential Section B: '1 from at least 3 of 4 categories' Neurosensory and perceptual Motor impairments	Must have two or more, grouped with cognitive: perceptual and sensory disturbances, ataxia, muscle weakness, fasciculations, photo-phobia, hypersensitivity to noise	Not included	Not included
Autonomic dysfunction	Not essential, but must be present if no cognitive dysfunction Orthostatic intolerance Orthostatic symptoms: light-headedness, fainting, increased fatigue, cognitive worsening, headaches or nausea	Not essential Section D: 1 from this category Orthostatic intolerance Palpitations with or without cardiac arrhythmias Light-headedness Laboured breathing	Not essential At least one symptom from two of the categories marked a, b and c: Category a: Orthostatic intolerance Light-headedness Extreme pallor Nausea Irritable bowel syndrome Bladder dysfunction Palpitations with or without cardiac arrhythmias Exertional dyspnoea	Not included	Not included

Neuroendocrine manifestations	Not essential Chills or night sweats	Not essential Section D: 1 from this category Loss of thermostatic stability	Not essential At least one symptom from two of the categories marked a, b and c: b. Loss of thermostatic stability Intolerance of extremes of heat and cold Marked weight change	Not included	Not included
Immune manifestations	Not essential Swollen or tender lymph nodes in the neck or armpit Frequent or recurring sore throat Allergies or sensitivities to foods, odours, chemicals, medications	Not essential Section C: 1 from at least 3 of 5 categories Flu-like symptoms Susceptibility to viral infections Sensitivities to food	Not essential At least one symptom from two of the categories marked a, b and c: c. Tender lymph nodes Recurrent sore throat Recurrent flu-like symptoms General malaise New sensitivities to food medications and/or chemicals	Not essential Grouped in 'four or more' symptoms required Tender lymph nodes A sore throat that is frequent or recurring	Not included

One paper suggests that for every 15 people diagnosed using the Oxford Criteria, 14 would not meet the requirements in the Canadian Criteria (44). As a result, it has been recommended that the Oxford Criteria be 'retired' (52).

To determine the effectiveness of a treatment, a physiotherapist must be able to appraise the evidence base and be confident that participants in a study are representative of the relevant population. A systematic review (53) looked at randomized controlled trials (RCTs) published over the last two decades that evaluated interventions from physiotherapists and classified the studies into groups depending on whether PEM was included in diagnostic criteria. Out of 18 RCTs, only one used criteria that stipulated PEM as essential, 14 used criteria that listed PEM as optional and three used criteria that did not include PEM at all. The review found that any positive intervention effects were diminished when criteria became more specific, and concluded that when PEM was used as an essential diagnostic criterion there was no evidence for the effectiveness of any physiotherapy intervention.

Timeframe for diagnosis

Diagnosis is based on subjective history, but many symptoms of ME/CFS may be experienced in a normal acute response to infection and last for days or weeks (4), or be caused by any number of other diseases. Without tests or markers, diagnosis is based on exclusion.

The recommended timeframe for diagnosis varies across the world. In the UK the National Institute of Health and Care Excellence (NICE) provides guidance that if symptoms of fatigue, PEM, unrefreshing sleep and cognitive difficulties persist beyond six weeks in adults and four weeks in children, and other medical conditions that can cause similar symptoms have been investigated and ruled out, then ME/CFS could be a suspected diagnosis (10), while in the USA, the Centers for Disease Control and Prevention (CDC) gives a timeframe of six months (54).

While these timeframes are the recommendation, many people may have to wait much longer for an official diagnosis. For example, a UK charity conducted a survey in which over 60% of respondents reported waiting a year or more for diagnosis from when their symptoms started (4). Surveys of general medical practitioners have found that reasons for delay of diagnosis include inadequate training and knowledge, lack of confidence, feeling that the label of ME/CFS could be harmful and difficulty understanding management options once the diagnosis was made (55) (56). In the UK in 2018–19, 59% of medical schools covered ME/CFS in their curriculum, with teaching duration averaging one hour over the full five-year course (57).

Early diagnosis is beneficial as people with ME/CFS could be provided with education and advice on managing symptoms and avoiding exacerbation. Some people who developed severe ME/CFS or very severe ME/CFS (see chapter 3) believed that if they had been given a diagnosis earlier they might have avoided such severity of symptoms (58).

Severity of ME/CFS

The International Consensus Criteria (ICC) (41) proposed the importance of categorizing different levels of disease severity to try to create better uniformity in research, direct treatment and determine disease burden (59). The Bells Disability Scale can be used to quantify the level of severity in a person with ME/CFS (see chapter 18) and self-reported levels of severity can be correlated with objective measures (59).

There is consensus that there are several levels of severity of ME/CFS (41) (4) (1) but no consistency on the definitions of each level. While it can be helpful to understand the differing types of severity, attempting to divide ME/CFS into strict categories cannot truly portray the lived experience of ME/CFS.

A combined version of severity levels is proposed as a pragmatic tool for clinical practice:

- *Mild:* Meets criteria for ME/CFS with a significantly reduced activity level. May be able to work and carry out activities of daily living without assistance.
- *Moderate:* Approximately 50% reduction in pre-illness activity levels. Has significant restrictions on mobility if outside. May require help with activities of daily living.
- *Severe:* Mostly housebound, may require a wheelchair or spends most of day in bed. Requires help with personal care and activities of daily living.
- *Very Severe:* Mostly bedbound, needing help with basic functions on a 24-hour basis.

It should be noted that the use of 'mild' is an inaccurate description of the impact of ME/CFS on quality of life, considering a 'reduced activity level' may mean a person is unable to work, or unable to care for their children without support, or no longer able to take part in their hobbies and interests.

Working with people who have severe and very severe ME/CFS presents further complexities, which are discussed in chapter 3.

Fluctuating severity: relapse and remission

It is common for symptoms of ME/CFS to fluctuate in terms of their severity and their impact on daily life (41). People with ME/CFS may experience periods of improved symptom severity or even temporary complete remission (1) but repeated relapses may also occur, often triggered by factors such as (4) (34) (60):

- physical, cognitive or emotional exertion
- sensory stimulation
- new infections
- vaccinations
- surgery and general anaesthetics
- temperature extremes
- alcohol
- the menstrual cycle, pregnancy and menopause
- side effects of pharmaceuticals
- environmental contaminants.

A longitudinal study, which is in preprint at the time of writing and therefore has not yet been peer-reviewed, analysed the DNA of two people with ME/CFS over 11 months and found changes in relation to primary immune function and metabolic, neurological and mito-chondrial function that varied in relation to each person's fluctuating symptoms (61).

Physiotherapy management strategies will need to account for the level of severity of ME/CFS and the potential fluctuating symptoms over time.

Prognosis and impact on quality of life

No definitive study of prognosis currently exists (1). An often quoted systematic review reported that 5% of people with 'chronic fatigue' and 'chronic fatigue syndrome' fully recover (62); however the studies included in this review have issues in relation to diagnostic criteria (see section: Diagnosis), small sample sizes and 'inappropriate definitions of recovery' (1).

Measuring recovery is problematic considering the fluctuating nature of symptoms and their impact on quality of life and function. People with ME/CFS may describe themselves as 'recovered' when in reality their symptoms have stabilized, but their level of function is still significantly reduced compared to before their illness (1).

Kim: 'ME/CFS has had a devasting impact on my life. I had to leave my lifelong vocation, which in turn has had a major financial impact. I've spent long periods housebound and was sometimes confined to bed. I couldn't join in with social or family events.'

In terms of disability, some estimates state that 50% of people with ME/CFS are unemployed, 75% are housebound most of the time and 25% are bedbound most of the time (63) (60). ME/CFS has been found to have a greater impact on function and quality of life in comparison to other chronic diseases such as cancer, depression and rheumatoid arthritis (3), and a significant correlation has been found on the impact on quality of life between the person with ME/CFS and their closest family members (64).

Without effective treatments, people with ME/CFS may experience symptoms for years, decades or, potentially, for their entire lifetime. Due to factors such as significant disability and illness, absence of effective treatments, social and physical isolation, lost careers, lost independence and potential disruption to plans to have children, people with ME/CFS are at an increased risk of suicide (65) (66) (58). On top of this, people with ME/CFS are more reluctant to engage with healthcare because of prolonged 'misattribution of ME/CFS to physical deconditioning or psychiatric disorders' (65).

Treatment for ME/CFS
Research into treatment for ME/CFS has been limited and there are currently no approved treatments specifically for ME/CFS (1). Specific symptoms may be managed or reduced through pharmacological and non-pharmacological measures, with the primary aim of any management to reduce the disease burden and improve quality of life (1).

There have been very few randomized controlled trials of pharmacological treatments for ME/CFS (67). Medications may help to reduce specific symptoms such as pain, sleep dysfunction or orthostatic intolerance (67). Use of supplements, vitamins, minerals and ions appears to be common in people with ME/CFS (68), although the evidence base for the effectiveness of any of them is weak or so far absent (4). A list of common medications, supplements and vitamins is included in the Appendix.

Ana: 'Living with ME/CFS has completely devastated my life and stripped me of what it feels like to be human.'

Non-pharmacological management options primarily involve education regarding energy management with the aim to minimize symptom exacerbation and maximize individual function and quality of life (1). Further discussion of energy management techniques can be found in chapters 16 and 17.

Symptom-specific treatments and management options relevant to a physiotherapist are discussed in each chapter of this book.

Physiotherapy management of ME/CFS

A physiotherapist should be aware of ME/CFS when working with any person, whether they are directly addressing ME/CFS symptoms or working with them on an unrelated matter.

When addressing symptoms directly related to ME/CFS

Physiotherapists may work with people with ME/CFS to provide a wide variety of interventions and services:

- energy management advice
- pain management
- postural management and maintenance for those who are bedbound
- aids and adaptations
- guidance on physical activity as part of energy management plan.

Further information around all of these measures is discussed in detail throughout this book.

When ME/CFS is a co-morbidity

A physiotherapist may work with a person who has ME/CFS in any setting for any reason. In this instance, any treatment plan must prioritize ME/CFS and be adapted in order to avoid causing PEM. A physiotherapist must therefore be able to understand and identify PEM, establish the means to monitor for any signs of symptom exacerbation, and adapt their treatment approach so that it is suitable for the person.

As exercise is a core treatment intervention of a physiotherapist and also a likely physical trigger of PEM, it is vitally important that a physiotherapist is fully aware of the impact of exercise on people with ME/CFS. This is discussed in depth in chapter 17.

SUMMARY

▸ ME/CFS is a condition that affects multiple systems and causes significant levels of disability.

▸ There remains no clear consensus on terminology, diagnosis or categorization of severity, and high quality evidence is currently lacking.

▸ Symptoms vary in terms of severity and can fluctuate for each person.

▸ There is no recognized direct treatment for ME/CFS. Individual symptoms may be managed with both pharmacological and non-pharmacological interventions.

APPLICATION TO PRACTICE

▸ A physiotherapist should routinely screen for an ME/CFS diagnosis in a person's medical history and treat it as a precaution for any intervention.

▸ Physiotherapy interventions cannot 'cure' ME/CFS but, like any other long-term condition, physiotherapists can still provide care for symptom management and support for maintaining function with the goal to improve quality of life.

▸ The aim of this book is to support physiotherapists in delivering safe and appropriate interventions for people with ME/CFS.

References

1. Bateman, L., Bested, A.C., Bonilla, H.F., Chheda, B.V., *et al.* (2021) 'Myalgic encephalomyelitis/chronic fatigue syndrome: essentials of diagnosis and management.' *Mayo Clinic Proceedings 96* (11).

2. Institute of Medicine (2015) *Beyond Myalgic Encephalomyelitis/Chronic Fatigue Syndrome: Redefining an Illness.* Washington, DC: The National Academies Press.

3. Nacul, L.C., Lacerda, E.M., Campion, P., Pheby, D., *et al.* (2011) 'The functional status and well being of people with myalgic encephalomyelitis/chronic fatigue syndrome and their carers.' *BMC Public Health 27* (11).

4. Shepherd, C. & Chaudhuri, A. (2019) *ME/CFS/PVFS: An Exploration of the Key Clinical Issues.* Gawcott: The ME Association

5. Lindan, R. (1956) 'Benign myalgic encephalomyelitis.' *Canadian Medical Association Journal 5* (7).

6. Holmes, G.P., Kaplan, J.E., Gantz, N.M., Komaroff, A.L., *et al.* (1988) 'Chronic fatigue syndrome: a working case definition.' *Annals of Internal Medicine 108* (3).

7. Jenkins, R. (1991) 'Post-viral fatigue syndrome. Epidemiology: lessons from the past.' *British Medical Bulletin 47* (4).

8. Jason, L.A., Sunnquist, M., Kot, B. & Brown, A. (2015) 'Unintended consequences of not specifying exclusionary illnesses for systemic exertion intolerance disease.' *Diagnostics 5*, 272–286.

9. Twisk, F.N. (2015) 'Accurate diagnosis of myalgic encephalomyelitis and chronic fatigue syndrome based upon objective test methods for characteristic symptoms.' *World Journal of Methodology 5* (2).

10. National Institute for Health and Care Excellence (2021) 'Myalgic encephalomyelitis (or encephalopathy)/chronic fatigue syndrome: diagnosis and management.' Accessed on 2/12/2022 at www.nice.org.uk/guidance/ng206.

11. Centers for Disease Control and Prevention (2022) 'Myalgic encephalomyelitis/chronic fatigue syndrome.' Accessed on 7/12/2022 at www.cdc.gov/me-cfs/index.html.

12. Mirin, A.A., Dimmock, M.E. & Jason, L.A. (2020) 'Research update: The relation between ME/CFS disease burden and research funding in the USA.' *Work 66* (2).

13. Mirin, A.A. (2021) 'Gender disparity in the funding of diseases by the U.S. National Institutes of Health.' *Journal of Women's Health (Larchmt) 30* (7).

14. Albright, F., Light, K., Light, A., Bateman, L. & Cannon-Albright, L.A. (2011) 'Evidence for a heritable predisposition to chronic fatigue syndrome.' *BMC Neurology 11* (62).

15. Perez, M., Jaundoo, R., Hilton, K., Del Alamo, A., *et al.* (2019) 'Genetic predisposition for immune system, hormone, and metabolic dysfunction in myalgic encephalomyelitis/chronic fatigue syndrome: a pilot study.' *Frontiers in Pediatrics 7.*

16. Dibble, J.J., McGrath, S.J. & Ponting, C.P. (2020) 'R1Genetic risk factors of ME/CFS: a critical review.' *Human Molecular Genetics 29.*

17. Jason, L.A., Cotler, J., Islam, M.F., Furst, J. & Katz, B. (2022) 'Predictors for developing severe myalgic encephalomyelitis/chronic fatigue syndrome following infectious mononucleosis.' *Journal of Rehabilitation Medicine 4* (1).

18. Decode ME Study (2020) *Decode ME Study.* Accessed on 7/12/2022 at www.decodeme.org.uk.

19. Komaroff, A.L. & Bateman, L. (2021) 'Will COVID-19 lead to myalgic encephalomyelitis/chronic fatigue syndrome?' *Frontiers in Medicine (Lausanne) 18* (7).

20. Naess, H., Sundal, E., Myhr, K.M. & Nyland, H.I. (2010) 'Postinfectious and chronic fatigue syndromes: clinical experience from a tertiary-referral centre in Norway.' *In Vivo 24* (2).

21. Gherardi, R.K., Crépeaux, G. & Authier, F.J. (2019) 'Myalgia and chronic fatigue syndrome following immunization: macrophagic myofasciitis and animal studies

support linkage to aluminum adjuvant persistency and diffusion in the immune system.' *Autoimmunity Reviews 18* (7).

22. Capelli, E., Zola, R., Lorusso, L., Venturini, L., Sardi, F. & Ricevuti, G. (2010) 'Chronic fatigue syndrome/myalgic encephalomyelitis: an update.' *International Journal of Immunopathology and Pharmacology 23* (4).

23. Dietert, R.R. & Dietert, J.M. (2008) 'Possible role for early-life immune insult including developmental immunotoxicity in chronic fatigue syndrome (CFS) or myalgic encephalomyelitis (ME).' *Toxicology 247* (1).

24. Skufca, J., Ollgren, J., Ruokokoski, E., Lyytikäinen, O. & Nohynek, H. (2017) 'Incidence rates of Guillain Barré (GBS), chronic fatigue/systemic exertion intolerance disease (CFS/SEID) and postural orthostatic tachycardia syndrome (POTS) prior to introduction of human papilloma virus (HPV) vaccination among adolescent girls.' *Papillomavirus Research 3*.

25. Komaroff, A.L. (2019) 'Advances in understanding the pathophysiology of chronic fatigue syndrome.' *JAMA 322* (6).

26. Jason, L.A., Porter, N., Herrington, J., Sorenson, M. & Kubow, S. (2009) 'Kindling and oxidative stress as contributors to myalgic encephalomyelitis/chronic fatigue syndrome.' *Journal of Behavioral Neuroscience 7* (2).

27. Morris, G. & Maes, M. (2013) 'A neuro-immune model of myalgic encephalomyelitis/chronic fatigue syndrome.' *Metabolic Brain Disease 28* (4).

28. Papadopoulos, A. & Cleare, A. (2012) 'Hypothalamic–pituitary–adrenal axis dysfunction in chronic fatigue syndrome.' *Nature Reviews Endocrinology 8*.

29. Proal, A. & Marshall, T (2018) 'Myalgic encephalomyelitis/chronic fatigue syndrome in the era of the human microbiome: persistent pathogens drive chronic symptoms by interfering with host metabolism, gene expression, and immunity.' *Frontiers in Pediatrics 4* (6).

30. Lim, E.J., Ahn, Y.C., Jang, E.S., Lee, S.W., Lee, S.H. & Son, C.G. (2020) 'Systematic review and meta-analysis of the prevalence of chronic fatigue syndrome/myalgic encephalomyelitis (CFS/ME).' *Journal of Translational Medicine 18* (1).

31. Jason, L.A., Richman, J.A., Rademaker, A.W., Jordan, K.M., *et al.* (1999) 'A community-based study of chronic fatigue syndrome.' *Archives of Internal Medicine 159* (18).

32. Thomas, N., Gurvich, C., Huang, K., Gooley, P.R. & Armstrong, C.W. (2022) 'The underlying sex differences in neuroendocrine adaptations relevant to myalgic encephalomyelitis chronic fatigue syndrome.' *Frontiers in Neuroendocrinology 66*.

33. Cheema, A.K., Sarria, L., Bekheit, M., Collado, F., *et al.* (2022) 'Unravelling myalgic encephalomyelitis/chronic fatigue syndrome (ME/CFS): gender-specific changes in the microRNA expression profiling in ME/CFS.' *Journal of Cellular and Molecular Medicine 24* (10).

34. Rowe, P.C., Underhill, R.A., Friedman, K.J., Gurwitt, A., *et al.* (2017) 'Myalgic encephalomyelitis/chronic fatigue syndrome diagnosis and management in young people: a primer.' *Frontiers in Pediatrics 19* (5).

35. Lewis, I., Pairman, J., Spickett, G. & Newton, J.L. (2013) 'Is chronic fatigue syndrome in older patients a different disease? A clinical cohort study.' *European Journal of Clinical Investigation 43* (3).

36. Kidd, E., Brown, A., McManimen, S., Jason, L.A., Newton, J.L. & Strand, E.B. (2016) 'The relationship between age and illness duration in chronic fatigue syndrome.' *Diagnostics (Basel) 6* (2).

37. Chou, K.L. (2013) 'Chronic fatigue and affective disorders in older adults: evidence from the 2007 British National Psychiatric Morbidity Survey.' *Journal of Affective Disorders 145* (3).

38. Dinos, S., Khoshaba, B., Ashby, D., White, P.D., *et al.* (2009) 'A systematic review of chronic fatigue, its syndromes and ethnicity: prevalence, severity, co-morbidity and coping.' *International Journal of Epidemiology 38* (6).

39. Bhui, K.S., Dinos, S., Ashby, D., Nazroo, J., Wessely, S. & White, P.D. (2011) 'Chronic fatigue syndrome in an ethnically diverse population: the influence of psychosocial adversity and physical inactivity.' *BMC Medicine 21* (9).
40. Bayliss, K., Riste, L., Fisher, L., Wearden, A., *et al.* (2014) 'Diagnosis and management of chronic fatigue syndrome/myalgic encephalitis in black and minority ethnic people: a qualitative study.' *Primary Health Care Research & Development 15* (2).
41. Carruthers, B.M., van de Sande, M.I., De Meirleir, K.L., Klimas, N.G., *et al.* (2011) 'Myalgic encephalomyelitis: International Consensus Criteria.' *Journal of Internal Medicine 270.*
42. Chu, L., Valencia, I.J., Garvert, D.W. & Montoya, J.G. (2018) 'Deconstructing post-exertional malaise in myalgic encephalomyelitis/chronic fatigue syndrome: a patient-centered, cross-sectional survey.' *PLOS ONE 13* (6).
43. Nacul, L., O'Boyle, S., Palla, L., Nacul, F.E., *et al.* (2020) 'How myalgic encephalomyelitis/chronic fatigue syndrome (ME/CFS) progresses: the natural history of ME/CFS.' *Frontiers in Neurology 11* (826).
44. Nacul, L., Lacerda, E.M., Kingdon, C.C., Curran, H. & Bowman, E.W. (2019) 'How have selection bias and disease misclassification undermined the validity of myalgic encephalomyelitis/chronic fatigue syndrome studies?' *Journal of Health Psychology 24* (12).
45. Centers for Disease Control and Prevention (2015) *IOM 2015 Diagnostic Criteria.* Accessed on 7/12/2022 at www.cdc.gov/me-cfs/healthcare-providers/diagnosis/iom-2015-diagnostic-criteria.html.
46. Carruthers, B.M., Jain, A.K., De Meirleir, K.L., Peterson, D.L., *et al.* (2003) 'Myalgic encephalomyelitis/chronic fatigue syndrome.' *Journal of Chronic Fatigue Syndrome 11* (1).
47. Fukuda, K., Straus, S.E., Hickie, I., Sharpe, M.C., Dobbins, J.G. & Komaroff, A.L. (1994) 'The chronic fatigue syndrome: a comprehensive approach to its definition and study.' *Annals of Internal Medicine 121.*
48. Sharpe, M.C., Archard, L.C. & Banatvala, J.E. (1991) 'A report: chronic fatigue syndrome: guidelines for research.' *Journal of the Royal Society of Medicine 84* (2).
49. Baraniuk, J.N. (2017) 'Chronic fatigue syndrome prevalence is grossly overestimated using Oxford criteria compared to Centers for Disease Control (Fukuda) criteria in a U.S. population study.' *Fatigue 5* (4).
50. Gotts, Z.M., Deary, V., Newton, J., Van der Dussen, D., De Roy, P. & Ellis, J.G. (2013) 'Are there sleep-specific phenotypes in patients with chronic fatigue syndrome? A cross-sectional polysomnography analysis.' *BMJ Open 3* (6).
51. Thapaliya, K., Staines, D., Marshall Gradisnik, S., Su, J. & Barnden, L. (2022) 'Volumetric differences in hippocampal subfields and associations with clinical measures in myalgic encephalomyelitis/chronic fatigue syndrome.' *Journal of Neuroscience Research 100* (7).
52. Smith, M.E.B., Nelson, H.D., Haney, E., Pappas, M., *et al.* (2014) 'Diagnosis and treatment of myalgic encephalomyelitis/chronic fatigue syndrome.' *Evidence Report/Technology Assessment (Full Rep.) 219.*
53. Wormgoor, M.E.A. & Rodenburg, S.C. (2021) 'The evidence base for physiotherapy in myalgic encephalomyelitis/chronic fatigue syndrome when considering post-exertional malaise: a systematic review and narrative synthesis.' *Journal of Translational Medicine 19* (1).
54. Centers for Disease Control and Prevention (2018) 'Proposed approach to ME/CFS diagnosis in children and adults.' Accessed on 8/12/2022 at www.cdc.gov/me-cfs/healthcare-providers/diagnosis/approach-to-diagnosis.html.
55. Bayliss, K., Goodall, M. & Chisholm, A. (2014) 'Overcoming the barriers to the diagnosis and management of chronic fatigue syndrome/ME in primary care: a meta synthesis of qualitative studies.' *BMC Family Practice 15* (44).

56. Chew-Graham, C., Dowrick, C., Wearden, A., Richardson, V. & Peters, S. (2010) 'Making the diagnosis of chronic fatigue syndrome/myalgic encephalitis in primary care: a qualitative study.' *BMC Primary Care 11* (16).

57. Muirhead, N. (2021) 'Medical school education on myalgic encephalomyelitis.' *Medicina 57* (542).

58. Williams, L.R. & Isaacson-Barash, C. (2021) 'Three cases of severe ME/CFS in adults.' *Healthcare (Basel) 9* (2).

59. van Campen, C.L.M.C., Rowe, P.C. & Visser, F.C. (2020) 'Validation of the severity of myalgic encephalomyelitis/chronic fatigue syndrome by other measures than history: activity bracelet, cardiopulmonary exercise testing and a validated activity questionnaire: SF-36.' *Healthcare (Basel) 8* (3).

60. Chu, L., Valencia, I.J., Garvert, D.W. & Montoya, J.G. (2019) 'Onset patterns and course of myalgic encephalomyelitis/chronic fatigue syndrome.' *Frontiers in Pediatrics 5.*

61. Helliwell, A.M, Stockwell, P.A, Edgar, C.D, Chatterjee, A. & Tate, W.P. (2022) 'Dynamic epigenetic changes during a relapse and recovery cycle in myalgic encephalomyelitis/chronic fatigue syndrome.' *International Journal of Molecular Sciences 23* (19).

62. Cairns, R. & Hotopf, M. (2005) 'A systematic review describing the prognosis of chronic fatigue syndrome.' *Occupational Medicine (London) 55.*

63. Collin, S.M., Crawley, E., May, M.T., Sterne, J.A., Hollingworth, W. & Database UK CFS/ME National Outcomes (2011) 'The impact of CFS/ME on employment and productivity in the UK: a cross-sectional study based on the CFS/ME national outcomes database.' *BMC Health Services Research 11.*

64. Vyas, J., Muirhead, N., Singh, R., Ephgrave, R. & Finlay, A.Y. (2022) 'Impact of myalgic encephalomyelitis/chronic fatigue syndrome (ME/CFS) on the quality of life of people with ME/CFS and their partners and family members: an online cross-sectional survey.' *BMJ Open 12 (5).*

65. Chu, L., Elliott, M., Stein, E. & Jason, L.A. (2021) 'Identifying and managing suicidality in myalgic encephalomyelitis/chronic fatigue syndrome.' *Healthcare (Basel) 9* (6).

66. Johnson, M.L., Cotler, J., Terman, J.M. & Jason, L.A. (2022) 'Risk factors for suicide in chronic fatigue syndrome.' *Death Studies 46* (3).

67. Castro-Marrero, J., Sáez-Francàs, N., Santillo, D. & Alegre, J. (2017) 'Treatment and management of chronic fatigue syndrome/myalgic encephalomyelitis: all roads lead to Rome.' *British Journal of Pharmacology 174* (5).

68. Weigel, B., Eaton-Fitch, N., Passmore, R., Cabanas, H., Staines, D. & Marshall-Gradisnik, S. (2021) 'A preliminary investigation of nutritional intake and supplement use in Australians with myalgic encephalomyelitis/chronic fatigue syndrome and the implications on health-related quality of life.' *Food & Nutrition Research 7* (65).

CHAPTER 2

Co-morbidities

PURPOSE OF THIS CHAPTER

There are several conditions that appear to be commonly associated with ME/CFS (1), many of which have overlapping symptoms, so it is important to be aware of potential co-morbidities and that a person with ME/CFS may present with multiple co-morbidities.

A person with ME/CFS may seek physiotherapy input for symptoms relating to a co-morbidity, yet treatment should always regard ME/CFS as a priority because of the potential for causing additional symptoms or an exacerbation of current symptoms with any intervention (post exertional malaise (PEM), discussed in chapter 6). Additionally, a person may not yet have a co-morbidity diagnosed, so a physiotherapist should be alert for signs and symptoms that may have been mistaken as part of ME/CFS, when they may in fact indicate another condition.

This chapter provides an outline of the key co-morbidities associated with ME/CFS. The list is presented alphabetically and is not exhaustive. Conditions discussed are:

- endometriosis
- fibromyalgia
- hypermobility syndromes
- irritable bowel syndrome
- mast cell activation syndrome (MCAS)
- migraines
- postural orthostatic tachycardia syndrome (POTS)
- spinal cord and brain stem co-morbidities
- temporomandibular disorders (TMDs).

This chapter aims to provide an overview of each condition rather than an in-depth guide on management. If relevant, further reading on any specific area is advised before management decisions are made.

Endometriosis

Endometriosis is an oestrogen dependent inflammatory disease (2) where tissue that is similar to the lining of the womb starts to grow in other parts of a woman's reproductive system such as the ovaries and fallopian tubes (3). Endometriosis is thought to affect 7–10% of women worldwide (4). The exact cause of endometriosis is not known, although several factors may be involved such as genetics and a dysfunction of the immune system (3). Symptoms include fertility problems and pain in the lower abdomen or pelvis that is worse during menstruation (3).

Endometriosis is considered a co-morbidity in women who have ME/CFS (5). For example, one study found 36.1% of 36 women with ME/CFS had endometriosis compared to 17% of a control group (5), and another found endometriosis was a diagnosis in 19% of 150 women with ME/CFS compared to 8% in a matched control group (6). Both of these studies used the Fukuda Criteria to select participants, which does not require PEM as essential for diagnosis (see chapter 1).

Equally, a cross-sectional survey (7) of 3680 women in the USA with diagnosis of endometriosis found 4.6% were also diagnosed with ME/CFS, compared to 0.03% of published rates in the general population of women in the USA at that time.

There is no cure for endometriosis, but treatment can focus on pain relief and fertility through analgesics, hormone treatment and surgery to remove the additional tissue growth (3). A person with ME/CFS presenting with pelvic pain or fertility problems should be referred on for review to establish whether they have this co-morbidity and to access relevant treatments.

Fibromyalgia

Fibromyalgia commonly co-exists with ME/CFS (8). Key symptoms of fibromyalgia are widespread muscle pain, fatigue, morning stiffness, non-restorative sleep and cognitive dysfunction (9).

Just like ME/CFS, the exact cause of fibromyalgia is still unknown, but its onset has been linked to viral infection or trauma, and one theory suggests that there may be an autoimmune dysfunction leading to low-grade inflammatory processes and oxidative stress (10).

Diagnosis of fibromyalgia requires specific scoring on the widespread pain index, with pain in at least four or five different regions that has been present for over three months (11). However, accurate diagnosis of fibromyalgia can be problematic in clinical settings leading to possible cases of misdiagnosis (12).

ME/CFS and fibromyalgia are diagnostically different conditions, as diagnosis of fibromyalgia does not require the presence of fatigue or PEM (13). Physiologically there are differences too: for example elevated levels of Substance P, a neurotransmitter that is associated with inflammatory processes and pain, have been found in people with fibromyalgia (14), whereas normal levels were found in people with ME/CFS (15).

It is important to note that having fibromyalgia as a co-morbidity with ME/CFS can increase the severity of ME/CFS symptoms, for example the presence of fibromyalgia can significantly increase the frequency and severity of PEM and therefore cause significantly worse physical functioning (8). Additionally, one study (16) demonstrated that balance was significantly worse in people with ME/CFS compared to healthy control groups, but the addition of a fibromyalgia diagnosis further reduced the performance of those with ME/CFS, especially in relation to vestibular function (16). This amplification of ME/CFS symptoms with fibromyalgia emphasizes that they are distinct clinical conditions (8).

Massage therapy has been found to provide short-term relief from pain, anxiety and depression in people with fibromyalgia (17) (18) although research is of low quality and the recommendation is that any intervention should be pain free and start at low intensity with careful monitoring of symptoms (19). However, one study found that the benefits of massage for fibromyalgia were actually diminished when there was a co-morbid diagnosis of ME/CFS (20).

Aerobic exercise and strength-training have been shown to have beneficial effects on the wellbeing and physical function of people with fibromyalgia, but the evidence is weaker in relation to pain and tender points (21). A systematic review and meta-analysis found moderate quality evidence of exercise reducing pain in fibromyalgia, but evidence was lacking on any long-term gains (22). Additionally, isometric exercise has been shown to cause increased sensitivity to pain in people with fibromyalgia (23), which is the opposite to what would be expected in the general population.

If fibromyalgia is a co-morbidity of ME/CFS then exercise may cause physical exertion and subsequent PEM, therefore the benefits found for fibromyalgia may not be seen in those who also have ME/CFS. The issues of exercise for ME/CFS are discussed in detail in chapter 17.

Hypermobility syndromes

Hypermobility is generally seen within heritable disorders of connective tissue (HDCT) (24) which include disorders such as:

- *Joint hypermobility syndrome*: excessive joint laxity that is symptomatic (25).
- *Ehlers–Danlos syndrome (EDS)*: the hallmarks of Ehlers–Danlos syndrome are skin elasticity, joint hypermobility and tissue fragility, with some severe forms also affecting internal connective tissue structures such as arteries and the intestine (26).
- *Marfan syndrome*: a multi-system connective tissue disorder often identifiable from childhood by skeletal abnormalities (27).

A retrospective cross-sectional study (28) of people seen by a specialist ME/CFS clinic in Sweden examined the prevalence of hypermobility (as well as craniocervical obstructions and signs of intercranial hypertension, which are discussed later in this chapter). Out of 229 people diagnosed with severe ME/CFS, general joint hypermobility was identified in 115 (50%), with 20% already having an established diagnosis of hypermobile EDS. Other studies have found a lower prevalence, with evidence of hypermobility found in 25% (29) or 20% (30) of people with ME/CFS, although this still compares to just 4% in the general population (30).

An overlap between symptoms is apparent when comparing ME/CFS and Ehlers–Danlos syndrome and it could be likely that a proportion of people diagnosed with ME/CFS may also have undiagnosed EDS (31). Fatigue is a frequent and clinically significant problem in people with EDS (32), although the cause of fatigue could be linked to sleep disorders, chronic pain, and dysfunction of cardiovascular, bladder and bowel systems (31).

EDS has been linked with Chiari malformations, upper cervical instability and tethered cord syndrome (33), which are all discussed in the 'Spinal cord and brain stem co-morbidities' section of this chapter.

Due to its higher prevalence in people with ME/CFS, joint hypermobility should be included in a physiotherapy assessment of a person with ME/CFS (34) (35), for example using a basic screen such as the nine-point Beighton scale (36).

Primary aims of treatment for hypermobility syndromes are to relieve and prevent joint pain (37). General exercise is often considered as a treatment to reduce pain intensity in people with hypermobility (38) but the evidence base is weak and lacks detail on specificity of intervention (39) with a focus on single joints rather than the whole body (38). Education on positioning or functional splints may also assist in protecting joints (37).

If hypermobility is present alongside ME/CFS then any exercise programme must consider the potential for physical exertion to trigger PEM, so typical approaches may need to be adjusted. Chapter 17 discusses adaptations and considerations in relation to exercise and ME/CFS.

Irritable bowel syndrome

Irritable bowel syndrome (IBS) is a disorder affecting the digestive system, with common symptoms being abdominal pain or bloating, changes in the appearance and/or frequency of a bowel movement, mucus in the stools and increased gas (40). There is no known cause of IBS, although theories include abnormal motility (movement of faecal matter through the bowel), hypersensitivity of the nervous system, genetic predisposition and psychosocial issues (41). IBS has been historically described as a functional disorder, which means no identifiable structural or biochemical abnormalities can explain the symptoms (42). However, more recent investigations have found evidence of organic changes such as increased gut permeability, changes to the neuroendocrine system and a dysfunction in the part of the autonomic nervous system that regulates the gastrointestinal tract, called the enteric nervous system (41). Dysfunction of the autonomic nervous system is a common issue in ME/CFS and is discussed in chapter 12.

IBS and ME/CFS are known co-morbidities (43) (1). One study (44) compared incidences of abdominal discomfort syndrome (which they associated with IBS) in 94 people with ME/CFS compared to 34 people with chronic fatigue. Abdominal discomfort was significantly higher in the ME/CFS group, with 59.6% experiencing symptoms compared to 17.7% in the fatigue group, leading the researchers to suggest that abdominal discomfort syndrome could be a characteristic subset of ME/CFS. However, this study used the Fukuda Criteria for participant selection, which does not require PEM as essential for diagnosis, therefore this may not be representative of the whole ME/CFS population.

There is no single treatment for IBS (40) but various pharmacological and dietary options exist. Pharmacological treatments include medication for pain relief from cramps and spasms, or medication to treat constipation or diarrhoea (1).

Probiotics are live bacteria and yeast that can be added to food or taken as supplements (45). A systematic review (46) of probiotic interventions for IBS and ME/CFS found excellent quality of evidence for probiotics to relieve the symptoms of IBS, but the evidence was limited and of poor quality when specifically in relation to people with ME/CFS.

Dietary changes may also be an option. Fermentable oligosaccharides, disaccharides, monosaccharides and polyols (FODMAP), ketogenic and gluten free diets are considered to have therapeutic effects for many conditions (47) and in particular relevance to ME/CFS there may be the potential for these diets to be 'mitoprotective', meaning they may prevent mitochondrial dysfunction (48). The FODMAP diet involves reducing wheat, milk and various fruits and vegetables (1) and the ketogenic diet involves very low carbohydrates and high fat intake (49). However, there is currently insufficient evidence that elimination diets can improve the symptoms of people with ME/CFS (50) and some diets may be inappropriate for people with ME/CFS (1), so management of any major dietary changes should be overseen by a dietician.

Faecal microbiome transplantation, or bacteriotherapy, has also been explored for people with ME/CFS in small studies (51) (52). Faecal transplantation, in which faecal matter is transferred from a healthy donor into the gastrointestinal tract, is usually used to treat bowel infections caused by Clostridium difficile (53) and gastrointestinal diseases such as inflammatory bowel disease, chronic constipation and IBS (54). With regards to ME/CFS, one study (51) found 70% of 60 people with ME/CFS diagnosed using Fukuda Criteria (without PEM as an essential symptom) improved their ME/CFS symptoms following faecal transplantation, although the symptoms that improved were defined as 'sleep deprivation, lethargy and fatigue', which may not represent every aspect of ME/CFS. Another study (52) of 42 people with ME/CFS diagnosed using the ICC criteria (which does stipulate PEM as essential) gave half the participants standard approaches for IBS, and the other half a faecal transplant. Two of the 21 people receiving the implants did not tolerate the procedure. The remainder appeared to have some improvement; however no valid outcome measure was used and results were based on clinical judgement alone. It is clear that further research is required to explore this area of potential treatment for people with ME/CFS.

It is important to note that abdominal symptoms and fatigue can be linked to serious medical conditions such as ovarian cancer and inflammatory bowel disease (1) so any person with ME/CFS experiencing unexplained digestive symptoms should be referred for a medical review.

Mast cell activation syndrome (MCAS)

Mast cells are a type of white blood cell involved in the immune system that activate in response to infection or environmental threats (55). Mast cells may become overproduced or overactive (56), and this dysfunction is known as mast cell activation disease, an umbrella term that includes mast cell activation syndrome (MCAS) as well as mastocytosis, a rare benign localized skin disorder, and hereditary α-tryptasemia (HaT), a genetic trait that is also linked to dysautonomia, chronic pain and connective tissue disorders (55).

MCAS is estimated to affect as many as 17% of the population, with the ratio of female to male at 3:1 (55). MCAS is considered to be a co-morbidity of conditions such as fibromyalgia, dysautonomia, irritable bowel syndrome and Ehlers–Danlos syndrome, as well as ME/CFS (55). The overlap with ME/CFS is noticeable when considering symptoms of MCAS (57):

- fatigue
- itching, rashes and skin discolouration
- abdominal issues including pain, bloating, diarrhoea, nausea and vomiting

- joint and muscle pain
- cognitive dysfunction
- shortness of breath, chest pain, light-headedness
- anaphylaxis.

Symptoms fluctuate over years and may worsen over time, causing significant impact on activities of daily living and quality of life (55). The potential triggers of symptoms are varied and include (57):

- food and beverages (including alcohol)
- medications
- stress
- fatigue
- environmental stimuli such as temperature, scents, chemical exposure (e.g. cleaning products), pressure/touch
- exercise
- illness or infection.

If MCAS is suspected, the person should be supported in finding a clinician specializing in allergy and immunology for further testing (55). Treatment options include medications such as antihistamines and using activity tracking to determine triggers.

Migraines

A migraine is a type of headache that if untreated lasts for 4 to 72 hours and may have some of the following characteristics (58):

- unilateral location
- pulsating
- moderate or severe intensity of pain
- aggravated by physical activity
- causes nausea and/or vomiting
- causes sensitivity to light and/or sound.

A migraine may also be associated with 'aura' symptoms, which are disturbances to sensory systems such as vision, speech, motor activity and sensation (58).

Migraines are considered a common co-morbidity of ME/CFS (1) and may be associated with a rapid drop in temperature, vomiting, diarrhoea and severe weakness (59).

A cross-sectional study of 143,000 people with ME/CFS in England found 39.2% reported migraines, in comparison to 21.3% in healthy controls (60). Conversely, a study (61) exploring fatigue symptoms in people with chronic migraine found that 66.7% would meet the Fukuda Criteria for diagnosis of ME/CFS. It is not clear whether this means these people have ME/CFS, or that the Fukuda Criteria are unable to differentiate between ME/CFS and chronic migraine.

Migraines are more prevalent in women in the general population (62), and as women are also more likely to have ME/CFS this could be one explanation for the higher numbers of people with ME/CFS experiencing migraines. They may be triggered by dietary changes, pre-menstrual hormones, sleep dysfunction and odours (63), all of which may also be linked to symptom exacerbation in ME/CFS (64).

Standard medications for migraine, both analgesic and preventative measures, can be applied to people with ME/CFS (1), so if migraines are a significant issue then a physiotherapist should refer the person on for medical management.

Postural orthostatic tachycardia syndrome (POTS)

Postural orthostatic tachycardia syndrome (POTS) is characterized by an abnormal increase in heart rate when moving from a lying position into a standing position, with the diagnostic criteria in adults stipulating an increase of over 30 beats per minute or above 120 beats per minute within the first ten minutes of standing (65). POTS can also be present in children and adolescents, with a slightly altered criteria of over 40 beats per minute or a maximum heart rate of over 130 beats per minute (66). POTS is more commonly seen in the younger population (15–40 years) and more predominantly in women (65).

For diagnosis, POTS symptoms must be present for at least three to six months, resolved with a supine position, be in the absence of a drop in blood pressure and have all other potential conditions causing tachycardia ruled out (65). Tests to confirm diagnosis include the tilt table test, active stand test and the NASA lean test (67), which are discussed in chapter 18.

Symptoms of POTS that are specific to adopting an upright posture include light-headedness, shortness of breath, chest pain, palpitations and weakness. Additional symptoms independent of posture include fatigue, sleep dysfunction, headache, gastrointestinal disturbances and difficulty concentrating (68).

It is currently unclear how POTS develops and the syndrome is thought to be multifactorial (66). One theory involves abnormally low extracellular fluid alongside low tone in the lower-extremity vascular structures (69) as idiopathic POTS symptoms have resolved with saline infusions. However, abnormal autonomic reflexes, raised adrenaline levels, damaged muscle pump, mast cell activation, iron deficiency and autoimmune dysfunction are all considered potential components of the condition (66), and POTS can have a variety of triggers such as fever, dehydration, anaemia, autonomic neuropathies, damage to the heart and hyperthyroidism (66). The exact occurrence of POTS in people with ME/CFS is difficult to determine, and research in this area is contradictory (70) with the prevalence of POTS in people with ME/CFS ranging from 19% to 70% (71).

More information on POTS in relation to ME/CFS can be found in chapter 12, alongside other types of orthostatic intolerance.

Spinal cord and brain stem co-morbidities

There are several conditions thought to be potential co-morbidities of ME/CFS that involve the brain stem and spinal cord (72), including those in Table 2.1:

Table 2.1 Potential spinal cord and brain stem co-morbidities of ME/CFS

Cervical stenosis	A narrowing of the diameter of the cervical spinal canal resulting in compression of the spinal cord
	Stenosis can be caused by traumatic, degenerative and inflammatory conditions and result in neurological symptoms such as numbness, weakness and balance problems
	Cervical spinal stenosis can also be asymptomatic (73)
Chiari malformations	Structural changes to the skull resulting in the lower part of the brain (cerebellum) pressing on the brain stem and spinal cord
	Symptomatic presentations include headaches, fatigue, dizziness, muscle weakness and problems with vision, hearing and swallowing
	Can also be asymptomatic and incidental (74) (75)

cont.

Craniocervical instability (CCI)/ atlantoaxial instability (AAI)	Instability at the junction between the skull and the upper cervical spine (CCI) or between the atlas and axis (AAI) caused by laxity or injury of the ligaments; the excessive movement can compress the brain stem and spinal cord Ligament laxity could be linked to aging, inflammatory diseases, hypermobility syndromes or traumatic injury Symptoms include headaches, dizziness, fatigue and neurological impairments (76) (77)
Intercranial hypertension	A build-up of pressure around the brain, which can be caused by sudden trauma to the brain (e.g. stroke), or be a chronic presentation linked to altered blood flow to the brain; Chiari malformations can also be a cause Symptoms include headaches, fatigue and visual disturbances (78)
Tethered cord syndrome	Fixation/tethering of the spinal cord at the lower back resulting in limited movement and neurological symptoms such as sensory and motor deficits in the lower limbs, and possibly bladder and bowel dysfunction Can be congenital, developmental or acquired (79)

There has been some research and anecdotal reporting of various brain stem and spinal cord co-morbidities contributing to the symptoms of ME/CFS (80). A retrospective cross-sectional study (28) of people seen by a specialist ME/CFS clinic in Sweden looked for a prevalence of hypermobility (see Hypermobility syndromes in this chapter) but also scanned for craniocervical obstructions and signs of intercranial hypertension. Of the 205 participants who consented to a brain MRI, 115 (56%) showed cerebellar tonsil protrusion, which can put pressure on the brain stem, and 171 (83%) had signs of possible intercranial hypertension. Of the 125 participants who consented to an MRI of the cervical spine, 100 (80%) had craniocervical obstructions. The researchers concluded that joint hypermobility and craniocervical obstructions may be a potential causative factor in developing ME/CFS; however they acknowledged that their research covered a group that was specific to their own clinic, which required a diagnosis of severe ME/CFS and may therefore not be representative of the whole ME/CFS population.

A series of three case studies (80) further explored the potential of cord compression being a cause of ME/CFS symptoms. The three people featured in the case series had symptoms of ME/CFS alongside orthostatic intolerance and were found to have cervical stenosis without signs of hypermobility. They were treated with spinal decompression surgery and all three demonstrated a marked improvement in their symptoms, with normal function occurring promptly post-surgery and showing long-term carry over. This is a small case series however, so the results cannot be generalized to the whole ME/CFS population. Any spinal surgery would have significant associated risks and must be very carefully considered in line with the available evidence base.

A cervical collar is a non-invasive method of supporting the neck and some people with ME/CFS have tried cervical collars with anecdotally reported improvement in symptoms (76). A small study (81) of ten people with postural orthostatic tachycardia syndrome (discussed in this chapter) found reduced orthostatic intolerance symptoms when using a Q-collar, although this study did not note whether they also had a diagnosis of ME/CFS.

As a physiotherapist, an awareness of the potential for brain stem and spinal cord co-morbidities in people with ME/CFS is essential during assessment of any neurological symptoms and if considering any manual techniques around the cervical spine.

Temporomandibular disorders (TMDs)

Temporomandibular disorders affect the temporomandibular joint (TMJ) and associated structures (82). The main symptom of TMD disorders is pain in the TMJ or muscles of mastication that may radiate to areas such as the jaw, teeth, ear, temples and cheeks. There may be clicking of the jaw, headaches and tinnitus (82). Diagnosing the source of pain and determining whether it is caused by muscle or articular structures is very difficult (83) and should be reviewed by an experienced clinician.

Temporomandibular disorders are considered to be a co-morbidity of ME/CFS (59). One study (84) took 51 people diagnosed with ME/CFS and found almost a third had a TMD, although the participants had been diagnosed using the Fukuda Criteria, which does not require PEM as essential for diagnosis, and TMD was identified using a screening tool, which cannot be used for diagnosis.

Low heart rate variability is suggestive of an autonomic nervous system dysfunction and has been found in people with TMD (85) as well as people with ME/CFS (see chapter 12). However, it is yet to be established whether the symptoms of TMD are a cause or a consequence of autonomic dysfunction.

Physiotherapy is a primary treatment for TMD and a systematic review and meta-analysis (86) found that physiotherapy interventions are effective at reducing pain and increasing active range of movement of the jaw. In a survey of 208 people in the United Kingdom with TMD, 72% of respondents reported physiotherapy to be effective for their symptoms, with treatments ranging through jaw exercises, ultrasound, manual therapy, acupuncture and laser therapy (87). However, studies into treatment for TMD are small, with variable outcome measures used, and some question over whether manual therapy has a direct impact on the structures involved or on the nervous system in general (86). Additionally, no studies have been carried out specifically on treatment for TMD in people with ME/CFS, so it is important to monitor for signs of PEM both during and after any intervention.

SUMMARY

There is no definitive list of co-morbidities for ME/CFS, and there can be many conditions that have symptoms which overlap with those of ME/CFS. As well as the conditions discussed in this chapter, there are a number of other suggested co-morbidities or differential diagnoses (72), including:

- ▶ gastroparesis
- ▶ coeliac disease
- ▶ Crohn's disease
- ▶ diverticulitis
- ▶ sleep apnoea
- ▶ endocrine disorders
- ▶ peripheral/small fibre neuropathy
- ▶ hypothyroidism
- ▶ metabolic syndrome
- ▶ interstitial cystitis
- ▶ overactive bladder
- ▶ vitamin deficiencies (B12, D)
- ▶ neurodivergence.

APPLICATION TO PRACTICE

▸ Typical treatment approaches for some co-morbidities may not always be compatible with ME/CFS due to PEM.

▸ Co-morbidities might impact on the severity of ME/CFS symptoms and vice versa.

References

1. Shepherd, C. & Chaudhuri, A. (2019) *ME/CFS/PVFS: An Exploration of the Key Clinical Issues*. Gawcott: The ME Association.
2. Burney, R.O. & Giudice, L.C. (2012) 'Pathogenesis and pathophysiology of endometriosis.' *Fertility and Sterility 98* (3).
3. NHS (2019) 'Endometriosis.' Accessed on 8/12/2022 at www.nhs.uk/conditions/endometriosis.
4. Baldi, A., Campioni, M. & Signorile, P.G. (2008) 'Endometriosis: pathogenesis, diagnosis, therapy and association with cancer (review).' *Oncology Reports 19* (4).
5. Boneva, R.S., Lin, J.S., Wieser, F., Nater, U.M., *et al.* (2019) 'Endometriosis as a comorbid condition in chronic fatigue syndrome (CFS): secondary analysis of data from a CFS case-control study.' *Frontiers in Pediatrics 21* (7).
6. Harlow, B.L., Signorello, L.B., Hall, J.E., Dailey, C. & Komaroff, A.L. (1998) 'Reproductive correlates of chronic fatigue syndrome.' *American Journal of Medicine 105* (3A).
7. Sinaii, N., Cleary, S.D., Ballweg, M.L., Nieman, L.K. & Stratton, P. (2002) 'High rates of autoimmune and endocrine disorders, fibromyalgia, chronic fatigue syndrome and atopic diseases among women with endometriosis: a survey analysis.' *Human Reproduction 17* (10).
8. McManimen, S.L. & Jason, L.A. (2017) 'Post-exertional malaise in patients with ME and CFS with comorbid fibromyalgia.' *SRL Neurological Neurosurgery 3* (1).
9. Häuser, W., Zimmer, C., Felde, E. & Köllner, V. (2008) 'What are the key symptoms of fibromyalgia? Results of a survey of the German Fibromyalgia Association.' *Schmerz (Pain) 22* (2).
10. Bazzichi, L., Giacomelli, C., Consensi, A., Giorgi, V., *et al.* (2020) 'One year in review 2020: fibromyalgia.' *Clinical and Experimental Rheumatology 123* (1).
11. Wolfe, F., Clauw, D.J., Fitzcharles, M.A., Goldenberg, D.L., *et al.* (2016) '2016 revisions to the 2010/2011 fibromyalgia diagnostic criteria.' *Seminars in Arthritis and Rheumatology 46* (3).
12. Wolfe, F., Schmukler, J., Jamal, S., Castrejon, I., *et al.* (2019) 'Diagnosis of fibromyalgia: disagreement between fibromyalgia criteria and clinician-based fibromyalgia diagnosis in a university clinic.' *Arthritis Care Research (Hoboken) 71* (3).
13. Nijs, J., Crombez, G., Meeus, M., Knoop, H., *et al.* (2012) 'Pain in patients with chronic fatigue syndrome: time for specific pain treatment?' *Pain Physician 15* (5).
14. Russell, I.J., Orr, M.D., Littman, B., Vipraio, G.A., *et al.* (1994) 'Elevated cerebrospinal fluid levels of substance P in patients with the fibromyalgia syndrome.' *Arthritis and Rheumatology 37* (11).
15. Evengard, B., Nilsson, C.G., Lindh, G., Lindquist, L., *et al.* (1998) 'Chronic fatigue syndrome differs from fibromyalgia: no evidence for elevated substance P levels in cerebrospinal fluid of patients with chronic fatigue syndrome.' *Pain 78* (2).
16. Serrador, J.M., Quigley, K.S., Zhao, C., Findley, T. & Natelson, B.H. (2018) 'Balance deficits in chronic fatigue syndrome with and without fibromyalgia.' *NeuroRehabilitation 42* (2).

17. Li, Y.H., Wang, F.Y., Feng, C.Q., Yang, X.F. & Sun, Y.H. (2014) 'Massage therapy for fibromyalgia: a systematic review and meta-analysis of randomized controlled trials.' *PLOS ONE 9* (2).

18. Yuan, S.L., Matsutani, L.A. & Marques, A.P. (2015) 'Effectiveness of different styles of massage therapy in fibromyalgia: a systematic review and meta-analysis.' *Manual Therapy 20* (2).

19. Kalichman, L. (2010) 'Massage therapy for fibromyalgia symptoms.' *Rheumatology International 30*.

20. Falaguera-Vera, F.J., Garcia-Escudero, M., Bonastre-Férez, J., Zacarés, M. & Oltra, E. (2020) 'Pressure point thresholds and ME/CFS comorbidity as indicators of patient's response to manual physiotherapy in fibromyalgia.' *International Journal of Environmental Research and Public Health 17* (21).

21. Busch, A.J., Schachter, C.L., Overend, T.J., Peloso, P.M. & Barber, K.A. (2008) 'Exercise for fibromyalgia: a systematic review.' *Journal of Rheumatology 35* (6).

22. Mascarenhas, R.O., Souza, M.B., Oliveira, M.X., Lacerda, A.C., *et al.* (2021) 'Association of therapies with reduced pain and improved quality of life in patients with fibromyalgia: a systematic review and meta-analysis.' *JAMA Internal Medicine 181* (1).

23. Staud, R., Robinson, M.E. & Price, D.D. (2005) 'Isometric exercise has opposite effects on central pain mechanisms in fibromyalgia patients compared to normal controls.' *Pain 118* (1–2).

24. Grahame, R. (1999) 'Joint hypermobility and genetic collagen disorders: are they related?' *Archives of Disease in Childhood 80* (2).

25. Grahame, R. (2009) 'Joint hypermobility syndrome pain.' *Current Science 13*.

26. Steinmann, B., Royce, P. & Superti-Furga, A. (2002) 'The Ehlers–Danlos Syndrome.' In P.M. Royce & B. Steinmann (eds) *Connective Tissue and Its Heritable Disorders*. New York: Wiley.

27. Dean, J. (2007) 'Marfan syndrome: clinical diagnosis and management.' *European Journal of Human Genetics 15*.

28. Bragée, B., Michos, A., Drum, B., Fahlgren, M., Szulkin, R. & Bertilson, B.C. (2020) 'Signs of intracranial hypertension, hypermobility, and craniocervical obstructions in patients with myalgic encephalomyelitis/chronic fatigue syndrome.' *Frontier of Neurology 28* (11).

29. Nijs, J., De Meirleir, K. & Truyen S. (2004) 'Hypermobility in patients with chronic fatigue syndrome: preliminary observations.' *Journal of Musculoskeletal Pain 12* (1).

30. Nijs, J., Aerts, A. & De Meirleir, K. (2006) 'Generalized joint hypermobility is more common in chronic fatigue syndrome than in healthy control subjects.' *Journal Manipulative Physiological Therapeutics 29* (1).

31. Hakim, A., De Wandele, I., O'Callaghan, C., Pocinki, A. & Rowe, P. (2017) 'Chronic fatigue in Ehlers–Danlos syndrome - hypermobile type.' *American Journal of Medical Genetics: Seminars in Medical Genetics 175C*.

32. Voermans, N.C., Knoop, H., van de Kamp, N., Hamel, B.C., Bleijenberg, G. & van Engelen, B.G. (2010) 'Fatigue is a frequent and clinically relevant problem in Ehlers–Danlos syndrome.' *Seminars in Arthritis and Rheumatology 40* (3).

33. Henderson, Sr., F.C., Austin, C., Benzel, E., Bolognese, P., et al. (2017) 'Neurological and spinal manifestations of the Ehlers–Danlos syndromes.' *American Journal of Medical Genetics 175C*.

34. Nijs, J., Meeus, M. & De Meirleir, K. (2006) 'Chronic musculoskeletal pain in chronic fatigue syndrome: recent developments and therapeutic implications.' *Manual Therapies 11* (3).

35. Rowe, P.C., Barron, D.F., Calkins, H., Maumenee, I.H., Tong, P.Y. & Geraghty, M.T. (1999) 'Orthostatic intolerance and chronic fatigue syndrome associated with Ehlers–Danlos syndrome.' *Journal of Pediatrics 135* (4).

36. Beighton, P., Solomon, L. & Soskolne, C.L. (1973) 'Articular mobility in an African population.' *Annals of the Rheumatic Diseases 32* (5).

37. Keer, R. & Simmonds, J. (2011) 'Joint protection and physical rehabilitation of the adult with hypermobility syndrome.' *Current Opinion in Rheumatology 23* (2).

38. Palmer, S., Davey, I., Oliver, L., Preece, A., Sowerby, L. & House, S. (2021) 'The effectiveness of conservative interventions for the management of syndromic hypermobility: a systematic literature review.' *Clinical Rheumatology 40* (3).

39. Palmer, S., Bailey, S., Barker, L., Barney, L. & Elliott, A. (2014) 'The effectiveness of therapeutic exercise for joint hypermobility syndrome: a systematic review.' *Physiotherapy 100* (3).

40. NHS (2021) 'Irritable bowel syndrome.' Accessed on 8/12/2022 at www.nhs.uk/conditions/irritable-bowel-syndrome-ibs.

41. Jahng, J. & Kim, Y.S. (2016) 'Irritable bowel syndrome: is it really a functional disorder? A new perspective on alteration of enteric nervous system.' *Journal of Neurogastroenterology and Motility 22* (2).

42. Longstreth, G.F., Thompson, W.G., Chey, W.D., Houghton, L.A., Mearin, F. & Spiller, R.C. (2006) 'Functional bowel disorders.' *Gastroenterology 130* (5).

43. Riedl, A., Schmidtmann, M., Stengel, A., Goebel, M., *et al.* (2008) 'Somatic comorbidities of irritable bowel syndrome: a systematic analysis.' *Journal of Psychosomatic Research 64* (6).

44. Maes, M., Leunis, J.C., Geffard, M. & Berk, M. (2014) 'Evidence for the existence of myalgic encephalomyelitis/chronic fatigue syndrome (ME/CFS) with and without abdominal discomfort (irritable bowel) syndrome.' *Neuroendocrinology Letters 35* (6).

45. NHS (2018) 'Probiotics.' Accessed on 8/12/2022 at www.nhs.uk/conditions/probiotics.

46. Corbitt, M., Campagnolo, N., Staines, D. & Marshall-Gradisnik, S. (2018) 'A systematic review of probiotic interventions for gastrointestinal symptoms and irritable bowel syndrome in chronic fatigue syndrome/myalgic encephalomyelitis (CFS/ME).' *Probiotics and Antimicrobial Proteins 10* (3).

47. Reddel, S., Putignani, L. & Del Chierico, F. (2019) 'The impact of low-FODMAPs, gluten-free, and ketogenic diets on gut microbiota modulation in pathological conditions.' *Nutrients 11*.

48. Craig, C. (2015) 'Mitoprotective dietary approaches for myalgic encephalomyelitis/chronic fatigue syndrome: caloric restriction, fasting, and ketogenic diets.' *Medical Hypotheses 85* (5).

49. Masood, W., Annamaraju, P. & Uppaluri, K.R. (2022) *Ketogenic Diet.* Treasure Island (FL): StatPearls Publishing.

50. Campagnolo, N., Johnston, S., Collatz, A., Staines, D. & Marshall-Gradisnik, S. (2017) 'Dietary and nutrition interventions for the therapeutic treatment of chronic fatigue syndrome/myalgic encephalomyelitis: a systematic review.' *Journal of Human Nutrition and Dietetics 30* (3).

51. Borody, T., Nowak, A., Torres, M., Campbell, J., Finlayson, S. & Leis, S. (2012) 'Bacteriotherapy in chronic fatigue syndrome (CFS): a retrospective review.' *American Journal of Gastroenterology 107*.

52. Kenyon, J.N., Coe, S. & Izadi, H (2019) 'A retrospective outcome study of 42 patients with chronic fatigue syndrome, 30 of whom had irritable bowel syndrome. Half were treated with oral approaches, and half were treated with faecal microbiome transplantation.' *Human Microbiome Journal 13*.

53. Johns Hopkins Medicine (2022) 'Fecal transplantation (bacteriotherapy).' Accessed on 8/12/2022 at www.hopkinsmedicine.org/gastroenterology_hepatology/clinical_services/advanced_endoscopy/fecal_transplantation.html.

54. Aroniadis, O.C. & Brandt, L.J. (2013) 'Fecal microbiota transplantation: past, present and future.' *Current Opinion in Gastroenterology 29* (1).

55. Selleck, B. & Selleck, C. (2021) 'A primer on mast cell activation disease for the nurse practitioner.' *Journal for Nurse Practitioners 17* (7).

56. Akin, C. (2017) 'Mast cell activation syndromes.' *Journal of Allergy and Clinical Immunology 140* (2).

57. Jennings, S.V., Slee, V.M., Zack, R.M., Verstovsek, S, *et al.* (2018) 'Patient perceptions in mast cell disorders.' *Immunology and Allergy Clinics of North America 38* (3).
58. International Headache Society (2021) 'IHS Classification ICHD-3.' Accessed on 9/12/2022 at https://ichd-3.org/1-migraine.
59. Carruthers, B.M., van de Sande, M.I., De Meirleir, K.L., Klimas, N.G., *et al.* (2011) 'Myalgic encephalomyelitis: International Consensus Criteria.' *Journal of Internal Medicine 270.*
60. Nacul, L.C., Lacerda, E.M., Pheby, D., Campion, P., *et al.* (2011) 'Prevalence of myalgic encephalomyelitis/chronic fatigue syndrome (ME/CFS) in three regions of England: a repeated cross-sectional study in primary care.' *BMC Medical 28* (9).
61. Peres, M.F., Zukerman, E., Young, W.B. & Silberstein, S.D. (2002) 'Fatigue in chronic migraine patients.' *Cephalalgia 22* (9).
62. Nappi, R.E. & Nappi, G. (2012) 'Neuroendocrine aspects of migraine in women.' *Gynecological Endocrinology 28* (1).
63. Fukui, P.T., Gonçalves, T.R., Strabelli, C.G., Lucchino, N.M., *et al.* (2008) 'Trigger factors in migraine patients.' *Arquivos de Neuro-Psiquiatria 66* (3A).
64. Ravindran, M.K., Zheng, Y., Timbol, C., Merck, S.J. & Baraniuk, J.N. (2011) 'Migraine headaches in chronic fatigue syndrome (CFS): comparison of two prospective cross-sectional studies.' *BMC Neurology 11.*
65. Fedorowski, A. (2019) 'Postural orthostatic tachycardia syndrome: clinical presentation, aetiology and management.' *Journal of Internal Medicine 285* (4).
66. Chen, G., Du, J., Jin, H. & Huang, Y. (2020) 'Postural tachycardia syndrome in children and adolescents: pathophysiology and clinical management.' *Frontiers in Pediatrics 20* (8).
67. Hyatt, K.H., Jacobson, L.B. & Schneider, V.S. (1975) 'Comparison of 70 degrees tilt, LBNP, and passive standing as measures of orthostatic tolerance.' *Aerospace Medicine and Human Performance 46* (6).
68. Bourne, K.M., Lloyd, M.G. & Raj, S.R. (2021) 'Diagnostic Criteria for Postural Tachycardia Syndrome: Consideration of the Clinical Features Differentiating PoTS from Other Disorders of Orthostatic Intolerance.' In N. Gall, L. Kavi & M.D. Lobo (eds) *Postural Tachycardia Syndrome.* Cham: Springer International Publishing.
69. Jacob, G., Shannon, J.R., Black, B., Biaggioni, I., *et al.* (1997) 'Effects of volume loading and pressor agents in idiopathic orthostatic tachycardia.' *Circulation 86* (2).
70. Newton, J.L., Okonkwo, O., Sutcliffe, K., Seth, A., Shin, J. & Jones, D.E.J. (2007) 'Symptoms of autonomic dysfunction in chronic fatigue syndrome.' *QJM: An International Journal of Medicine 100* (8).
71. Freeman, R. (2002) 'The chronic fatigue syndrome is a disease of the autonomic nervous system. Sometimes.' *Clinical Autonomic Research 12* (4).
72. U.S. ME/CFS Clinician Coalition (2020) 'Diagnosing and treating myalgic encephalomyelitis / chronic fatigue syndrome V2.' Accessed on 7/12/2022 at https://mecfscliniciancoalition.org/wp-content/uploads/2021/06/MECFS-Clinician-Coalition-Diagnosis-and-Treatment-Handout-V2.pdf.
73. Lee, M.J., Cassinelli, E.H. & Riew, K.D. (2007) 'Prevalence of cervical spine stenosis: anatomic study in cadavers.' *Journal of Bone and Joint Surgery 89* (2).
74. Proctor, M.R., Scott, R.M., Oakes, W.J. & Muraszko, K.M. (2011) 'Chiari malformation.' *Neurosurgical Focus 31* (3).
75. NHS (2019) 'Chiari malformation.' Accessed on 7/12/2022 at www.nhs.uk/conditions/chiari-malformation.
76. Johnson, C. (2019) 'Could craniocervical instability be causing ME/CFS, fibromyalgia & POTS? Pt I – The spinal series.' Accessed on 7/12/2022 at www.healthrising.org/blog/2019/02/27/brainstem-compression-chronic-fatigue-syndrome-me-cfs-fibromyalgia-pots-craniocervical-instability.
77. Henderson, F.C. (2016) 'Cranio-cervical instability in patients with hypermobility connective disorders.' *Journal of Spine 5* (299).

78. NHS (2019) 'Intracranial hypertension.' Accessed on 7/12/2022 at www.nhs.uk/conditions/intracranial-hypertension.
79. NORD (2010) 'Tethered cord syndrome.' Rare Disease Database. Accessed on 7/12/2022 at https://rarediseases.org/rare-diseases/tethered-cord-syndrome.
80. Rowe, P.C., Marden, C.L., Heinlein, S. & Edwards, C.C. (2018) 'Improvement of severe myalgic encephalomyelitis/chronic fatigue syndrome symptoms following surgical treatment of cervical spinal stenosis.' *Journal of Translational Medicine 16*, (21).
81. Nardone, M., Guzman, J., Harvey, P.J., Floras, J.S. & Edgell, H. (2020) 'Effect of a neck compression collar on cardiorespiratory and cerebrovascular function in postural orthostatic tachycardia syndrome (POTS).' *Journal of Applied Physiology 128* (4).
82. National Institute for Health and Care Excellence (2021) 'Temporomandibular disorders (TMDs).' Accessed on 7/12/2022 at https://cks.nice.org.uk/topics/temporomandibular-disorders-tmds.
83. Herb, K., Cho, S. & Stiles, M.A. (2006) 'Temporomandibular joint pain and dysfunction.' *Current Pain and Headache Reports 10* (6).
84. Robinson, L., Durham, J., Maclachlan, L. & Newton, J. (2015) 'Autonomic function in chronic fatigue syndrome with and without painful temporomandibular disorder.' *Fatigue: Biomedicine, Health & Behavior 3*.
85. Chinthakanan, S., Laosuwan, K., Boonyawong, P., Kumfu, S., Chattipakorn, N. & Chattipakorn, S.C. (2018) 'Reduced heart rate variability and increased saliva cortisol in patients with TMD.' *Archives of Oral Biology 90*.
86. Paço, M., Peleteiro, B., Duarte, J. & Pinho, T. (2016) 'The effectiveness of physiotherapy in the management of temporomandibular disorders: a systematic review and meta-analysis.' *Journal of Oral & Facial Pain and Headache 30* (3).
87. Rashid, A., Matthews, N.S. & Cowgill, H. (2013) 'Physiotherapy in the management of disorders of the temporomandibular joint: perceived effectiveness and access to services: a national United Kingdom survey.' *British Journal of Oral and Maxillofacial Surgery 51*.

CHAPTER 3

Severe and Very Severe ME/CFS

PURPOSE OF THIS CHAPTER

Severe and very severe ME/CFS involves symptoms so extreme that the person is mostly housebound or mostly bedbound, and therefore has a greater impairment of general function and poorer quality of life compared to those who are not housebound (1).

It is estimated that approximately 25% of people with ME/CFS are classed as being severe or very severe (2). The exact numbers are difficult to determine due to the lack of data. A scoping review (3) aimed to identify papers relating to severe or very severe ME/CFS and found that out of over two thousand papers there were only 21 that met their criteria. People with severe ME/CFS and very severe ME/CFS are significantly under-represented in research because they are unable to leave their homes to attend a research site, or their symptoms are too severe for them to be well enough to participate in any capacity (4).

People with severe ME/CFS and very severe ME/CFS are also less likely to be seen by healthcare providers because they are unable to leave their homes, often only encountering health professionals such as physiotherapists during a crisis requiring hospital admission (5). Lack of expertise in such a specialist area may cause some health professionals to be reluctant to engage (6). These barriers to accessing healthcare are a serious concern considering this is a population who would most benefit from the continuing care of diverse and specialist clinicians.

If people with severe ME/CFS and very severe ME/CFS can only access services provided at home, then community-based professionals such as physiotherapists may be at the forefront of their care.

Physiotherapists who are used to working with chronic conditions should have the skills and compassion to benefit people with severe ME/CFS and very severe ME/CFS, but to provide adequate care they must understand the depth of suffering that is being endured (7). The significant disability and extremes of symptoms may surprise physiotherapists who have not encountered people with severe ME/CFS before (5), which is why severe and very severe ME/CFS warranted its own chapter in this book.

This chapter describes the nature of severe and very severe ME/CFS and the key adaptations to practice that a physiotherapist must consider in order to minimize symptom exacerbation.

What is severe and very severe ME/CFS?

The presentation of ME/CFS has been roughly divided into levels of severity based on the impact on function and level of disability (8) (9) (10). The severity of ME/CFS can be defined as ranging from mild to very severe, discussed further in chapter 1. People with mild and moderate ME/CFS have significantly reduced activity levels but may be able to carry out activities of daily living independently and access the community. Those with 'severe' and 'very severe' ME/CFS may only be able to carry out very basic activities of daily living independently and will need assistance with all tasks (2) including nutritional support that may even require tube feeding (11).

Symptoms of severe and very severe ME/CFS

The diverse range of symptoms linked to ME/CFS are also found in people with severe and very severe ME/CFS but are more prevalent and much more extreme (5), resulting in a more significant impact on quality of life and function (Table 3.1). One paper notes that 'the vocabulary to describe the experience of people with severe ME/CFS is inadequate' (6).

In addition to these ME/CFS symptoms, there are also the complications of being homebound and bedbound that can add to the disease burden and should be considered as part of the management plan (5), for example osteoporosis, pressure ulcers, compromised respiratory function, risk of contractures and malnutrition. These complications could be supported by physiotherapists; however consideration for the need to avoid symptom exacerbation with any intervention is crucial. Simply interacting with a person with severe or very severe ME/CFS may be enough to cause a worsening of symptoms and so a physiotherapist may have to make significant adaptations to their conduct, which is discussed later in this chapter.

Table 3.1 Symptoms of severe and very severe ME/CFS

Motor impairments	Profound weakness and extreme fatigue affecting mobility
	Housebound and/or bedbound
	May need assistance to mobilize or manoeuvre in bed
	May have impairment of speech or swallow
Cognitive dysfunction	Severe cognitive impairment; the person may struggle to communicate or understand written materials
Pain	Widespread pain, severe headaches/migraines
Orthostatic intolerance	Often unable to tolerate any upright position
Hypersensitivity	Extreme intolerance to light, sound, touch, chemicals and smell
	Exposure can increase symptoms
Gastrointestinal dysfunction	Nausea and abdominal pain
	Food intolerances, impaired swallow, or being too incapacitated to eat and drink can impair adequate nutrition
	May be at risk of life-threatening levels of malnutrition and may require tube feeding (11)
Sleep dysfunction	Altered sleep cycles and fractured sleep

People with severe and very severe ME/CFS may experience these extremes of symptoms for years or even decades (5). They may also have frequent hospital admissions. One survey of the experiences of 282 people with ME/CFS found the most common reason for admission was linked to orthostatic intolerance symptoms such as dizziness and fainting (12). But there was general dissatisfaction reported about the experience of being in hospital. For example, 42% of survey respondents had been dismissed as having a psychosomatic issue and 41% stated they had avoided seeking medical assistance because they did not think they would be taken seriously.

Given the significant impact on quality of life it is not a surprise that secondary depression and anxiety may be present in people with severe and very severe ME/CFS, as with any chronic condition (5). The extreme symptoms of severe and very severe ME/CFS mean people will have had to give up their education or employment (13), their independence and future plans such as having children (14) and as a result are likely to be experiencing grief (5). Sadly, there is an increased risk of suicide in people with severe and very severe ME/CFS (5) (14) and physiotherapists should be alert to this risk and offer support in the most appropriate way, keeping in mind that people with ME/CFS may be reluctant to engage with healthcare because of prolonged 'misattribution of ME/CFS to physical deconditioning or psychiatric disorders' (15).

Due to the extreme nature of these symptoms, people with severe ME/CFS are reliant on carer support for most or all activities of daily living, and therefore the potential for carer stress is also an important consideration (5). Carers experience a similar level of emotional burden (16) and their quality of life can be significantly impacted (17).

Physiological changes in severe and very severe ME/CFS

Research into the physiological changes involved with ME/CFS continues to find abnormalities across a wide spectrum of bodily systems, and some research has started to look into the differences between mild/moderate and severe/very severe ME/CFS (18) (19) (20) (21) (22) (23) (24).

Intolerance to physical exertion

Results from two-day cardiopulmonary exercise tests show a consistent decrease in performance from mild to severe ME/CFS in terms of peak oxygen consumption, oxygen consumption at the ventilatory threshold, peak workload and workload at the ventilatory threshold (23). People with severe ME/CFS have also been found to have higher rates of respiratory acidification (22). This demonstrates why people with severe/very severe ME/CFS tolerate physical exertion even less than those with mild/moderate ME/CFS. Chapter 6 explores the outcome of exercise testing in more detail.

Cerebral blood flow and orthostatic intolerance

In healthy people cerebral blood flow reduces by up to 6% when they are tilted fully upright (25). In people with mild to moderate ME/CFS, cerebral blood flow was found to be reduced by 26% in a 70-degree head-up tilt position (24). People with severe ME/CFS reached a 27% reduction in cerebral blood flow after only 20 degrees of tilt (24) and even demonstrated a 24.5% reduction just by sitting upright (18). Reduced cerebral blood flow when adopting an upright position may cause symptoms relating to orthostatic intolerance and is discussed in detail in chapter 12.

Cellular bioenergetic function

In cellular bioenergetics, while all severities of ME/CFS showed reduced mitochondrial function, people with severe ME/CFS were found to have higher rates of respiratory acidification and reduced glycolysis (22). Mitochondrial function in ME/CFS is discussed more in chapter 6.

Lower levels of an enzyme involved with energy production in tissues such as skeletal muscle, the heart and brain were found in people with ME/CFS compared to healthy controls (21). While these levels still tended to stay within 'normal' limits in people with mild ME/CFS, significantly lower levels were seen in people with severe ME/CFS, suggesting a specific abnormality in energy production for those with severe ME/CFS. The researchers note that these results could not be completely explained by reduced physical activity.

Immune function

A small immunological study found significant alterations in innate and adaptive immune cells in severe ME/CFS over a six-month period in comparison to healthy controls and those with moderate ME/CFS (19). This may suggest an enhanced and ongoing immune response in people with severe ME/CFS, and a greater potential for cytotoxic activity.

Cellular stress markers

One study (20) measured levels of a protein secreted in response to physiological stressors, in particular mitochondrial disorders. They found no significant differences between healthy controls and people with mild/moderate ME/CFS or multiple sclerosis. But a multivariate analysis found cases of severe ME/CFS had significantly increased levels and the researchers suggest levels of this protein could become a biomarker for symptom severity in ME/CFS as it may be signalling levels of cellular stress.

Overall, this research suggests there are physiological differences between mild/moderate and severe/very severe ME/CFS; however most studies are of small sample size and more research is needed to fully determine whether these differing physiological changes are the cause of such extreme symptoms in people with severe ME/CFS or are as a result of the significant inactivity these symptoms have imposed.

Adaptation to practice
Planning for an appointment

For people who are housebound, the most obvious requirement for an appointment is that it is carried out at the person's home (5) (6). Telephone or video calls could be an alternative, but this type of interaction does require a level of cognitive exertion. The timing of an appointment should also be considered, for example due to erratic sleep patterns (6). As every person is unique, it is best to find out first what location and time of day are most suitable for each individual.

The unpredictable nature and severity of symptoms means that there may be last-minute changes to the person's availability or ability to tolerate an interaction, so it is beneficial to confirm that the appointment can still go ahead just prior to the arranged time and be prepared for potential changes or cancellations.

Subjective information gathering can be a taxing process for anyone with ME/CFS (see chapter 8) and especially so for those with severe or very severe ME/CFS. People with severe ME/CFS may also have speech and communication difficulties (5) so therefore consider how to obtain as much information as possible outside the visit, either through past medical notes or written communication with the person or their caregivers.

Find out before the visit what measures may need to be taken to account for hypersensitivities or intolerances (5). People with severe ME/CFS may not tolerate light and may be lying in a darkened room (6), so a clinician should be prepared for low light conditions and not expect to be able to take notes easily. If light is required, a person with ME/CFS could use an eye-mask or a hood to minimize their disruption. Check beforehand whether scent intolerances are an issue and consider avoiding smoking, use of fragrance or even wearing clothes laundered in scented products (6).

People with severe or very severe ME/CFS may be more vulnerable to infection so if the clinician is showing signs of viral infection on the day of the visit, they should postpone (6). Even if there are no signs of infection, check before the visit whether the person and their caregiver have an infection control protocol, for example whether personal protective equipment is required.

During an initial assessment

People with severe or very severe ME/CFS are unlikely to tolerate a prolonged interaction (6) so consider the length of appointment and make sure it is focused on key priorities. Gathering subjective information beforehand either through direct written communication with the person, or through their caregiver, will save time and avoid unnecessary cognitive exertion. A person with severe or very severe ME/CFS may only be able to tolerate a short interaction before requiring a rest, so this should be built in to the assessment plan. A full assessment is unlikely to be possible in one session.

Establishing a therapeutic relationship is key as a clinician may be involved in a person's journey over a long period of time (6). Previous experiences with healthcare providers may have been poor or limited (13). People with severe or very severe ME/CFS have sometimes been misdiagnosed with a mental illness, or their carers accused of neglect or abuse (5). So the first step to building trust is to listen to the person and believe them, then find a way to demonstrate that understanding (7) (6).

The assessment

A general overview of assessment can be found in chapter 14 and many adaptations will apply regardless of the severity of ME/CFS. But consider the following particularly in relation to severe and very severe ME/CFS:

- Structure the assessment to allow for rest periods to minimize symptom exacerbation (6).
- Adapt questions to take into account cognitive dysfunction (see chapter 8).

- Consider the volume and tone of your voice in respect of any sound sensitivities (6).
- Run through primary symptoms and try to establish whether any may be due to medical conditions that require review, for example undiagnosed orthostatic intolerances, unrecognized sensory hypersensitivities, gastrointestinal issues etc. (5). A deterioration in specific symptoms may be due to a co-morbidity that could be medically managed, so check whether there has been a recent thorough medical review (6).
- Find out what activities the person is able to manage themselves, what they need support with, and whether any activities are causing exacerbation of symptoms or exceeding their available energy (5).
- Complications from being bedbound include development of contractures and issues with skin integrity (5). A brief check of joint range of movement and skin can be carefully carried out, but be aware of hypersensitivity to touch and check that they can tolerate passive handling or monitor their response closely.
- Feelings of grief and/or depression may be common due to their circumstances, so check whether the person has been offered emotional support in the past, or if they would find this beneficial (7), while making it clear that you understand their condition is real and has a physiological basis.
- If the person with severe or very severe ME/CFS has their care provided by family or a partner, be alert for any signs of caregiver stress or breakdown and provide information on community support and respite services if required (5).
- If the person does not have a caregiver, check whether they are managing with basic care needs such as obtaining and preparing food, and refer on for support if required and agreed by the person (5).
- Find out what current support is provided in terms of finance, and which agencies are already involved (5).

Ana: 'For most of my adult life I have had to live in a quiet dark room in order to survive. I am completely unable to raise my limbs against gravity, which means that I need help with every aspect to stay alive.'

Physiotherapy management for severe and very severe ME/CFS

It is unlikely that intensive input will be required for people with severe ME/CFS; instead they may benefit from a regular review over a prolonged period of time (6). If operating within a service that does not allow for long-term care and management, be sure to give the person and their caregivers the information they need to access your service again in future if required.

More regular input may be appropriate for a person experiencing a change in the severity of symptoms, for example improvements following a relapse, where a physiotherapist may be able to assist with the pacing and management of activities that are being reintroduced. An example of this can be seen at the end of this book in Ana's story.

Activity and environment management

Ensure the person and their caregivers understand post exertional malaise (PEM) and why it is important to avoid this as much as is feasible (5). Work through the daily routine to see if adequate rest has been scheduled and consider levels of stimulation in their environment and activities. Chapter 15 discusses energy management in more detail.

Consider aids and adaptations to reduce energy expenditure for activities of daily living, for example wheelchairs, walking aids, specialized beds, bedpans or perching stools (5), or refer to occupational therapy services if this is outside your scope of practice.

Look at the environment and suggest modifications to minimize sensory triggers as appropriate, for example light and sound levels, or visual stimuli such as bright colours and patterns (5). The person may have already tried many techniques or changes, so find out first what has and has not worked for them in the past.

Maintenance and prevention

Consider gentle range of movement exercises (5), whether passive, active-assisted or active depending on the person's capabilities and their ability to tolerate such intervention, in order to prevent contractures, improve blood flow and help with pain management. Take into account whether a person is also hypermobile (see chapter 2) and be sure to educate the person and/or their caregiver on appropriate handling techniques.

Be mindful that prolonged tension on neural tissues can trigger an immune response (26) which could exacerbate symptoms. For example, one study found a passive straight leg raise held for 15 minutes was enough to trigger pain, cognitive dysfunction and other general symptoms in people with ME/CFS both during the manoeuvre and up to 24 hours after (27).

Be sure to monitor how the person tolerates any intervention; take into consideration that PEM is generally a delayed response (see chapter 6). Review whether there was any impact of your intervention for the following 72 hours before deciding whether to incorporate it into the support plan. Adaptations to any plan may be required considering the fluctuating nature of the condition. Monitoring is essential due to the severity of the symptoms, but a rigorous activity and symptom diary may be difficult for a person with severe or very severe ME/CFS to maintain. Using family or carers to provide information may be helpful, or a more simplified system of tracking symptom severity such as a basic numerical rating scale could be more manageable.

Positional support
Advise on postural management strategies for those who are bedbound to prevent joint contractures and pressure areas (5), which may involve provision of positional aids or education for carers on passive movements, appropriate positioning and regular positional changes. Check appropriate equipment is in place for maintenance of skin integrity and consider referral to appropriate community nursing support if required.

Pain management
If pain is a significant problem, consider pain management techniques such as gentle massage or a review of their medication. Chapter 10 discusses pain management in more detail.

Referrals to other agencies
Provide information or refer to appropriate services for financial assistance if required (5). Provide information on relevant support groups and charities for the person with ME/CFS and for their carers (5).

Refer to services to offer support with mental and emotional health if indicated (5).

Hospital admissions
As mentioned earlier in this chapter, people with severe and very severe ME/CFS may sometimes require hospital admission. A specialist

hospital service for people with severe and very severe ME/CFS is a rarity, and hospitals therefore provide very challenging environments considering the nature of severe and very severe ME/CFS symptoms.

A physiotherapist, whether as a linked advocate for the person coming in from the community or as an inpatient physiotherapist working directly with the person on the ward, can take on a key role as advocate for the person with severe or very severe ME/CFS with the aim to minimize symptom exacerbation as much as possible. This could include (5):

- educating hospital staff about the nature of severe and very severe ME/CFS and the adaptations to practice that will be required
- making adaptations to minimize the sensory disturbances from light and sound in the environment as much as possible
- limiting unnecessary staff interactions to minimize sensory stimulation
- working with the person to make an information pack about their individual needs that can be taken to all medical appointments so that information does not have to be repeated
- highlighting precautions for surgery – for example ensuring adequate hydration and avoiding medications that could exacerbate orthostatic intolerances or interact with any other co-morbidities (28)
- considering transportation to/from hospital, for example planning the route in advance and making arrangements for the person to be admitted to a ward without delay.

SUMMARY

▸ Severe and very severe ME/CFS describes people who are mostly house or bedbound and suffer with significant disability, requiring assistance for most or all of their activities of daily living.
▸ Symptoms of severe and very severe ME/CFS are similar to general symptoms of ME/CFS but tend to be more extreme and more prevalent, alongside secondary complications of prolonged inactivity.

APPLICATION TO PRACTICE

▸ Make adaptations to all interactions and environments to account for sensory sensitivities.

▸ Utilize aids and adaptations to minimize energy usage.

▸ Aim to prevent secondary complications through positioning, education and passive movement if tolerated.

▸ Act as an advocate to help educate their carers, families and other healthcare providers.

References

1. Pendergrast, T., Brown, A., Sunnquist, M., Jantke, R., *et al.* (2016) 'Housebound versus nonhousebound patients with myalgic encephalomyelitis and chronic fatigue syndrome.' *Chronic Illness 12* (4).
2. Conroy, K., Bhatia, S., Islam, M. & Jason, L.A. (2021) 'Homebound versus bedridden status among those with myalgic encephalomyelitis/chronic fatigue syndrome.' *Healthcare 9* (2).
3. Strassheim, V., Lambson, R., Hackett, K.L. & Newton, J.L. (2017) 'What is known about severe and very severe chronic fatigue syndrome? A scoping review.' *Fatigue: Biomedicine, Health & Behavior 5* (3).
4. Baxter, H. (2022) 'Ensuring the voice of the very severely affected myalgic encephalomyelitis/chronic fatigue syndrome patient is heard in research: a research model.' *Healthcare (Basel) 10* (7).
5. Montoya, J.G., Dowell, T.G., Mooney, A.E., Dimmock, M.E. & Chu, L. (2021) 'Caring for the patient with severe or very severe myalgic encephalomyelitis/chronic fatigue syndrome.' *Healthcare 9*.
6. Kingdon, C., Giotas, D., Nacul, L. & Lacerda, E. (2020) 'Health care responsibility and compassion: visiting the housebound patient severely affected by ME/CFS.' *Healthcare 8* (197).
7. Fennell, P.A., Dorr, N. & George, S.S. (2021) 'Elements of suffering in myalgic encephalomyelitis/chronic fatigue syndrome: the experience of loss, grief, stigma, and trauma in the severely and very severely affected.' *Healthcare 9*.
8. Carruthers, B.M., van de Sande, M.I., De Meirleir, K.L., Klimas, N.G., *et al.* (2011) 'Myalgic encephalomyelitis: International Consensus Criteria.' *Journal of Internal Medicine 270*.
9. Shepherd, C. & Chaudhuri, A. (2019) *ME/CFS/PVFS: An Exploration of the Key Clinical Issues*. Gawcott: The ME Association.
10. Nacul, L., O'Boyle, S., Palla, L., Nacul, F.E., *et al.* (2020) 'How myalgic encephalomyelitis/chronic fatigue syndrome (ME/CFS) progresses: the natural history of ME/CFS.' *Frontiers in Neurology 11*.
11. Baxter, H., Speight, N. & Weir, W. (2021) 'Life-threatening malnutrition in very severe ME/CFS.' *Healthcare 9*.
12. Timbol, C.R. & Baraniuk, J.N. (2019) 'Chronic fatigue syndrome in the emergency department.' *Open Access Emergency Medicine 11*.
13. Strassheim, V., Newton, J.L. & Collins, T. (2021) 'Experiences of living with severe chronic fatigue syndrome/myalgic encephalomyelitis.' *Healthcare 9*.
14. Williams, L.R. & Isaacson-Barash, C. (2021) 'Three cases of severe ME/CFS in adults.' *Healthcare 9*.

15. Chu, L., Elliott, M., Stein, E. & Jason, L.A. (2021) 'Identifying and managing suicidality in myalgic encephalomyelitis/chronic fatigue syndrome.' *Healthcare (Basel)* 9 (6).

16. Nacul, L.C., Lacerda, E.M., Campion, P., Pheby, D., *et al.* (2011) 'The functional status and well being of people with myalgic encephalomyelitis/chronic fatigue syndrome and their carers.' *BMC Public Health 11* (402).

17. Brittain, E., Muirhead, N., Finlay, A.Y. & Vyas, J. (2021) 'Myalgic encephalomyelitis/chronic fatigue syndrome (ME/CFS): major impact on lives of both patients and family members.' *Medicina (Kaunas) 57* (1).

18. Campen, C.M.V., Rowe, P.C. & Visser, F.C. (2020) 'Reductions in cerebral blood flow can be provoked by sitting in severe myalgic encephalomyelitis/chronic fatigue syndrome patients.' *Healthcare 8* (394).

19. Hardcastle, S.L., Brenu, E.W. & Johnston, S. (2015) 'Longitudinal analysis of immune abnormalities in varying severities of chronic fatigue syndrome/myalgic encephalomyelitis patients.' *Journal of Translational Medicine 13* (299).

20. Melvin, A., Lacerda, E. & Dockrell, H.M. (2019) 'Circulating levels of GDF15 in patients with myalgic encephalomyelitis/chronic fatigue syndrome.' *Journal of Translational Medicine 17* (409).

21. Nacul, L., de Barros, B., Kingdon, C.C., Cliff, J.M. *et al.* (2019) 'Evidence of clinical pathology abnormalities in people with myalgic encephalomyelitis/chronic fatigue syndrome (ME/CFS) from an analytic cross-sectional study.' *Diagnostics 9* (41).

22. Tomas, C., Elson, J.L., Strassheim, V., Newton, J.L. & Walker, M. (2020) 'The effect of myalgic encephalomyelitis/chronic fatigue syndrome (ME/CFS) severity on cellular bioenergetic function.' *PLOS ONE 15* (4).

23. van Campen, C.M.C., Rowe, P.C. & Visser, F.C (2020) 'Two-day cardiopulmonary exercise testing in females with a severe grade of myalgic encephalomyelitis/chronic fatigue syndrome: comparison with patients with mild and moderate disease.' *Healthcare 8* (192).

24. van Campen, C.M.C., Rowe, P.C. & Visser, F.C. (2020) 'Cerebral blood flow is reduced in severe myalgic encephalomyelitis/chronic fatigue syndrome patients during mild orthostatic stress testing: an exploratory study at 20 degrees of head-up tilt testing.' *Healthcare 8* (169).

25. van Campen, C.L.M.C., Verheugt, F.W.A. & Visser, F.C. (2018) 'Cerebral blood flow changes during tilt table testing in healthy volunteers, as assessed by Doppler imaging of the carotid and vertebral arteries.' *Clinical Neurophysiology Practice 23* (3).

26. Ellis, R., Carta, G., Andrade, R.J. & Coppieters, M.W. (2022) 'Neurodynamics: is tension contentious?' *Journal of Manual & Manipulative Therapy 30* (1).

27. Rowe, P.C., Fontaine, K.R., Lauver, M., Jasion, S.E., Marden, C.L. & Moni, M. (2016) 'Neuromuscular strain increases symptom intensity in chronic fatigue syndrome.' *PLOS ONE 11* (7).

28. Lapp, C. (2020) 'Recommendations for persons with myalgic encephalomyelitis/chronic fatigue syndrome (ME/CFS) who are anticipating surgery or anesthesia.' Accessed on 8/12/2022 at https://drlapp.com/resources/advice-for-pwcs-anticipating-anesthesia-or-surgery.

CHAPTER 4

Paediatric ME/CFS

PURPOSE OF THIS CHAPTER

Children and young people can be affected by ME/CFS, with profound consequences for their access to education and quality of life. A physiotherapist may be able to assist a young person in areas such as energy management, postural management and guidance on adaptations to allow for educational access. A physiotherapist may also cause an inadvertent exacerbation of symptoms by using treatment approaches that can trigger post exertional malaise (PEM).

It is therefore important for any physiotherapist who works with children and young people to have an awareness of ME/CFS, whether they are working with the child directly for the condition or for an unrelated matter, so that the most appropriate treatment and management options are implemented, and adaptations are made to practice in order to minimize harmful triggers of PEM.

This chapter will discuss diagnostic criteria, impact upon education and management options, and how ME/CFS presents in children and young people.

What is the cause of ME/CFS in children and young people?

The predisposition, involvement of a trigger and subsequent persisting physiological processes that are currently known about ME/CFS are all discussed in chapter 1. While similar causes are presumed to occur in children, particularly following an infectious trigger, most research into the pathophysiology of ME/CFS has been conducted in adults so it is difficult to conclude that exactly the same processes are occurring in children and young people (1).

Who develops ME/CFS?

As discussed in chapter 1, there appears to be a peak of onset of ME/ CFS between the ages of 11 to 19 years in children and 33 to 39 years in adults (2) (3) (4).

ME/CFS is more common in adult females, and this is replicated in adolescent females aged between 12 and 18 years with reported rates between 74% and 82% (5). However, a more equal occurrence of ME/ CFS has been found between the sexes in children aged less than 12 years old (5). These findings suggest that the hormonal changes during puberty may trigger the female-dominant prevalence (6).

Symptoms

Symptoms of ME/CFS are summarized in chapter 1 and discussed in detail throughout this book. As well as the hallmark feature of ME/ CFS PEM (discussed in chapter 6), the most prominent symptoms in children are reported as headaches, orthostatic intolerance, cognitive impairments and sleep disturbances (7) (1).

Orthostatic intolerance, which is an inability to tolerate an upright position, is considered to be a common presentation in children with ME/CFS (1). Small studies have found higher instances of postural orthostatic tachycardia syndrome with or without hypotension in adolescents with ME/CFS compared to healthy controls (8) and adolescents who had experienced 'simple faint' (syncope) (9), although statistically significant differences are not always found (10). A reduction in blood flow to the brain in an upright position has also been found in young people with ME/CFS regardless of whether they exhibit signs of orthostatic intolerance (11), which has also been demonstrated consistently in adults (12). Further information on orthostatic intolerance can be found in chapter 12.

Joint hypermobility may also be more common in children with ME/CFS compared to healthy controls (13) and this should be considered during any physical assessment. More information on joint hypermobility can be found in chapter 2.

A study in the UK and the Netherlands analysed data from over 1500 adolescents and over 200 children under 12 with ME/CFS and found some differences in presentation in comparison to an adult cohort (5). Adolescents with ME/CFS were more likely to have headaches and less likely to have other types of pain compared to adults with ME/CFS, and children were more likely to have sore throats and less likely to have cognitive dysfunction. However, the set of diagnostic criteria used for this study was Fukuda, which does not require PEM as essential, so these findings are subject to the issues with diagnostic accuracy discussed in more detail in chapter 1.

Diagnosis

An overview of the various diagnostic criteria for ME/CFS can be found in chapter 1; however most case definitions and diagnostic criteria have been based on symptoms in the adult population (1) (14). Diagnostic criteria for ME/CFS specifically for children were proposed in 2006 (6), summarized in Table 4.1.

Table 4.1 Paediatric criteria

Timeframe of symptoms	Symptoms persisting or reoccurring for at least three months
Post exertional malaise	Essential
Fatigue	Unexplained chronic fatigue, unrelated to ongoing exertion, not relieved by rest, and resulting in a substantial reduction in previous levels of education, and social and personal activities
Sleep dysfunction	Essential
Pain	Essential. At least one from: a) myofascial and/or joint pain b) abdominal and/or head pain
Cognitive impairments	Essential. Two or more symptoms e.g.: • impaired memory • impaired attention/concentration • word finding difficulties
Neurological impairments	Not included
Autonomic dysfunction	Not essential. Included as 'at least one symptom from two of three categories': • orthostatic intolerance • palpitations with or without cardiac arrhythmias • dizziness • disturbed balance • shortness of breath

cont.

Neuroendocrine manifestations	Not essential. Included as 'at least one symptom from two of three categories': • recurrent feelings of feverishness and cold extremities • subnormal body temperature and marked diurnal fluctuations • sweating episodes • intolerance of extremes of heat and cold • marked weight change • loss of appetite or abnormal appetite
Immune manifestations	Not essential. Included as 'at least one symptom from two of three categories': • recurrent flu-like symptoms • sore or scratchy throat • repeated fevers and sweats • tender lymph nodes • new sensitivities to food, odours or chemicals

Alterations to the adult criteria include a change to how some symptoms are described in relation to a physical baseline, because as children go through constant physical development they may have no baseline against which to compare their physical or cognitive functioning (6). The timeframe for diagnosis was also reduced from the six months, stipulated in many criteria, down to three months. However, there is currently no consensus on the timeframe for diagnosis of ME/CFS in children and young people. While the Canadian Criteria (15) also suggest that symptoms should be present for three months in children for diagnosis compared to six months in adults, other diagnostic criteria do not stipulate a specific timeframe for diagnosis in children at all. While in the UK the National Institute of Health and Care Excellence (NICE) suggests that ME/CFS could be a suspected diagnosis if symptoms persist beyond four weeks in children, compared to six weeks in adults (16).

Although recommendations for a timeframe of diagnosis exist, they are not necessarily followed in clinical practice. One study found that in the UK the median time to assessment by a specialist service for children was 18 months (17).

Accurate diagnosis is important for several reasons. In research, if there is no consensus on criteria used, or criteria are not specific enough to exclude children with other conditions, then it becomes very difficult to compare the outcomes of studies robustly, for example in a meta-analysis (6).

In clinical practice, a lack of diagnostic certainty combined with poor awareness and training of medical professionals in paediatric ME/CFS have led to reports of children being misdiagnosed with psychiatric conditions such as school refusal, pervasive refusal syndrome and somatoform disorder (1) (18) (6). Parents have also been accused of Munchausen Syndrome by Proxy (now called 'factitious disorder imposed on another') and may be investigated by social services due to their child having to miss school, with some children even forcibly removed from their parents (19) (20) (18). Early and accurate diagnosis can therefore lessen the impact of ME/CFS on the child and their family (1).

Severity

Symptoms of ME/CFS in children and young people vary greatly, from mild through to very severe, and general definitions of these levels of severity can be found in chapter 1. Children with milder symptoms may be able to attend school with modifications (1). Those with severe and very severe ME/CFS experience symptoms so significantly debilitating they are mostly housebound or mostly bedbound (21) (22). There is an estimated 25% of people with ME/CFS classed as being severe or very severe (23); however, this figure relates to adults and no official data currently exists for children. Further information on severe and very severe ME/CFS in general can be found in chapter 3.

Regardless of the level of severity, ME/CFS can have a profound impact on the quality of life of children and young people (1), which is discussed later in this chapter.

Fluctuating severity

Symptoms of ME/CFS in children and adolescents can fluctuate considerably, both day-to-day and even within each day (1). Spontaneous remission and recovery have been reported, but also relapses can occur, due to factors such as (1):

- over-exertion
- illness/infection

- menstruation
- onset of puberty.

Such unpredictability in symptom severity can impede the ability to plan for school or social and family activities, and has further negative impacts on quality of life (1). Intermittent cessation of symptom severity may also lead to educators or health professionals developing an inaccurate impression from only seeing the child on 'good days', which may cause confusion or even scepticism as to the diagnosis (6).

Prognosis and impact on quality of life

Some studies have concluded that the prognosis for children and young people with ME/CFS is more favourable than for adults (1); however the evidence for this is based on small sample sizes and questionable diagnostic criteria. For example, a prospective community study of over 800 adolescents in Great Britain found an incidence rate of 30.3% of young people with 'fatigue', 1.1% with 'chronic fatigue' and 0.5% with 'chronic fatigue syndrome' as defined by the Fukuda Criteria (24). On follow-up four to six months later, all cases of 'chronic fatigue' and 'chronic fatigue syndrome' had recovered, leading the study to conclude that prognosis was 'good'. However, given the diagnostic criteria used for this study did not include PEM as essential, it is not possible to conclude whether any of the children who recovered had been experiencing the hallmark symptom of ME/CFS.

In contrast, an Australian study (14) of a cohort of 16 young people who had a diagnosis of ME/CFS found that after an average of four years 44% were unimproved or worse, 31% had improved but not completely and 25% had symptoms that were nearly or completely resolved. Another study (25) of 54 adolescents with ME/CFS reported near complete improvement in just over half of the group after two years, but ongoing significant symptoms and physical impairment in the other half. All of these studies used the Fukuda Criteria for diagnosis of ME/CFS, which do not include PEM as essential, therefore it is difficult to fully apply their findings to the ME/CFS population. There is further discussion on the issues around diagnostic criteria in chapter 1. It is important to note that there is no published data on prognosis for children with very severe ME/CFS (1).

The significant limitations on activity caused by ME/CFS result in profound social and intellectual isolation (22). Unsurprisingly, children and adolescents with ME/CFS have been found to have a lower quality of life than children with other paediatric conditions including asthma, diabetes, epilepsy, chronic digestive diseases and cystic fibrosis (26).

Impact of ME/CFS on education

Children and young people with ME/CFS are known to have frequent absences from school (1). For example, a retrospective survey of schools in England over five years found that ME/CFS was the cause of 42% of long-term sickness absence, which was in excess of all other medical causes (27).

As well as children having to miss school due to periods of increased symptom severity, the very act of attending school may cause a worsening of symptoms. A day in school involves getting up, getting dressed, getting to school, listening and digesting information in aural and visual form, walking between classrooms and around school sites, talking to other students and travelling home. Considering that triggers for PEM include physical, cognitive, sensory and emotional exertion (see chapter 6), it is clear how attending school may cause a number of issues for children and young people with ME/CFS.

The right to education is stipulated in Article 26 of the Universal Declaration of Human Rights (28). Children and young people with ME/CFS therefore need an adapted plan to continue to access education, otherwise there would be a breach of their human rights, as well as a loss of the educational and social benefits of attending school which may impact negatively on their quality of life (29). A physiotherapist may assist in providing the advice and guidance required to help a child with ME/CFS access education, and this is discussed later in this chapter.

Treatment of children and young people with ME/CFS

As discussed in chapter 1, there is no single treatment for ME/CFS. Management primarily involves addressing individual symptoms and does not differ from options for symptom management in the adult population. More information on specific symptoms and their management can be found throughout this book and can also apply to children and young people, with the necessary adaptations to working with a younger population such as appropriate presentation of information and consideration of their constant growth and development.

Regular assessment is advised to monitor for the development of any secondary illnesses, and to support the child and their family with changes to symptom severity over time (1).

Physiotherapy management of children and young people with ME/CFS

Energy management

Energy management involves managing activities within the energy envelope to avoid symptom exacerbation and is discussed at length in chapter 15.

Avoid implementation of any rigid programmes which involve a 'graded approach to education', where a child is encouraged to increase attendance at school regardless of their symptoms. An incremental increase in any activity does not reflect the nature of ME/CFS symptoms, in particular PEM.

While planning school activities can often take priority in the management of children and young people with ME/CFS, it is important to remember the benefits of social interaction and other activities that bring the child joy. Managing their time to dedicate all available energy to school may have a negative impact on their overall quality of life, so educational attendance should be seen as just one component of the child's energy expenditure. A physiotherapist should involve the child and their family when developing an energy management plan, taking into account personal priorities.

Supporting access to education

A physiotherapist could provide guidance and advice on possible adaptations to school, for example:

- Provide educational materials to school staff highlighting the key characteristics of ME/CFS and how physical, cognitive, sensory and emotional exertion may cause an exacerbation of symptoms.
- Suggest a quiet place is provided to allow for rest periods in a low sensory stimulus environment throughout the day.

- Allow the child to sit with their feet propped up in lessons if this is helpful.
- Ascertain whether long periods of sitting unsupported on the floor (for example in school assemblies) is tolerable, and if not suggest the child can be seated in a chair instead.
- Minimize movement between classrooms, which may require special passes to circumvent one-way systems.
- Provide information as to why general physical education sessions are not appropriate for a child with ME/CFS.
- Printed lesson handouts, recordings or a personal scribe can reduce the amount of attention and memory required during a lesson.
- Small class sizes or group work can minimize sensory stimulation compared to large classes.
- Exam concessions can make qualifications more accessible with less demands.
- Online schools remove the physical demands of travelling to attend school.

Greater challenges face children and young people with severe or very severe ME/CFS who are housebound or bedbound and physically unable to attend a place of education at all (22). Additionally, a child with severe or very severe ME/CFS may have significant cognitive dysfunction that would make engaging in a full lesson impossible, for example reduced attention and processing speed (22). Their capacity to engage may be in shorter bursts and at irregular timings, so the rigid structure of a school timetable may not be suitable for them (22). While robotics can allow children to attend live lessons without leaving their homes, online learning and online schools may allow more flexible educational access within a routine that suits the child.

Oliver: 'ME/CFS has affected all areas of my life. I can't go to school. I can't play football. I can't see my friends. I spend most of my time in my bedroom.'

A physiotherapist could provide assessment and advice on the learning environment at home, considering supportive seating, adequate positioning of screens, lighting and temperature.

Severe and very severe ME/CFS

For children who are bedbound, a physiotherapist may be able to provide input regarding postural management in order to prevent the secondary complications of immobility such as contractures and pressure sores (30). Further exploration of the management of someone with severe or very ME/CFS is found in chapter 3.

Additional physiotherapy input

A physiotherapist may be able to assist in the management of other symptoms of ME/CFS in children and young people, for example pain, orthostatic intolerance and fatigue. More information about each symptom along with management options can be found throughout this book, as well as considerations regarding exercise which are discussed at length in chapter 17.

SUMMARY

▸ Children and young people can be diagnosed with ME/CFS, and the condition will have a profoundly negative impact on their quality of life.

▸ Current research, definitions and diagnostic criteria are largely based on the adult population and may therefore not be applicable to children and young people.

▸ Symptoms and progression may differ in children and young people compared to adults, although not enough research has been carried out to allow for definite conclusions.

▸ A child's right to access education will be significantly challenged by ME/CFS.

APPLICATION TO PRACTICE

▸ Similar management strategies used for adults can also apply to children.

▸ Access to education is one priority and there are many areas to provide guidance and advice.

▸ When planning activities as part of an energy management plan, consider the child's quality of life and the importance of social/ joyful activities alongside education.

References

1. Rowe, P.C., Underhill, R.A., Friedman, K.J., Gurwitt, A., *et al.* (2017) 'Myalgic encephalomyelitis/chronic fatigue syndrome diagnosis and management in young people: a primer.' *Frontiers in Pediatrics 19* (5).
2. Bateman, L., Bested, A.C., Bonilla, H.F., Chheda B.V., *et al.* (2021) 'Myalgic encephalomyelitis/chronic fatigue syndrome: essentials of diagnosis and management.' *Mayo Clinic Proceedings 96* (11), 2861–2878.
3. Rowe, P.C., Underhill, R.A., Friedman, K.J., Gurwitt, A., *et al.* (2017) 'Myalgic encephalomyelitis/chronic fatigue syndrome diagnosis and management in young people: a primer.' *Frontiers in Pediatrics 19* (5).
4. Bakken, I.J., Tveito, K., Gunnes, N., Ghaderi, S., *et al.* (2014) 'Two age peaks in the incidence of chronic fatigue syndrome/myalgic encephalomyelitis: a population-based registry study from Norway 2008–2012.' *BMC Med 12* (167).
5. Collin, S.M., Nuevo, R., van de Putte, E.M., Nijhof, S.L. & Crawley, E. (2015) 'Chronic fatigue syndrome (CFS) or myalgic encephalomyelitis (ME) is different in children compared to in adults: a study of UK and Dutch clinical cohorts.' *BMJ Open 5* (10).
6. Jason, L.A., Jordan, K., Miike, T., Bell, D.S., *et al.* (2006) 'A pediatric case definition for myalgic encephalomyelitis and chronic fatigue syndrome.' *Journal of Chronic Fatigue Syndrome 13* (2–3).
7. Carruthers, B.M., van de Sande, M.I., De Meirleir, K.L., Klimas, N.G., *et al.* (2012) *Myalgic Encephalomyelitis – Adult & Paediatric: International Consensus Primer for Medical Practitioners.* Accessed on 12/01/2023 at www.investinme.org/ Documents/Guidelines/Myalgic Encephalomyelitis International Consensus Primer-2012-11-26.pdf.
8. Galland, B.C., Jackson, P.M., Sayers, R.M. & Taylor, B.J. (2008) 'A matched case control study of orthostatic intolerance in children/adolescents with chronic fatigue syndrome.' *Pediatric Research 63* (2).
9. Stewart, J.M., Gewitz, M.H., Weldon, A., Arlievsky, N., Li, K. & Munoz, J. (1999) 'Orthostatic intolerance in adolescent chronic fatigue syndrome.' *Pediatrics 103* (1).
10. Katz, B.Z., Stewart, J.M., Shiraishi, Y., Mears, C.J. & Taylor, R. (2012) 'Orthostatic tolerance testing in a prospective cohort of adolescents with chronic fatigue syndrome and recovered controls following infectious mononucleosis.' *Clinical Pediatrics 51* (9).
11. Tanaka, H., Matsushima, R., Tamai, H. & Kajimoto, Y. (2002) 'Impaired postural cerebral hemodynamics in young patients with chronic fatigue with and without orthostatic intolerance.' *Journal of Pediatrics 140* (4).
12. van Campen, C.L.M.C., Verheugt, F.W.A., Rowe, P.C. & Visser, F.C. (2020) 'Cerebral blood flow is reduced in ME/CFS during head-up tilt testing even in the absence of hypotension or tachycardia: a quantitative, controlled study using Doppler echography.' *Clinical Neurophysiology Practice 8* (5).
13. Barron, D.F., Cohen, B.A., Geraghty, M.T., Violand, R. & Rowe, P.C. (2002) 'Joint hypermobility is more common in children with chronic fatigue syndrome than in healthy controls.' *Journal of Pediatrics 141* (3).
14. Gill, A.C., Dosen, A. & Ziegler, J.B. (2004) 'Chronic fatigue syndrome in adolescents: a follow-up study.' *Archives of Pediatrics and Adolescent Medicine 158* (3).
15. Carruthers, B.M., Jain, A.K., De Meirleir, K.L., Peterson, D.L., *et al.* (2003) 'Myalgic encephalomyelitis/chronic fatigue syndrome.' *Journal of Chronic Fatigue Syndrome 11* (1).

16. National Institute for Health and Care Excellence (2021) 'Myalgic encephalomy-elitis (or encephalopathy)/chronic fatigue syndrome: diagnosis and management.' Accessed on 8/12/2022 at www.nice.org.uk/guidance/ng206.

17. Webb, C.M., Collin, S.M., Deave, T., Haig-Ferguson, A., Spatz, A. & Crawley, E. (2011) 'What stops children with a chronic illness accessing health care: a mixed methods study in children with chronic fatigue syndrome/myalgic encephalomy-elitis (CFS/ME).' *BMC Health Services Research 11* (11).

18. Colby, J. (2007) 'Special problems of children with myalgic encephalomyelitis/chronic fatigue syndrome and the enteroviral link.' *Journal of Clinical Pathology 60* (2).

19. Wynarczyk, N. (2019) 'ME awareness: social services can threaten families of children with chronic fatigue.' The ME Association. Accessed on 8/12/2022 at https://meassociation.org.uk/2019/05/me-awareness-social-services-can-threat-en-families-of-children-with-chronic-fatigue-05-may-2019.

20. Shepherd, C. & Chaudhuri, A. (2019) *ME/CFS/PVFS: An Exploration of the Key Clinical Issues.* Gawcott: The ME Association.

21. Pendergrast, T., Brown, A., Sunnquist, M., Jantke, R., *et al.* (2016) 'Housebound versus nonhousebound patients with myalgic encephalomyelitis and chronic fatigue syndrome.' *Chronic Illness 12* (4).

22. Newton, F.R. (2021) 'The impact of severe ME/CFS on student learning and K–12 educational limitations.' *Healthcare 9* (627).

23. Conroy, K., Bhatia, S., Islam, M. & Jason, L.A. (2021) 'Homebound versus bedridden status among those with myalgic encephalomyelitis/chronic fatigue syndrome.' *Healthcare 9* (106).

24. Rimes, K.A., Goodman, R., Hotopf, M., Wessely, S., Meltzer, H. & Chalder, T. (2007) 'Incidence, prognosis, and risk factors for fatigue and chronic fatigue syndrome in adolescents: a prospective community study.' *Pediatrics 119* (3).

25. van Geelen, S.M., Bakker, R.J., Kuis, W. & van de Putte, E.M. (2010) 'Adolescent chronic fatigue syndrome: a follow-up study.' *Archives of Pediatrics and Adolescent Medicine 164* (9).

26. Roma, M., Marden, C.L., Flaherty, M.A.K., Jasion, S.E., Cranston, E.M. & Rowe, P.C. (2019) 'Impaired health-related quality of life in adolescent myalgic enceph-alomyelitis/chronic fatigue syndrome: the impact of core symptoms.' *Frontiers in Pediatics 15* (7).

27. Dowsett, E.G. & Colby, J. (2011) 'Long-term sickness absence due to ME/CFS in UK schools.' *Journal of Chronic Fatigue Syndrome 3* (2).

28. United Nations (1948) *Universal Declaration of Human Rights.* Accessed on 9/12/2022 at www.un.org/en/about-us/universal-declaration-of-human-rights.

29. Similä, W.A. (2022) 'Health-related quality of life in young people with chronic fatigue syndrome/myalgic encephalomyelitis.' PhD thesis, Norwegian University of Science and Technology.

30. Speight, N. (2020) 'Severe ME in Children.' *Healthcare 8* (211).

CHAPTER 5

Management in Acute Post Viral Presentations

PURPOSE OF THIS CHAPTER

Viral infection is reported to be one the leading triggers of ME/CFS, as well as causing prolonged symptoms in the form of post viral fatigue and post viral fatigue syndrome. A physiotherapist in any service may be presented with a person who has post viral complications, including post exertional malaise (PEM). For example, the COVID-19 pandemic is resulting in a high number of people presenting to physiotherapists with acute and chronic complications, in inpatient, outpatient, community and paediatric services.

It is important that every physiotherapist has an awareness of the potential development of post viral complications, including PEM, because many physiotherapy interventions may be a trigger and cause an exacerbation of symptoms. A physiotherapist may even be the first health professional whom a person approaches with post viral problems, and therefore must be able to identify key symptoms and understand appropriate and effective management strategies.

This chapter will discuss the historical occurrence of ME/CFS following viral infections and pandemics including COVID-19, the nature of post viral complications such as post viral fatigue, post viral fatigue syndrome and Long Covid, and how to assess and manage a person with these conditions.

ME/CFS following viral infections

Symptoms linked to ME/CFS have been reported following infection with many types of virus including Epstein–Barr, Ross River, Ebola,

West Nile and Dengue, as well as infection from types of bacteria and parasite (1). For example, a prospective cohort study of 250 people seen with Epstein–Barr (glandular fever) in primary care in the UK reported that 9% went on to be diagnosed with 'chronic fatigue syndrome' (using Fukuda Criteria) (2). Similarly 11% of 253 people in Australia with Epstein–Barr, Q Fever and Ross River infections demonstrated a 'post-infective fatigue illness' after six months, which shared a similar presentation regardless of the infective agent (3).

Epidemics have allowed for data collection on concurrent infections, with reported increases in people struggling with severe long-lasting fatigue. Following the Spanish flu outbreak in 1918 there were reports that of every 1000 cases, about 200 (20%) did not make a full recovery (4). A long-term follow up of people recovering from severe acute respiratory syndrome (SARS) in Hong Kong found after four years that 40% of 233 survivors reported chronic fatigue symptoms and 27% would meet the Fukuda Criteria for ME/CFS (5).

The limitations of older studies investigating the occurrences of post viral ME/CFS is that the diagnostic criteria used are not the more recent versions that include PEM as the hallmark characteristic of ME/CFS and essential for diagnosis. It is therefore currently difficult to draw definitive conclusions on the prevalence of ME/CFS after viral infections.

COVID-19 and Long Covid

The novel coronavirus SARS-CoV-2 (COVID-19) was first identified at the end of 2019 and a pandemic was declared by the World Health Organization in March 2020 (6). Long-term symptoms following COVID-19 infection were reported, although at first data collection focused only on people who had been hospitalized (7), which led to an assumption that long-term symptoms were linked to severity of the disease (8). However, reports grew of people who had milder cases of the disease and still suffered long-term symptoms, for example in a global online survey of 3762 adults experiencing long-term symptoms, only 8.43% of respondents had been hospitalized (9).

A myriad of terms emerged to describe the long-term symptoms following COVID-19 infection such as long-haul COVID-19, post-COVID syndrome, chronic COVID syndrome and post-acute sequelae of SARS-CoV-2 infection (PASC) (10). Long Covid was a term first used through social media by people with the condition as a means to describe their experiences, before the term was gradually adopted by the media and some researchers (8). For the remainder of this chapter, Long Covid will be used to describe the long-term symptoms following COVID-19 infection.

Considering that ME/CFS is common after viral triggers, it is plausible that the COVID-19 pandemic could also cause a new cohort of people with ME/CFS. As more information about Long Covid began to surface, it became clear there was an overlap between many Long Covid symptoms and ME/CFS (11). A global online survey was carried out of 3762 adults experiencing long-term symptoms after confirmed or suspected COVID-19 infection between September and November 2020 (9) and several comparisons with ME/CFS could be made. For example, women made up nearly 79% of respondents; the most common symptoms at six months were fatigue, PEM and cognitive dysfunction; and a pattern of relapse and remission was described by over 85% of respondents. The most common triggers of symptom exacerbation were physical activity, stress, exercise and cognitive exertion. At the time of the survey 118 respondents had already received a diagnosis of ME/CFS.

However, the survey captured a total of 203 different symptoms across ten organ systems, including many symptoms not necessarily associated with ME/CFS such as seizures, changes to vision and hearing and facial paralysis. The term Long Covid may therefore include cases of ME/CFS but also cover a much wider population. For example, one review (12) proposed that people with Long Covid may be experiencing a cluster of symptoms or syndromes such as permanent organ damage, post intensive care syndrome and post viral fatigue syndrome. A systematic review in 2020 suggested four categories within Long Covid (13):

1. Symptoms continuing from the acute phase of COVID-19 infection.
2. Symptoms causing a new health condition.
3. Late onset symptoms as a consequence of COVID-19 which are separate to the acute phase.
4. Impact on a pre-existing health condition or disability.

To explore the link between Long Covid and ME/CFS, a systematic review in 2021 contrasted reported Long Covid symptoms in 21 research articles with ME/CFS symptoms defined across multiple case definitions (see chapter 1 for a review of ME/CFS diagnostic criteria) and found that almost every ME/CFS symptom was reported in at least one Long Covid paper (10). However, symptoms not listed on ME/CFS criteria such as rashes and loss of smell and/or taste were also reported by those with Long Covid (10).

Another study (14) explored how symptoms in Long Covid changed over time. In August 2020 they used the DePaul Symptom Questionnaire (see chapter 18) to capture the symptoms of 278 people with Long Covid, both at the time of reporting and approximately 21 weeks previously. The group had significantly improved in almost all symptoms apart from sensitivity to alcohol, loss of hair, cognitive dysfunction in the form of trouble forming words, difficulty focusing and absentmindedness. The study also compared symptoms of the Long Covid group to a cohort of 502 people with ME/CFS. In terms of symptom severity the ME/CFS group were significantly more impaired in 39 symptoms, but the Long Covid group were more impaired in the symptoms of chest pain, shortness of breath and an irregular heartbeat. The authors note that they did not differentiate between people with Long Covid who did or did not have organ damage following infection, which could explain the severity of chest complaints in the Long Covid group. COVID-19 has been found to have caused organ damage which may result in long-term symptoms, such as permanent lung injury (15) and cardiovascular complications (16) including the finding of persisting microclots, which are thought to block capillaries and impair oxygen exchange (17).

Long Covid has also been reported in children and young people, although the prevalence differs significantly between studies (18). Symptoms listed mirror those found in children and young people with ME/CFS (see chapter 4) such as headache, fatigue, sleep dysfunction and cognitive difficulties. However, as with the adult studies of Long Covid, other symptoms unrelated to ME/CFS are also reported, such as disturbances in smell and taste, and skin complaints.

Long Covid is therefore a broad term that captures all experiences of the long-term complications following COVID-19 infection. Of relevance to this chapter are the symptoms that do overlap with ME/CFS, in particular PEM, as the management strategies are the same for both groups with the priority of minimizing symptom exacerbation.

Post viral fatigue syndrome

A degree of fatigue after viral infection is common and known as 'post viral fatigue' (19) with a gradual recovery expected over a couple of weeks once the infection resolves (20).

Post viral fatigue syndrome (PVFS) can be diagnosed if fatigue persists and other symptoms manifest, including (19):

- post exertional malaise (symptoms exacerbated by physical, cognitive, sensory or emotional exertion)
- intermittent and recurrent flare of viral symptoms
- unable to maintain previous levels of activity
- unrefreshing sleep and/or excessive daytime sleepiness
- cognitive dysfunction
- orthostatic intolerance.

It is suggested that with appropriate management PVFS will resolve over a number of months (19). For example, a study exploring symptoms in people with Long Covid (14) found many symptoms similar to PVFS had improved over an average of a 21-week period. Although the study does not directly link symptoms to a diagnosis of PVFS, the findings could appear to demonstrate this time-course.

If symptoms of PVFS continue to persist and cause significant functional impairment with no improvement after several months, then ME/CFS could become a considered diagnosis (19) (see chapter 1). There is an obvious overlap between the symptoms of PVFS and ME/CFS. While ME/CFS can be commonly linked to a viral infection, it is not the only known trigger, therefore PVFS only refers to symptoms arising from a known viral infection.

One paper (20) hypothesizes a timescale of stages from acute infection to ME/CFS as:

- onset: the acute infection stage
- prodromal period (0–4 months): fatigue symptoms, recovery likely
- early disease (4–24 months): variable severity of symptoms, recovery possible
- established disease (24+ months): complicated disease with variable severity, recovery less likely.

This time-course is so far hypothetical. There is currently no clear concept of what factors will determine whether a person will completely recover following viral infection, develop PVFS or go on to develop ME/CFS. Discussion of the current understanding around predisposing factors can be found in chapter 1.

One suggested pathophysiological process that may cause or contribute to post viral fatigue syndrome is viral persistence, in which ongoing immune and inflammatory responses are caused by an ongoing viral infection, with local effects of the virus in muscles or the central nervous system (21) (22) (23). There may also be a dysfunction of the inflammatory response pathways, where symptoms are caused by elevated and prolonged pro-inflammatory processes triggered by the viral infection (24).

Viruses have the potential to affect the human microbiome, which is the abundance of bacteria, fungi and viruses that are present inside human beings (23). Viral-induced microbiome changes may cause disease in the human host (25) and the potential for viral infection to directly cause ME/CFS continues to be explored in research. Currently the evidence base suffers from too many inconsistencies in diagnostic criteria, sample processing and analysis, so robust comparisons and conclusions have not yet been possible (25).

The ongoing prevalence of COVID-19 infections and cases of Long Covid provides an opportunity for researchers to track how viral infections persist to cause post viral fatigue syndrome, as well as ME/CFS, and perhaps new understanding will emerge in the near future.

Adaptation to practice
Understanding the limitations of evidence when applying to practice

The emergence of Long Covid has highlighted the importance of appraising evidence before implementing findings to clinical practice.

Currently most studies of Long Covid have major limitations due to the lack of a uniform definition or diagnosis of Long Covid, variable timeframes following infection, reliance on patient-reported measures, selection bias and a lack of control groups (14) (18) (10). As discussed earlier in this chapter, Long Covid is a term that describes a diverse collection of symptoms and conditions, so there are therefore a wide range of potential treatment and management options presented in the literature. For example, one study (26) reports that a six-week pulmonary rehabilitation programme will improve exercise capacity, functional status, breathlessness, fatigue and quality of life of 'patients with Long Covid'. While the paper later notes that the results cannot be generalized to the total population, the abstract and title suggests that pulmonary rehabilitation, which is an exercise-based approach, is a safe and effective treatment for people with Long Covid. However, of the 58 participants in this study, 41 had reported breathlessness, 37 fatigue and 22 cognitive dysfunction, but there is no mention of PEM. Given physical exertion is one of the known triggers of PEM (discussed in chapter 6), it is likely that a progressive exercise programme would not only be ineffective for a person with Long Covid who experiences PEM: it may also cause an exacerbation of symptoms. Therefore, the results of this study should not be generalized to every person with Long Covid.

When working with people who experience PEM, whether as part of post viral fatigue syndrome, Long Covid or ME/CFS, a physiotherapist should always ensure their clinical practice is only influenced by research that specifically includes this cohort, especially when broader terminology is used such as Long Covid or 'chronic fatigue'.

> **Mo**: 'My recovery from COVID-19 did not follow 'normal' patterns and I never got back to what I could do before I was ill.'

Ultimately, research will always have limitations, and all treatment should be individualized, constantly monitored and evaluated.

Assessment of a post viral presentation

If a person attends a physiotherapy appointment and reports reduced physical and/or cognitive function with a recent history of infection, then post viral fatigue syndrome should be seriously considered. If the person has not had a recent medical review, then they should also be referred to rule out differential diagnoses.

History of infection and recovery

The physiotherapist should find out more about the history of infection and details of the recovery process. Did they feel fully recovered before returning to their normal baseline of activities or did they not have the opportunity to rest due to commitments?

It should also be investigated as to whether the infectious agent has known complications, for example COVID-19 has been linked to cardiopulmonary damage (15) (16), formation of microclots (17) and postural orthostatic tachycardia syndrome (POTS) (27). If relevant medical assessments have not been carried out and symptoms may be indicative of secondary complications then refer for appropriate medical review.

Are there signs of post viral fatigue syndrome?

Symptoms of post viral fatigue syndrome are diverse and a person may not have linked them together to explain their presenting problem, therefore it is important to ask whether the person has experienced or is experiencing any of the key features of post viral fatigue syndrome.

Post exertional malaise

PEM is characterized by a worsening of current symptoms or addition of new symptoms following a trigger, which may be physical, cognitive, sensory or emotional. As discussed in chapter 6, PEM can be unpredictable, manifest as a variety of symptoms and due to its delayed nature the trigger can often be difficult to define. A person seeking physiotherapy input may also not be familiar with the terminology and therefore not directly report it as an issue.

There may be obvious links between doing 'too much' and a symptom relapse, or they may describe how their symptoms have responded well when they have reduced their activity or rested more. For example:

'I went for a ten-minute walk and it wiped me out for the rest of the week.'

'I enjoyed seeing my friends for the afternoon, but I felt so unwell afterwards.'

'I tried going back to work but only lasted two days and then crashed badly.'

It would be helpful for the person to keep an activity and symptom diary to track patterns and identify potential triggers. More information on assessment of PEM can be found in chapter 14.

Intermittent and recurrent flare of viral symptoms

Look for signs of a relapse and remission pattern. Some people may describe this as 'boom or bust' where there are periods of remission allowing for increased activity followed by periods of symptom exacerbation, likely caused by the increased activity.

Viral symptoms such as malaise, sore throat and tender glands can be a sign of PEM.

Unable to maintain previous levels of activity

The person may not have returned to their normal level of activity after an infection, for example they may not be able to work the same number of hours that they previously were able to achieve. Or they may be able to do most things but are struggling to sustain them, for example they have returned to work but are having to use the weekends to recover, or they are no longer able to do any extra hobbies or social activities.

Unrefreshing sleep

Do they feel refreshed after a good night's sleep? Are there issues falling asleep, or frequent waking? See chapter 14 for more information on what to ask about sleeping patterns.

Cognitive dysfunction

Are there any signs of cognitive dysfunction? The person may describe problems with attention or concentration, difficulties with memory, or use the term 'brain fog'. More information on cognitive dysfunction in relation to ME/CFS can be found in chapter 8.

Orthostatic intolerance

Orthostatic intolerance is an inability to maintain heart rate or blood pressure against gravity and is discussed in detail in chapter 12. The person may report that their symptoms are worse when they stand up, perhaps noticing shortness of breath, palpitations or dizziness on standing. A quick screening procedure for orthostatic intolerance is the active stand test or NASA lean test, both of which are described in chapter 18.

Management of acute post viral fatigue/ post viral fatigue syndrome

Management of post viral fatigue and post viral fatigue syndrome follows the basics of (19):

- plenty of rest
- pacing activities to minimize energy expenditure (energy management)
- hydration and nutrition
- maximizing sleep.

If symptoms seem out of control and are greatly impacting on a person's function, then introduce the concept devised by the charity ME Action of 'Stop – Rest – Pace' (28) (29):

- Stop: avoid pushing limits and over-exertion.
- Rest: use rest as a management strategy.
- Pace: use energy management techniques to adapt activities without causing symptoms.

Energy management provides the means to allow a person to function within their available energy without exacerbating symptoms. More information about the importance of rest (including what constitutes therapeutic rest) and energy management can be found in chapter 15.

Increasing activity levels

It is important to understand that an improvement in symptoms may allow for an increase in activity levels, as opposed to the notion that increasing activity levels may have a therapeutic effect on symptoms or provide a cure for the condition.

Given that post viral fatigue syndrome may improve naturally over time, a person may find they are gradually able to increase their activity levels without causing symptom exacerbation. Some people may make a complete recovery, others may find they reach a limit of what they can manage and are unable to move beyond it without triggering symptoms. Reasons for such differences in recovery are not yet understood.

A physiotherapist can work alongside the person to help them monitor and manage their symptoms, and plan and prioritize their energy expenditure. Any increase in activity levels should be done in line with the person's abilities, priorities and symptom stability, with regular monitoring and evaluation to ensure additions to their workload have not triggered PEM.

A rigid incremental increase in activity levels may push a person beyond their limitations and cause PEM. Such an approach is not appropriate for people with post viral fatigue syndrome in the presence of PEM. It is typically applied to general cases of deconditioning, which is not reflective of the complex physiological processes that occur in post viral fatigue syndrome or ME/CFS. Deconditioning is discussed further in chapter 7.

When ME/CFS is suspected

There is no clear differentiation between the diagnosis of post viral fatigue syndrome and ME/CFS and no clear consensus on the diagnostic process or criteria for ME/CFS. (Further information on diagnosis of ME/CFS is in chapter 1.) A physiotherapist should be aware of the key symptoms and timeframe (in general, symptoms must be present for more than six months, but there are variations in this timescale across the different criteria), and if an acute presentation of post viral fatigue syndrome continues to persist they may consider referring the person to a medical practitioner for formal diagnosis.

> **Kim**: 'I already had ME/CFS, but infection with COVID-19 has made me more severe, reactivated shingles and given me new orthostatic intolerance symptoms.'

Regardless of diagnosis the management strategies remain the same between post viral fatigue syndrome and ME/CFS, with the over-riding priority for a physiotherapist to minimize PEM and find ways to maximize quality of life.

SUMMARY

▶ A viral infection can lead to longer term complications such as post viral fatigue syndrome and/or ME/CFS.

▶ A viral pandemic is likely to cause a sudden increase in people presenting with post viral fatigue symptoms across many areas of physiotherapy services.

▶ 'Long Covid' is a broad term that includes people presenting with post viral fatigue syndrome and ME/CFS, as well as other potential complications following COVID-19 infection. Of relevance to the information in this chapter is the presence of PEM.

APPLICATION TO PRACTICE

▶ Any person presenting with a decrease in function and a history of viral infection should be screened for signs of post viral fatigue syndrome.

▶ A physiotherapist in any setting may come across a person with post viral complications and should therefore have a basic awareness of the signs and symptoms, in particular PEM.

▶ The presence of PEM must take priority in all management and treatment planning.

▶ The evidence base for broad terms such as Long Covid should be carefully appraised for relevance to a cohort with PEM, before applying findings to clinical practice.

References

1. Komaroff, A.L. & Bateman, L. (2021) 'Will COVID-19 lead to myalgic encephalomyelitis/chronic fatigue syndrome?' *Frontiers in Medicine (Lausanne) 18* (7).
2. White, P.D., Thomas, J.M., Amess, J., Crawford, D.H., *et al.* (1998) 'Incidence, risk and prognosis of acute and chronic fatigue syndromes and psychiatric disorders after glandular fever.' *British Journal of Psychiatry 173.*
3. Hickie, I., Davenport, T., Wakefield, D., Vollmer-Conna, U., *et al.* (2006) 'Dubbo Infection Outcomes Study Group: post-infective and chronic fatigue syndromes precipitated by viral and non-viral pathogens: prospective cohort study.' *BMJ 333* (7568).
4. Islam, M.F., Cotler, J. & Jason, L.A. (2020) 'Post-viral fatigue and COVID-19: lessons from past epidemics.' *Fatigue: Biomedicine, Health & Behavior 8* (2).
5. Lam, M.H., Wing, Y.K., Yu, M.W., Leung, C.M., *et al.* (2009) 'Mental morbidities and chronic fatigue in severe acute respiratory syndrome survivors: long-term follow-up.' *Archives of Internal Medicine 169* (22).
6. Pollard, C.A., Morran, M.P. & Nestor-Kalinoski, A.L. (2020) 'The COVID-19 pandemic: a global health crisis.' *Physiological Genomics 52* (11).
7. Subramanian, A., Nirantharakumar, K., Hughes, S., Myles, P., *et al.* (2022) 'Symptoms and risk factors for long COVID in non-hospitalized adults.' *Nature Medicine 28* (8).
8. Callard, F. & Perego, E. (2021) 'How and why patients made Long Covid.' *Social Science & Medicine 268.*
9. Davis, H.E., Assaf, G.S., McCorkell, L., Wei, H., *et al.* (2021) 'Characterizing long COVID in an international cohort: 7 months of symptoms and their impact.' *eClinicalMedicine 38.*

10. Wong, T.L. & Weitzer, D.J. (2021) 'Long COVID and myalgic encephalomyelitis/chronic fatigue syndrome (ME/CFS): a systemic review and comparison of clinical presentation and symptomatology.' *Medicina (Kaunas) 57* (5).

11. Siberry, V.G.R. & Rowe, P.C. (2022) 'Pediatric Long COVID and myalgic encephalomyelitis/chronic fatigue syndrome: overlaps and opportunities.' *Pediatric Infectious Disease Journal 41* (4).

12. The National Institute for Health Research (2021) 'Living with COVID19 Second Review.' Accessed on 12/01/2023 at https://evidence.nihr.ac.uk/themedreview/living-with-covid19-second-review.

13. Ceravolo, M.G., Arienti, C., de Sire, A., Andrenelli, E., *et al.* 2020. 'International Multiprofessional Steering Committee of Cochrane Rehabilitation REH-COVER action. Rehabilitation and COVID-19: the Cochrane Rehabilitation 2020 rapid living systematic review.' *European Journal of Physical and Rehabilitation Medicine 56* (5).

14. Jason, L.A., Islam, M., Conroy, K., Cotler, J., *et al.* (2021) 'COVID-19 symptoms over time: comparing long-haulers to ME/CFS.' *Fatigue 9* (2).

15. Wang, F., Kream, R.M. & Stefano, G.B. (2020) 'Long-term respiratory and neurological sequelae of COVID-19.' *Medical Science Monitor 1* (26).

16. Becker, R.C. (2020) 'Anticipating the long-term cardiovascular effects of COVID-19.' *Journal of Thrombosis and Thrombolysis 50* (3).

17. Kell, D.B., Laubscher, G.J. & Pretorius, E. (2022) 'A central role for amyloid fibrin microclots in long COVID/PASC: origins and therapeutic implications.' *Biochemical Journal 479* (4).

18. Zimmermann, P., Pittet, L.F. & Curtis, N. (2021) 'How common is Long COVID in children and adolescents?' *Pediatric Infectious Disease Journal 40* (12).

19. Shepherd, C. (2021) 'Long Covid and ME/CFS.' ME Association. Accessed on 9/12/2022 at https://ccisupport.org.nz/wp-content/uploads/2021/08/Long-covid-and-MECFS-May-2021.pdf.

20. Nacul, L., O'Boyle, S., Palla, L., Nacul, F.E., *et al.* (2020) 'How myalgic encephalomyelitis/chronic fatigue syndrome (ME/CFS) progresses: the natural history of ME/CFS.' *Frontiers in Neurology 11* (11).

21. Mowbray, J.F. & Yousef, G.E. (1991) 'Immunology of postviral fatigue syndrome.' *British Medical Bulletin 47* (4).

22. de la Torre, J.C., Borrow, P. & Oldstone, M.B. (1991) 'Viral persistence and disease: cytopathology in the absence of cytolysis.' *British Medical Bulletin 47* (4).

23. Proal, A. & Marshall, T. (2018) 'Myalgic encephalomyelitis/chronic fatigue syndrome in the era of the human microbiome: persistent pathogens drive chronic symptoms by interfering with host metabolism, gene expression, and immunity.' *Frontiers in Pediatrics 4* (6).

24. Islam, M.F., Cotler, J. & Jason, L.A. (2020) 'Post-viral fatigue and COVID-19: lessons from past epidemics.' *Fatigue: Biomedicine, Health & Behavior 8* (2).

25. Newberry, F., Hsieh, S.Y., Wileman, T. & Carding, S.R. (2018) 'Does the microbiome and virome contribute to myalgic encephalomyelitis/chronic fatigue syndrome?' *Clinical Science (London) 132* (5).

26. Nopp, S., Moik, F., Klok, F.A., Gattinger, D., *et al.* (2022) 'Outpatient pulmonary rehabilitation in patients with Long COVID improves exercise capacity, functional status, dyspnea, fatigue, and quality of life.' *Respiration 1* (9).

27. Raj, S.R., Arnold, A.C., Barboi, A., Claydon, V.E., *et al.* (2021) 'American Autonomic Society: Long-COVID postural tachycardia syndrome: an American Autonomic Society statement.' *Clinical Autonomic Research 31* (3).

28. ME Action (2022) 'Stop Rest Pace.' Accessed on 9/12/2022 at www.meaction.net/stoprestpace.

29. Décary, S., Gaboury, I., Poirier, S., Garcia, C., *et al.* (2021) 'Humility and acceptance: working within our limits with Long COVID and myalgic encephalomyelitis/chronic fatigue syndrome.' *Journal of Orthopaedic & Sports Physical Therapy 51* (5).

SYMPTOMS and MANAGEMENT

CHAPTER 6

Post Exertional Malaise

PURPOSE OF THIS CHAPTER

Post exertional malaise (PEM) is the hallmark characteristic of ME/CFS and involves additional symptoms and/or the exacerbation of current symptoms in response to exertion (1). Physiotherapy interventions may cause PEM, therefore it is essential that physiotherapists have an awareness of what may trigger PEM and an understanding of how to adapt their approach in order to avoid it.

This chapter details the symptoms, triggers and timeframe of PEM, the current theories that explain the processes behind it, how to adapt interactions and interventions to avoid it, and what management tools exist to help people to minimize PEM in their daily life.

What Is PEM?

PEM describes the onset of new symptoms or an exacerbation of current symptoms in response to physical, cognitive, sensory and emotional exertion and is considered the hallmark feature of ME/CFS (1)(2). Similar terms include 'post exertional neuroimmune exhaustion' (PENE) or 'post exertional symptom exacerbation' (PESE) (3).

The term 'post exertional malaise' was created in 1994 in conjunction with the development of the Centers for Disease Control and Prevention (CDC) Criteria for diagnosis of ME/CFS (otherwise known as the Fukuda Criteria) (4). Without clear explanation of what this term meant, or inclusion in the list of symptoms essential for diagnosis, the CDC Criteria were criticized for not being specific enough to ME/CFS and the term PEM has been used inconsistently by clinicians and researchers (3).

Research has been conducted to try to define PEM more accurately, with alternative suggestions for the term such as PENE or PESE (3)(5).

An International Consensus Criteria in 2011 (6) listed post exertional neuroimmune exhaustion (PENE) as a compulsory symptom for diagnosis of ME/CFS, describing it as 'a pathological inability to produce sufficient energy on demand with prominent symptoms primarily in the neuroimmune regions'. The characteristics of PENE are described as:

- marked rapid physical and/or cognitive fatiguability in response to exertion
- post exertional symptom exacerbation
- post exertional exhaustion that may occur immediately or delayed by hours or days
- prolonged recovery, lasting longer than 24 hours but can last days, weeks or longer.

Kim: 'I have to carefully pace myself each and every day to avoid PEM. Heat, cold, viruses and external matters all have an impact, some foreseeable and some not. During PEM I lose the ability to look and listen and walk and talk. It is only alleviated by rest and quiet.'

Although 'malaise' is not an accurate description of the experience of PEM, for the purposes of consistency this book will continue to use 'PEM' to describe the onset of new symptoms or exacerbation of current symptoms following exertion, as it is the terminology most used in current literature relating to ME/CFS.

Some qualitative research has been carried out to try to understand the experience of PEM (5)(3), but this data will be limited by size and potential selection bias, and may not be reflective of every individual's experience of PEM.

Symptoms of PEM

There are no set symptoms that define PEM. Each person with ME/CFS may experience PEM differently to others, and their individual PEM symptoms may depend on the nature of the triggering event. An international survey of over 1500 people with ME/CFS (5) listed symptoms affecting cardiovascular, neurological, musculoskeletal, metabolic, autonomic, immune and gastrointestinal systems. The most common symptoms reported were:

- reduced stamina and/or functional capacity (99.4%)

- physical fatigue (98.9%)
- cognitive exhaustion (97.4%)
- problems thinking (97.4%)
- unrefreshing sleep (95.0%)
- muscle pain (87.9%)
- insomnia (87.3%)
- muscle weakness/instability (87.3%)
- temperature dysregulation (86.9%)
- flu-like symptoms (86.6%).

Some symptoms of PEM, like fatigue and muscle ache, may be commonly experienced mildly by the general population after an exertional activity such as strenuous exercise (3). For example, following a cardiopulmonary exercise test (CPET) a group of healthy participants reported fatigue, weakness and painful muscles and joints (2). These symptoms were short lived, did not impact on activities of daily living, and most participants had returned to their baseline of activity within a day of completing the test.

However, in people with ME/CFS the severity of PEM symptoms can be disproportionate to the extent of the trigger (1). Additionally, although the general population or people with other medical conditions may experience 'fatigue' after exertion, they do not experience the constellation or severity of symptoms reported by people with ME/CFS (3). For example, when people with ME/CFS undertook a CPET they reported symptoms including cognitive dysfunction and decrease in function and flu-like symptoms, and the average time for these symptoms to resolve was 4.5 days (2).

Oliver: 'I have to constantly plan ahead so I can function without triggering PEM.'

The experience of PEM therefore is the hallmark for people with ME/CFS and the response to exertion can cause severe and widespread symptoms.

Triggers of PEM

The nature of PEM is that it is triggered by exertion. What constitutes 'exertion' is important to understand, as it covers a wide range of experiences. The trigger may not always be identifiable, for example in the international survey 84.9% reported that in some instances there was no identifiable trigger for their symptom exacerbation (5). A physiotherapist may be able to help with trigger identification through use of a symptom and activity diary, although it should be noted that the very act of having to keep a diary may cause cognitive exertion and be a trigger of PEM itself. Exertional triggers of PEM can take the following forms.

Physical
Physical exertion may be interpreted as exercise; however, physical exertion for people with ME/CFS may occur during typical everyday activities such as walking, climbing the stairs, taking a shower or even just sitting up in bed. For example, in the international survey of over 1500 people with ME/CFS (5) 78.2% described 'basic activities of daily living' as a trigger of PEM and 64.5% cited simply changing position was enough of a trigger. PEM may be triggered by positional changes against gravity, which can be linked with orthostatic intolerances that are discussed in chapter 12.

Cognitive
Cognitive exertion has been shown to trigger similar levels of PEM symptoms compared to physical exertion (7), for example researchers have used simulated driving as a means to trigger PEM (7) (8). Cognitive exertion may be caused by simple activities such as reading for leisure or communicating with others. See chapter 8 for more information on cognitive dysfunction in people with ME/CFS.

Sensory
People with ME/CFS may be hypersensitive to a range of sensory stimulation, such as light, noise and smell, and over 80% of survey respondents reported sensory overload as a trigger for their PEM (5). More information on hypersensitivity can be found in chapter 11.

Emotional
Strong emotions can also be a trigger for PEM (3) with 93.2% of survey respondents reporting they experienced PEM after emotional stress and 88.3% reporting emotional events as a cause (5). Emotional triggers could be from positive or negative events, and link with cognitive and sensory overload.

Onset and duration of PEM

The onset of PEM may immediately follow an exertional trigger or it can be a delayed response of several hours or days (1). In an international survey of over 1500 people with ME/CFS the most commonly reported time of onset was one to two days (5).

Duration of PEM symptoms has been reported to last several hours, several days or even several months (3). In the same survey (5) 58% of respondents reported symptoms lasting between three and six days and 46.7% between one week and one month. A total of 1029 (67.1%) people described a crash that never resolved, suggesting the overall severity of their symptoms had permanently worsened following a trigger.

There is no set time of onset or duration of PEM for each individual with ME/CFS nor always a predictable response to a specific trigger (3).

Normal physiological responses to physical exertion

As physiotherapists predominantly deal with physical activity, the remainder of this chapter will focus on physical exertion. In order to understand why a person with ME/CFS cannot tolerate physical exertion it is first helpful to understand the typical response in a healthy body.

A simplified version of these responses is as follows: to meet the demands of any physical activity the heart, blood cells and lungs must supply oxygen-rich blood to the tissues of the required muscles, and those muscles then use oxygen alongside glucose, fats and sometimes protein to produce energy in the form of adenosine triphosphate (ATP). This process is called aerobic metabolism (9) and can produce 34 molecules of ATP from one molecule of glucose (10). One of the by-products of aerobic metabolism is carbon dioxide, which is removed from the blood using the same systems.

When energy demands increase, so too does the requirement for oxygen and subsequently the amount of carbon dioxide produced, with an expected increase in heart rate, blood pressure and respiratory rate accordingly.

When the oxygen supply can no longer meet the energy demands, metabolism switches to anaerobic, which does not need oxygen to produce energy and the level of carbon dioxide exceeds the level of oxygen. Anaerobic metabolism is not as efficient as aerobic metabolism, generating only two molecules of ATP per molecule of glucose and producing lactic acid and carbon dioxide as a by-product (10). The point at which aerobic metabolism transitions to anaerobic metabolism is called various terms, such as 'lactate threshold', 'heart rate deflection point' and 'ventilatory anaerobic threshold' (VAT) (9).

Objectively these processes can be measured using a cardiopulmonary exercise test (CPET) (11). Equipment that captures and analyses expired gas is fitted to a participant alongside monitors for heart rate and blood pressure. The participant is then asked to work to a point of maximal exertion, usually on a static exercise bike with increasing resistance provided.

In sports and rehabilitation the aerobic capacity can be improved by training at or around the anaerobic threshold (12) (9). These beneficial effects also occur across population groups, for example aerobic exercise can increase aerobic capacity in people with mild to moderate stroke (13), chronic heart failure (14) and chronic obstructive pulmonary disease (COPD) (15).

Physiological response to physical exertion in ME/CFS

Cardiopulmonary exercise tests have been used to investigate the physiological responses to exercise in people with ME/CFS. After a single test, some studies have shown no differences between people with ME/CFS and matched controls in terms of peak heart rate and peak VO_2 (maximum oxygen consumption), which suggests that there is no 'deconditioning' of the participants with ME/CFS (16) (17). Other studies have found differences after a single CPET, demonstrating people with ME/CFS had a blunted heart rate response (chronotropic intolerance), reduced anaerobic threshold and higher levels of lactic acid production in comparison to controls who were age and sex matched (18) (19) (20).

The disparity in findings may be explained by differences in the aerobic fitness of participants and not necessarily the physiological characteristics of ME/CFS (21). However, the processes involved with ME/CFS and PEM become clearer with a 'two-day CPET', which involves a second CPET repeated 24 hours after the first one.

In the general population the result of a repeated test usually closely matches or improves upon the first in terms of performance. People with chronic lung and heart disease, and fatigue-producing conditions such as HIV and multiple sclerosis, can also reproduce or even improve upon their results from the previous day (22). But people with ME/CFS have shown a marked deterioration on the second CPET in all measures of performance such as reduced heart rate response, entering anaerobic metabolism more quickly than the previous test, reduced VO_2 Max, and increased blood lactate levels (18)(19)(23)(20). Such deterioration in function over a two-day CPET has so far only been seen in people with ME/CFS and is indicative of the processes behind PEM (19).

The decline in performance has been replicated in another form of physical exertion in people with ME/CFS. Repeated maximal muscle contraction tests in hand grip (24) and of quadriceps (25) show how healthy controls can match previous results, whereas again people with ME/CFS have a reduction in performance. The mechanisms behind this potential peripheral fatigue are discussed in detail in chapter 7.

Other adverse physiological effects of physical exertion have been found in people with ME/CFS during exercise testing, including:

- reduced oxygenation of the prefrontal cortex (26)
- impaired cognitive processing (27)(2)
- altered gut microbiome and increased bacterial transloca-tion (28)
- decreased pain threshold (29).

Further discussion of the effects of exercise on people with ME/CFS can be found in chapter 17.

What causes PEM?

There are currently several theories exploring the cause of PEM in people with ME/CFS.

Mitochondrial dysfunction

One theory for the inability to meet energy demands is that ME/CFS involves a form of mitochondrial dysfunction. Mitochondria are responsible for energy production and are integral to normal cellular function (30). Mitochondria contain enzymes that oxidate sugar, fats and proteins to produce energy in the form of adenosine triphosphate (ATP) in a process called mitochondrial respiration (31)(30).

Mitochondria are not only important for producing energy; they also contribute to cellular stress responses and regulate communication between cells and tissues (32) and additionally are thought to be involved in neurogenesis, which is the process of new neurons being formed in the brain (33).

Mitochondrial dysfunction can occur through genetic disorders (primary mitochondrial disorder) where there is an issue in the gene coding specifically for mitochondrial respiration and related proteins (34). Mitochondrial dysfunction can also occur as a consequence of neurodegenerative, genetic and metabolic diseases (secondary mitochondrial dysfunction) (34) (32) (33) including Alzheimer's disease (35), cholestatic liver disease (36), Parkinson's disease (37) and even from the effects of aging (33).

Mitochondrial dysfunction has been found in people with ME/CFS. For example, a study of 138 people with ME/CFS (almost all confirmed with criteria that includes PEM as essential) looked at the availability of ATP and the efficiency of the mitochondria. In comparison to normal function in 53 healthy controls, the study identified mitochondrial dysfunction in every ME/CFS participant (38). Significant differences have been seen in mitochondrial respiratory function between people with ME/CFS and healthy controls (39) (40), although one study found no difference in individual mitochondrial activity, suggesting the dysfunction in respiration may lie somewhere else in the energy production chain (41). Mitochondrial dysfunction has been found in people with both severe and moderate ME/CFS, but while all have reduced mitochondrial function compared to healthy controls, those with severe ME/CFS also had higher rates of respiratory acidification (39).

A systematic review (40) of studies comparing mitochondrial function between people with ME/CFS and healthy controls found such a variance in testing protocols and outcome measures between studies that there was not enough consistency for a true analysis and that it is currently too difficult to establish the exact role of mitochondria in relation to ME/CFS.

DNA studies in people with ME/CFS have found no evidence of primary mitochondria disorders (40). This suggests that mitochondrial dysfunction may be a consequence of ME/CFS, rather than a primary cause (40).

Given mitochondrial dysfunction can be seen in a number of conditions that do not exhibit PEM, it is difficult to conclude that mitochondrial dysfunction alone is the reason that people with ME/CFS experience PEM. In comparison to other disorders that feature mitochondrial dysfunction, one study found that while the oxidative capacity of the mitochondria was no different between people with ME/CFS and those with other disorders, there was a reliable difference seen in terms of ATP production and mitochondrial respiration activities that would allow for discrimination between ME/CFS and other mitochondrial dysfunction disorders (42).

One theory to explain the role of mitochondria in ME/CFS suggests that immune-inflammatory processes may inhibit mitochondrial respiration and cause damage to mitochondria, resulting in reduced energy production and subsequent symptoms of PEM and fatigue (43).

As yet no research exists to support any conclusion as to the exact role of mitochondrial dysfunction in relation to PEM.

Cardiac neural regulation abnormalities

Normal changes in heart rate necessary to meet the demands of an increased physical workload are controlled by the sympathetic nervous system. People with ME/CFS may have abnormalities in cardiac neural regulation that explain why their cardiovascular system is unable to adapt to the energy demands of physical exertion, which may be a manifestation of autonomic nervous system dysregulation (18). The role of the autonomic nervous system in ME/CFS is discussed in more detail in chapter 12.

Ana: 'Talking or moving my body in bed can be enough to exacerbate my symptoms.'

Metabolic abnormalities

Changes to metabolic processes have been found in people with ME/CFS in relation to PEM. One study (44) found evidence of hypermetabolism occurring during a period of PEM, indicating an increased state of metabolic activity. Another study (45) found significant metabolic disturbances within the first 24 hours following maximal physical exertion in people with ME/CFS compared to controls, as well as the presence of four metabolites that have yet to be identified and may have significant relevance to the processes involved in ME/CFS. This study also found alterations in energy-production pathways, particularly in relation to glutamate metabolism, which has a major role in the central nervous system as an excitatory neurotransmitter.

Abnormalities have been found too in the red blood cells of people with ME/CFS (46). As red blood cells transport oxygen around the body, an abnormality in these cells could reduce the oxygen supply with subsequent difficulties in aerobic metabolism.

Adaptation to practice
Avoiding post exertional malaise

Given PEM may be triggered by physical, cognitive, sensory or emotional exertion, there are many aspects of a physiotherapy interaction and intervention that may inadvertently cause PEM (see Table 6.1 for examples).

Table 6.1 Physiotherapy interactions that may cause PEM

Physical	Any aspect of physical assessment
	Exercise
	Position of person (e.g. upright against gravity in comparison to supported seat/bed)
	Passive stretches (47)
	Travel to the appointment (if applicable)
Cognitive	Listening to and answering questions
	Filling in questionnaires
	Listening to verbal advice/instruction
	Reading and comprehending written materials
Sensory	Visual stimulus from body language/clothing and environment (e.g. lighting)
	Auditory stimulus from volume/tone of voice and environment
	Touch from manual handling/manual therapy techniques
	Scent of perfume/washing powder/deodorant/smoke/air fresheners
Emotional	Fear of not being believed (due to previous experience)
	Distress from discussing severity of disability
	Anxiety and anticipation of appointment
	Overload from a positive or negative interaction

The nature of a trigger and the severity of any resulting PEM will differ between each person. A physiotherapist should consider how to adapt their practice to minimize the exposure to triggers and therefore minimize the potential of triggering PEM. Suggestions of how to adapt practice in relation to each specific trigger can be found throughout this book, including an overview in chapter 14.

Physiotherapy management of PEM
Assessing PEM

The two-day cardiopulmonary exercise test is so far the closest objective measure available to identify PEM (19). Unfortunately the very nature of the test involves pushing a person into PEM and may cause serious symptom exacerbation, and the means to carry out a CPET are not available in most standard physiotherapy services. For people with severe ME/CFS it is highly unlikely they would be able to participate in the test.

PEM may be identified with a detailed subjective assessment. Key areas to be looking for include a pattern of symptom exacerbation and recovery. People may describe 'good days' where they are able to achieve more, followed by a period of 'bad days', but they may not be able to identify a specific trigger. They may describe PEM as a 'relapse', 'flare', 'crash' or 'payback' (3).

When assessing for PEM it is helpful to build a week-by-week picture of activities and symptoms, remembering that cognitive, emotional and sensory exertion can be as much of a cause of PEM as physical. The aim is to establish triggering activities with the resultant symptoms and how long they may last for but, as discussed in this chapter, the nature of PEM is very variable and there may not be a simple pattern. Symptom severity and exertional tolerance may fluctuate depending on a number of factors, for example many women report that the menstrual cycle, pregnancy and menopause have exacerbated their symptoms (48). Rather than mapping out a rigid set of symptoms and triggers it is more likely that a thorough subjective assessment with activity tracking will give an outline of areas that can be addressed.

Measuring PEM is discussed further in chapter 14 and chapter 18.

Avoiding/minimizing PEM in daily life

The key physiotherapy management of PEM is in assisting the person to structure their activities in order to avoid it as much as possible. More information regarding energy management can be found in chapter 15. A heart rate monitor may be a useful objective tool to help people avoid or minimize anaerobic metabolism and therefore minimize their physical exertion, and this is discussed in detail in chapter 16.

Management during PEM

During a period of PEM a physiotherapy intervention may not be appropriate and the advice may be to allow the person to rest and recover before any further interaction occurs. Alternatively a person may benefit from input to manage acute symptoms such as pain, or to identify that the person is currently in a PEM flare and needs to reduce their activity levels.

Following an episode of PEM it may be helpful to reflect on what the trigger could have been and work with the person to find ways of minimizing this in future. Realistically, many aspects of daily life may be unavoidable or of high priority to the person, and therefore unfortunately the potential for PEM could be unavoidable. Suggestions on aids and adaptations to minimize energy expenditure may be of value.

Faith: 'I try to avoid new experiences because it is hard to evaluate the likelihood or severity of PEM they may cause.'

SUMMARY

▸ Post exertional malaise (PEM) is the addition of symptoms, or an exacerbation of current symptoms, following exertion.
▸ Triggers can be physical, cognitive, emotional and sensory.
▸ PEM can be a delayed response so it may not always be apparent that an activity has caused it at the time.
▸ People with ME/CFS have shown a deterioration in performance on repeated cardiopulmonary exercise tests, compared to healthy controls and other fatigue-producing diseases, who can match or improve on previous tests.

APPLICATION TO PRACTICE

▸ The priority in any setting is to avoid triggering PEM, so appropriate measures must always be in place to monitor for signs of PEM.
▸ Every physiotherapy intervention should be adapted to reduce physical, cognitive, sensory and emotional exertion in order to minimize or avoid causing PEM.
▸ Physiotherapists can help people with ME/CFS to identify triggers and adapt their activities of daily living in order to minimize PEM.

References

1. Bateman, L., Bested, A.C., Bonilla, H.F., Chheda, B.V., *et al.* (2021) 'Myalgic encephalomyelitis/chronic fatigue syndrome: essentials of diagnosis and management.' *Mayo Clinic Proceedings 96* (11).
2. Mateo, L.J., Chu, L., Stevens, S., Stevens, J., *et al.* (2020) 'Post-exertional symptoms distinguish myalgic encephalomyelitis/chronic fatigue syndrome subjects from healthy controls.' *Work 66* (2).
3. Chu, L., Valencia, I.J., Garvert, D.W. & Montoya, J.G. (2018) 'Deconstructing post-exertional malaise in myalgic encephalomyelitis/chronic fatigue syndrome: a patient-centered, cross-sectional survey.' *PLOS ONE 13* (6).
4. Fukuda, K., Straus, S.E., Hickie, I., Sharpe, M.C., Dobbins, J.G. & Komaroff, A.L. (1994) 'The chronic fatigue syndrome: a comprehensive approach to its definition and study.' *Annals of Internal Medicine 121.*
5. Holtzman, C.S., Bhatia, S., Cotler, J. & Jason, L.A. (2019) 'Assessment of post-exertional malaise (PEM) in patients with myalgic encephalomyelitis (ME) and chronic fatigue syndrome (CFS): a patient-driven survey.' *Diagnostics (Basel) 9* (1).
6. Carruthers, B.M., van de Sande, M.I., De Meirleir, K.L., Klimas, N.G., *et al.* (2011) 'Myalgic encephalomyelitis: International Consensus Criteria.' *Journal of Internal Medicine 270*, 327–338.
7. Keech, A.C., Sandler, C.X., Vollmer-Conna, U., Cvejic, E., Lloyd, A.R. & Barry, B.K. (2015) 'Capturing the post-exertional exacerbation of fatigue following physical and cognitive challenge in patients with chronic fatigue syndrome.' *Journal of Psychosomatic Research 79* (6).
8. Cvejic, E., Sandler, C.X., Keech, A., Barry, B.K., Lloyd, A.R. & Vollmer-Conna, U. (2017) 'Autonomic nervous system function, activity patterns, and sleep after physical or cognitive challenge in people with chronic fatigue syndrome.' *Journal of Psychosomatic Research 103.*
9. Ghosh, A.K. (2004) 'Anaerobic threshold: its concept and role in endurance sport.' *Malaysian Journal of Medical Sciences 11* (1).
10. Staughton, J. (2021) 'Aerobic metabolism vs anaerobic metabolism.' Accessed on 9/12/2022 at www.scienceabc.com/pure-sciences/aerobic-metabolism-vs-anaerobic-metabolism.html.
11. Albouaini, K., Egred, M., Alahmar, A. & Wright, D.J. (2007) ' Cardiopulmonary exercise testing and its application.' *Postgraduate Medical Journal 83* (985).
12. Davis, J.A., Frank, M.H., Whipp, B.J. & Wasserman, K. (1979) 'Anaerobic threshold alterations caused by endurance training in middle-aged men.' *Journal of Applied Physiology 46* (6).
13. Pang, M.Y., Eng, J.J., Dawson, A.S. & Gylfadóttir, S. (2006) 'The use of aerobic exercise training in improving aerobic capacity in individuals with stroke: a meta-analysis.' *Clinical Rehabilitation 20* (2).
14. Sullivan, M.J., Higginbotham, M.B. & Cobb, F.R. (1989) 'Exercise training in patients with chronic heart failure delays ventilatory anaerobic threshold and improves submaximal exercise performance.' *Circulation 79* (2).
15. Punzal, P.A., Ries, A.L., Kaplan, R.M. & Prewitt, L.M. (1991) 'Maximum intensity exercise training in patients with chronic obstructive pulmonary disease.' *Chest 100* (3).
16. Sargent, C., Scroop, G.C., Nemeth, P.M., Burnet, R.B. & Buckley, J.D. (2002) 'Maximal oxygen uptake and lactate metabolism are normal in chronic fatigue syndrome.' *Medicine & Science in Sports & Exercise 34* (1).
17. Nelson, M.J., Buckley, J.D. & Thomson, R.L. (2019) 'Diagnostic sensitivity of 2-day cardiopulmonary exercise testing in myalgic encephalomyelitis/chronic fatigue syndrome.' *Journal of Translational Medicine 17* (80).
18. Davenport, T.E., Lehnen, M., Stevens, S.R., VanNess, J.M., Stevens, J. & Snell, C.R. (2019) 'Chronotropic intolerance: an overlooked determinant of symptoms

and activity limitation in myalgic encephalomyelitis/chronic fatigue syndrome?' *Frontiers in Pediatrics 7* (82).

19. Davenport, T.E., Stevens, S.R., Stevens, J., Snell, C.R. & Van Ness, J.M. (2020) 'Properties of measurements obtained during cardiopulmonary exercise testing in individuals with myalgic encephalomyelitis/chronic fatigue syndrome.' *Work 66* (2).

20. Lien, K., Johansen, B., Veierød, M.B., Haslestad, A.S., *et al.* (2019) 'Abnormal blood lactate accumulation during repeated exercise testing in myalgic encephalomyelitis/chronic fatigue syndrome.' *Physiological Reports 7* (11).

21. Cook, D.B., VanRiper, S., Dougherty, R.J., Lindheimer, J.B., Falvo, M.J. & Chen, Y. (2022) 'Cardiopulmonary, metabolic, and perceptual responses during exercise in myalgic encephalomyelitis/chronic fatigue syndrome (ME/CFS): a multi-site clinical assessment of ME/CFS (MCAM) sub-study.' *PLOS ONE 17* (3).

22. Larson, B., Davenport, T.E., Stevens, S., Stevens, J., Van Ness, M.J. & Snell, C. (2019) 'Reproducibility of measurements obtained during cardiopulmonary exercise testing in individuals with fatiguing health conditions: a case series.' *Cardiopulmonary Physical Therapy Journal 30* (4).

23. Keller, B.A., Pryor, J.L. & Giloteaux, L. (2014) 'Inability of myalgic encephalomyelitis/chronic fatigue syndrome patients to reproduce VO_2peak indicates functional impairment.' *Journal of Translational Medicine 23* (12).

24. Jäkel, B., Kedor, C. & Grabowski, P. (2021) 'Hand grip strength and fatigability: correlation with clinical parameters and diagnostic suitability in ME/CFS.' *Journal of Translational Medicine 19* (159).

25. Paul, L., Wood, L., Behan, W.M. & Maclaren, W.M. (1999) 'Demonstration of delayed recovery from fatiguing exercise in chronic fatigue syndrome.' *European Journal of Neurology 6* (1).

26. Neary, P.J, Roberts A.D., Leavins, N., Harrison, M.F., Croll, J.C. & Sexsmith, J.R. (2008) 'Prefrontal cortex oxygenation during incremental exercise in chronic fatigue syndrome.' *Clinical Physiology and Functional Imaging 28* (6).

27. LaManca, J.J., Sisto, S.A., DeLuca, J., Johnson, S.K., *et al.* (1998) 'Influence of exhaustive treadmill exercise on cognitive functioning in chronic fatigue syndrome.' *American Journal of Medicine 28* (105).

28. Shukla, S.K., Cook, D., Meyer, J., Vernon, S.D., *et al.* (2015) 'Changes in gut and plasma microbiome following exercise challenge in myalgic encephalomyelitis/chronic fatigue syndrome (ME/CFS).' *PLOS ONE 10* (12).

29. Van Oosterwijck, J., Nijs, J., Meeus, M., Lefever, I., *et al.* (2010) 'Pain inhibition and postexertional malaise in myalgic encephalomyelitis/chronic fatigue syndrome: an experimental study.' *Journal of Internal Medicine 268* (3).

30. Osellame, L.D., Blacker, T.S. & Duchen, M.R. (2012) 'Cellular and molecular mechanisms of mitochondrial function.' *Best Practice & Research: Clinical Endocrinology & Metabolism 26* (6).

31. Hoeks, J., Hesselink, M. & Schrauwen, P. (2012) 'Mitochondrial Respiration.' In F.C. Mooren (ed.) *Encyclopedia of Exercise Medicine in Health and Disease.* Berlin: Springer.

32. Nunnari, J. & Suomalainen, A. (2012) 'Mitochondria: in sickness and in health.' *Cell 148* (6).

33. Khacho, M., Clark, A., Svoboda, D.S., MacLaurin, J.G., *et al.* (2017) 'Mitochondrial dysfunction underlies cognitive defects as a result of neural stem cell depletion and impaired neurogenesis.' *Human Molecular Genetics 26* (17).

34. Chinnery, P.F. (2000) 'Primary Mitochondrial Disorders Overview.' In H.H. Ardinger *et al.* (eds) *GeneReviews.* Washington, DC: University of Washington.

35. Wang, W., Zhao, F. & Ma, X. (2020) 'Mitochondria dysfunction in the pathogenesis of Alzheimer's disease: recent advances.' *Molecular Neurodegeneration 15* (30).

36. Arduini, A., Serviddio, G., Tormos, A.M., Monsalve, M. & Sastre, J. (2012) 'Mitochondrial dysfunction in cholestatic liver diseases.' *Frontiers in Bioscience 4* (6).

37. Greenamyre, J.T., MacKenzie, G., Peng, T.I. & Stephans, S.E. (1999) 'Mitochondrial dysfunction in Parkinson's disease.' *Biochemical Society Symposia 66.*
38. Booth, N.E., Myhill, S. & McLaren-Howard, J. (2012) 'Mitochondrial dysfunction and the pathophysiology of myalgic encephalomyelitis/chronic fatigue syndrome (ME/CFS).' *International Journal of Clinical and Experimental Medicine 5* (3).
39. Tomas, C., Elson, J.L., Strassheim, V., Newton, J.L. & Walker, M. (2020) 'The effect of myalgic encephalomyelitis/chronic fatigue syndrome (ME/CFS) severity on cellular bioenergetic function.' *PLOS ONE 15* (4).
40. Holden, S., Maksoud, R., Eaton-Fitch, N., Cabanas, H., Staines, D. & Marshall-Gradisnik, S. (2020) 'A systematic review of mitochondrial abnormalities in myalgic encephalomyelitis/chronic fatigue syndrome/systemic exertion intolerance disease.' *Journal of Translational Medicine 18* (1).
41. Tomas, C., Brown, A.E., Newton, J.L. & Elson, J.L. (2019) 'Mitochondrial complex activity in permeabilised cells of chronic fatigue syndrome patients using two cell types.' *PeerJ 7.*
42. Smits, B., van den Heuvel, L., Knoop, H., Küsters, B., *et al.* (2011) 'Mitochondrial enzymes discriminate between mitochondrial disorders and chronic fatigue syndrome.' *Mitochondrion 11* (5).
43. Morris, G. & Maes, M. (2014) 'Mitochondrial dysfunctions in myalgic encephalomyelitis/chronic fatigue syndrome explained by activated immuno-inflammatory, oxidative and nitrosative stress pathways.' *Metabolic Brain Disease 29* (1).
44. McGregor, N.R., Armstrong, C.W., Lewis, D.P. & Gooley, P.R. (2019) 'Post-exertional malaise is associated with hypermetabolism, hypoacetylation and purine metabolism deregulation in ME/CFS cases.' *Diagnostics (Basel) 9* (3).
45. Germain, A., Giloteaux, L., Moore, G.E., Levine, S.M., *et al.* (2022) 'Plasma metabolomics reveals disrupted response and recovery following maximal exercise in myalgic encephalomyelitis/chronic fatigue syndrome.' *JCI Insight 7* (9).
46. Saha, A.K., Schmidt, B.R., Wilhelmy, J., Nguyen, V., *et al.* 2019. 'Red blood cell deformability is diminished in patients with chronic fatigue syndrome.' *Clinical Hemorheology and Microcirculation 71* (1).
47. Rowe, P.C., Fontaine, K.R., Lauver, M., Jasion, S.E., Marden, C.L. & Moni, M. (2016) 'Neuromuscular strain increases symptom intensity in chronic fatigue syndrome.' *PLOS ONE 11* (7).
48. Chu, L., Valencia, I.J., Garvert, D.W. & Montoya, J.G. (2019) 'Onset patterns and course of myalgic encephalomyelitis/chronic fatigue syndrome.' *Frontiers in Pediatrics 5* (7).

CHAPTER 7

Fatigue

PURPOSE OF THIS CHAPTER

Fatigue is the one symptom used in every diagnostic criteria of ME/CFS and tends to be a priority in research studies. For example, a systematic review (1) of randomized controlled trials evaluating physiotherapeutic interventions found that almost all studies included outcome measures on fatigue.

But the definition of fatigue remains vague, the mechanisms behind it are poorly understood and many methods to measure it do not accurately capture the type of fatigue uniquely experienced by people with ME/CFS (2). One intervention typically used to address fatigue in most other fatigue-producing conditions is exercise, yet for people with ME/CFS exertion is likely to worsen fatigue.

This chapter explores what is meant by fatigue in terms of ME/CFS, which processes might be involved in causing fatigue and what physiotherapy interventions might be beneficial or counter-productive.

What is fatigue?

'Fatigue' describes a decrease in mental and physical performance and is a term that can be used alongside a wide variety of disease states as well as something regularly experienced by the general population. All people suffer from fatigue through daily life in response to increased energy expenditure, and this fatigue would be expected to improve with rest and not impact on overall quality of life or activities of daily living (3).

As a symptom fatigue can be caused by a wide range of conditions, for example (4):

- metabolic/endocrine diseases
- neurological disorders
- cardiac/pulmonary diseases
- mental health disorders
- infectious diseases
- vitamin deficiencies
- medication side effects
- cancer
- pregnancy.

'Fatigue' is a broad term that can describe a subjective experience, such as a perception of exhaustion, of activities requiring effort beyond the expected amount or general weariness (3). However, 'fatigue' can also describe an objective failure in performance (3), such as impaired physical functioning.

Measuring fatigue

A lack of clear definition of fatigue makes the measurement of this symptom very difficult. There are over fifty subjective measures of 'fatigue', many of which do not accurately represent the type of fatigue uniquely experienced by people with ME/CFS (2). A summary of commonly used fatigue scales in ME/CFS research can be found in chapter 18.

Objective tools to measure fatigue, such as measurement of mechanical and electromyographic responses of skeletal muscle during voluntary and evoked contractions, can also lead to differing conclusions depending on the definition and parameters of fatigue used (5).

Fatigue and ME/CFS

Fatigue is one of the primary symptoms of ME/CFS in all diagnostic criteria. There is no specific definition of 'fatigue' given in any of the criteria, but its characteristics are required to be persistent or recurrent, unexplained by any other condition or exertion, can be physical and mental and interferes with activities of daily living (6) (7) (8) (9).

Qualitative research (10) gathered descriptors of the specific symptom of fatigue experienced by people with ME/CFS in response to exertion, with the most common descriptions being:

- exhaustion
- tiredness
- drained of energy
- heaviness in the limbs
- foggy in the head.

The fatigue experienced by the people with ME/CFS in this study was categorized into two dimensions: physical and cognitive. More in-depth discussion of fatigue in relation to cognitive dysfunction is in chapter 8.

The cause of fatigue in ME/CFS is unclear. Fatigue can be as a result of the other key symptoms of ME/CFS:

- post exertional malaise (PEM)
- sleep dysfunction
- pain
- neurological impairments
- autonomic dysfunction (including orthostatic intolerances)
- immune and neuroendocrine dysfunction.

For a physiotherapist the nature and repercussions of fatigue are of most relevance when they impact on physical function. Therefore the remainder of this chapter will focus on the physical impact of fatigue. It is important to recognize that fatigue remains a broad term and may be just as debilitating in relation to other areas of ME/CFS, in particular cognitive function. These areas are explored in turn across other chapters of this book.

Types of physical fatigue

The cause of physical fatigue could be 'peripheral fatigue', linked to the muscle itself, or 'central fatigue' which originates from the central nervous system (11). While they may interact and influence each other, there are different processes behind these two types of fatigue, so they are discussed separately in this chapter.

Peripheral fatigue

Peripheral fatigue describes the inability of muscle fibres to contract (11). Peripheral fatigue occurs in the general population after physical exertion, but should be fairly short lived with substantial recovery expected within a few minutes following high intensity exercise (12).

Adenosine triphosphate (ATP) is required to generate a muscle contraction. ATP is produced by aerobic or anaerobic metabolism, which is discussed further in chapter 6. How a muscle fibre utilizes energy, and the metabolic processes utilized to replenish it, can determine how long a muscle contraction can be maintained (13). Different types of muscle fibres can produce ATP aerobically (type 1), anaerobically (type 2b) or by both processes (type 2a) and therefore will fatigue at different rates (14). Muscles may fatigue more quickly in conditions that exhibit mitochondrial dysfunction due to a reduced supply of ATP, although direct evidence of this is reported to be lacking (13).

Kim: 'Fatigue doesn't get near to describing the impact on my body. I feel physically, emotionally and socially shipwrecked and utterly dependent on others for basic needs.'

Neurologically, a muscle contraction normally occurs when a motor neuron interacts with a muscle fibre at the neuromuscular junction. Ion channels on the membrane of muscle fibres control the rush of sodium in and potassium out, resulting in the depolarization of the muscle membrane and an eventual action potential, causing fibres to contract (15). One process behind peripheral fatigue is thought to be the depression of sodium and potassium channels, disrupting the movement of ions and resulting in no action potential and therefore no contraction. This is described as a reduction in the 'excitability' of the muscle fibre membrane and has been seen after intense muscle activity in healthy people (16).

What causes the depression of sodium and potassium channels is unclear, but a suggested factor is an accumulation of 'reactive oxygen species' (ROS) (17), which are free radicals that can cause cellular damage but are normal biproducts of aerobic metabolism. Increased levels of ROS are common after exercise in the general population and are thought to be a factor in impaired muscle contraction, resulting in weakness and peripheral fatigue (18). The body has a number of mechanisms to deal with elevated ROS such as 'heat shock proteins' which activate antioxidants that reduce damage (19). An imbalance resulting in elevated ROS can negatively impact cell structures such as membranes, lipids and proteins, and this detrimental effect is called 'oxidative stress' (20).

Oxidative stress has been found in the general population following infection, stress, aging, exposure to various pollutants and exercise (21). The damage caused by oxidative stress has been linked to conditions such as cancer, cardiovascular disease, neurological diseases, respiratory disease, rheumatoid arthritis and kidney disease (20), all of which feature fatigue as primary symptoms.

Peripheral fatigue in ME/CFS

People with ME/CFS appear to have muscles that are weaker and quicker to fatigue in comparison to the general population (22). Reduced peak isometric strength and endurance has been consistently found during maximal sustained contractions in biceps (23), tibialis (24) and hand grip (25) when comparing people with ME/CFS against healthy age-matched controls.

People with ME/CFS also show abnormalities in terms of recovery from peripheral fatigue. During a hand-grip test separated by one hour of rest, healthy controls were able to match their previous results whereas people with ME/CFS showed a reduction in strength on the second attempt (25). Another study (26) tested repeated maximal contraction of the quadriceps and found that people with ME/CFS had reduced power in their muscle contraction in comparison to controls, and while people with ME/CFS appeared to fatigue at a similar rate to healthy controls, their recovery took longer. The test was repeated 24 hours later and the control group were able to match their previous results; however people with ME/CFS demonstrated a further reduction in performance. This deterioration in physical performance is seen in wider cardiopulmonary exercise testing and is indicative of PEM, the hallmark feature of ME/CFS which is discussed in chapter 6.

Potential abnormalities in mitochondrial function have been found in people with ME/CFS (27) resulting in impaired ATP production and a build-up of acidosis, which could explain peripheral fatigue. However, there is so far not enough consistency in mitochondrial studies to draw full conclusions as to their role in the symptoms of ME/CFS (28). More details on mitochondrial dysfunction can be found in chapter 6.

Abnormalities in relation to the neuromuscular mechanisms of muscular fatigue mentioned earlier in this chapter have been observed in people with ME/CFS, such as an excessive production of reactive oxygen species (ROS) and subsequent dysregulation of sodium and potassium channels that inhibits action potentials (29). Alterations in muscle membrane excitability have been found in people with ME/CFS in both active (11) and resting muscles (30).

Heat shock proteins, the defence mechanism against ROS, have also been found at a lower level in people with ME/CFS, and the body's response to increased ROS is delayed and reduced in comparison to healthy controls (31). As such, evidence of elevated oxidative stress levels has been found in people with ME/CFS (32) (33) (34).

However, it is important to note that many studies looking at muscle physiology in people with ME/CFS have inconsistencies within their participant groups, and there are opposing findings that show no differences in muscle function between people with ME/CFS and healthy controls (35). Such discrepancies have led some to suggest that there may be specific 'subsets' of people with ME/CFS, some with cellular dysfunction within skeletal muscle and some without (30). This could explain the variability of symptoms between people with ME/CFS.

In summary, some people with ME/CFS have physiological processes that cause impaired contractility, causing heightened peripheral muscle fatigue and reduced exercise tolerance (36). They also appear to take longer to recover from a period of peripheral fatigue, with poorer performance on repeated intervention. However, these findings are not universal, and it is not clear whether these peripheral abnormalities are the primary cause of physical fatigue, or influenced by central fatigue.

Central fatigue

Central fatigue describes the reduced ability of the central nervous system to activate a muscle (37). This reduction in muscle activation means that central fatigue can actually reduce or delay peripheral fatigue, because the muscle itself performs less activity (38).

The starting point for any muscle contraction is the central nervous system. The action potentials from motor neurons that interact with muscle fibres originate from the motor control areas of the cerebral cortex (brain) and the motor-neurons in the spinal cord (15). Muscle fatigue can be attributed to a failure in these central processes (15).

Physical exertion coincides with increased activity in the prefrontal cortexes and areas of the brain responsible for motor planning and execution, and this activity appears to correlate with a subjective perception of effort (39). This perception may be influenced by afferent stimuli from the peripheral system, providing feedback on metabolic, thermal and mechanical changes in the skeletal muscles (40). However, some research contradicts this theory and some researchers propose that the perception of effort is primarily generated by areas of the brain (40) or it may be a combination of both central and peripheral factors (41).

Some researchers suggest physical performance in the general population could be moderated more by a diminished drive from the central nervous system to the working muscle, than a loss of muscle contraction at the periphery (42). The application of this theory in exercise science involves attempts to engage the central nervous system to over-ride perceptions of fatigue, including motivational practices such as listening to music during exercise, which has been found to be successful at delaying reported fatigue and improving performance (43).

Central fatigue is a reported process in fatigue-producing diseases, for example people with multiple sclerosis (44), amyotrophic lateral sclerosis (45), Charcot-Marie-Tooth (46) and Guillain–Barré syndrome (47). However, central fatigue cannot be the sole explanation for the symptoms linked to any of these conditions (44).

Central fatigue and ME/CFS

Several findings indicate that central fatigue is demonstrated by people with ME/CFS following physical exertion, with studies demonstrating an abnormal voluntary control of muscles (48), diminished central motor drive during maximal muscle contraction (23) (49) and abnormal levels of neurotransmitters linked to fatigue (50). People with ME/CFS have also demonstrated slower reaction times and movement times, suggesting a deficit in the motor preparatory areas of the brain (51) (52). A systematic review and meta-analysis found that people with ME/CFS have an increased perception of effort during exercise testing in comparison to healthy controls (41).

These findings suggest the central nervous system could play a significant role in the fatigue experienced by people with ME/CFS. However, most studies in this area are of small sample size with some contradictory findings, inconsistent application of diagnostic criteria for participants and often much speculation required to apply findings to theory (50). As central fatigue is a process seen in many other conditions, as well as the general population, the process cannot fully explain the unique experiences of people with ME/CFS.

Deconditioning and physical fatigue

One cause of physical fatigue is deconditioning, a term to describe a progressively reduced exercise capacity. A decrease in physical activity leads to more easily fatigued muscles, which in turn leads to a further decrease in physical activity, creating a negative cycle of deconditioning with a profound effect on quality of life (53). Deconditioning has also been attributed to increasing the perception of effort (41). Combating deconditioning is usually a top priority for physiotherapists in all clinical settings.

Reduced physical activity leads to reductions in the cross-sectional area of muscle fibres, oxidative capacity and force output, meaning muscles become quicker to fatigue (54). Deconditioning can also result in abnormal muscle fibre composition, creating a greater proportion of the fatigue-prone type 2b fibres (55). After just four to six weeks of bed rest there can be up to a 40% loss of muscle strength (56) with the greatest decline seen in the first two weeks of bedrest followed by a plateau of reduced strength and atrophy (57). This deconditioning is seen in people with many chronic diseases that result in inactivity, such as coronary heart disease or chronic obstructive pulmonary disease (54).

However, deconditioning can be reversed (56). Exercise is used as an effective method to prevent or reverse deconditioning in presentations such as post-operative deconditioning in the elderly (58), people with spinal cord injury (59) and stroke (60).

Deconditioning, fatigue and ME/CFS

People with ME/CFS are likely to carry out less physical activity during daily life in comparison to the general population (22) and are therefore at risk of becoming deconditioned. Several physiological findings that are associated with deconditioning have been found in people with ME/CFS:

- changes to muscle composition, with an abnormal increase in type 2b fibres (61)
- an increase in resting heart rate (62)
- reduced left ventricular size and mass (62)
- lower peak VO$_2$ max (compared to healthy controls) (62).

While cardiopulmonary differences have been discovered during cardiopulmonary exercise testing in people with ME/CFS, many can be attributed to differences in aerobic fitness and not necessarily the physiological characteristics of ME/CFS (63).

However, there are inconsistencies in the evidence that proposes deconditioning is a defining characteristic of ME/CFS. A cardiopulmonary exercise test only gathers data about the person during the time of the test itself, so cannot produce information about the person's condition in general as it does not account for whether they are currently in a period of symptom stability or a flare. Some exercise tests have shown no difference in aerobic fitness between people with ME/CFS and healthy controls (64) (62) or even demonstrated that a person with ME/CFS had better fitness than a matched control (65). Another study found a high rest-to-peak change in cardiac output in some people with ME/CFS, whereas a low change is considered the hallmark feature of deconditioning (66). Deconditioning has also been ruled out as a cause for the orthostatic intolerances often found associated with ME/CFS as part of autonomic dysfunction (67), which is discussed further in chapter 12.

In one large-scale multisite exercise study, people with ME/CFS were matched against controls for levels of fitness and, while many of the cardiopulmonary deficits were similar, differences between people with ME/CFS and their matched controls remained in ventilatory efficiency, breathing patterns and rated perceived exertion (63). Although perceived exertion and sense of effort is raised in people with ME/CFS, which could be linked to deconditioning, a systematic review highlighted that the altered perceptions remain even when people with ME/CFS are matched against healthy controls who have the same level of activity (41).

Further inconsistencies have been seen in cardiopulmonary exercise tests (CPET) when they are repeated 24 hours later. People with ME/CFS have shown a marked deterioration in performance on the second test (68) (69) (70) whereas healthy sedentary controls and people with disorders that are associated with deconditioning, such as chronic lung and heart disease, HIV and multiple sclerosis, can reproduce or even improve upon their results from the previous day (71) (69). This deterioration in performance in people with ME/CFS is inconsistent with deconditioning (66) and instead may reflect the hallmark feature of ME/CFS, PEM. Detailed discussion of PEM and further information regarding CPET testing can be found in chapter 6.

While deconditioning may be a consequence of reduced activity due to the symptoms of ME/CFS, the inconsistencies in studies of aerobic fitness mean that deconditioning cannot explain the intolerance to exertion, let alone the constellation of symptoms found with ME/CFS, and therefore deconditioning should be considered a potential secondary complication as opposed to a primary cause (66) (62) (65).

Of most importance to note is that while exercise may typically address deconditioning in other populations, for people with ME/CFS exercise is likely to trigger PEM and worsen symptoms and may therefore be counter-productive. There is more discussion of exercise below.

Adaptation to practice
Assessment
Fatigue is a vague term that may be used to describe a variety of symptoms by different people, so it is important to be more thorough during subjective questioning of a person with ME/CFS with regards to this symptom to ascertain exactly what they are experiencing and how it may impact on their quality of life and function.

As fatigue may be a symptom linked to any number of other medical conditions it is also important to make sure that a thorough assessment takes place to rule out a differential diagnosis, with referrals for appropriate tests and medical reviews where indicated.

Some medications may be prescribed to treat fatigue and a list of examples can be found in the Appendix.

Physiotherapy management of fatigue
Energy management
Energy management, also known as activity management or pacing, involves managing a person's activities to stay within their energy envelope (72) and is considered to be an effective method of reducing symptom exacerbation including fatigue (73) (74) (75). Energy management is discussed in more detail in chapter 15.

What about exercise?
In most diseases the power of exercise-based interventions to improve physical fatigue is clear. For example, resistance training has been

shown to improve muscle strength and mass, as well as prevent deterioration with age (76). High intensity intermittent training has been shown to triple the exercise capacity of people with COPD (77), and improve exercise capacity and heart function with no adverse events in people with cardiac disease (78).

Historically, research into treatment for people with ME/CFS focused on exercise as a means to address deconditioning and therefore improve fatigue (79); and an approach termed 'graded exercise therapy', which involves progressively increasing the frequency, duration and intensity of exercise, was reported to improve the subjective fatigue and physical function of people with ME/CFS (80) (81). However, the graded exercise therapy approach has been heavily criticized for low evidence quality and reported harms, and it has been removed from clinical guidelines in the USA (82) and the UK (83). As discussed in this chapter, deconditioning is a secondary consequence as opposed to a cause of ME/CFS, and physical exertion is known to trigger symptom exacerbation via PEM, resulting in a decline in performance. An attempt to combat deconditioning through exercise may therefore trigger new symptoms or exacerbate current symptoms and lead to further intolerance to exertion, meaning the approach becomes counter-productive. More discussion of this, and how to consider other forms of exercise, can be found in chapter 17.

> **Mo**: 'My fatigue is overwhelming. Sometimes I have to nap in the afternoons, but I have so many responsibilities I often have to just push through, and this makes me worse.'

SUMMARY

- ▸ 'Fatigue' is a vague term that may cover a range of physical and cognitive symptoms.
- ▸ Physical fatigue may be caused by physiological changes in the periphery or dysfunction in the central nervous system – or both.
- ▸ Some people with ME/CFS take longer to recover from a period of physical fatigue, with poorer performance on repeated intervention even in comparison to other fatigue-producing conditions.
- ▸ Deconditioning may be a secondary consequence of ME/CFS but it is not the cause.

APPLICATION TO PRACTICE

▶ Typical approaches to fatigue and deconditioning that work for other groups will not be suitable for people with ME/CFS.

▶ Physiotherapists should focus on symptom management by avoiding exacerbations and helping people with ME/CFS to pace their available energies for maximum function and quality of life.

References

1. Wormgoor, M.E.A. & Rodenburg, S.C. (2021) 'The evidence base for physiotherapy in myalgic encephalomyelitis/chronic fatigue syndrome when considering post-exertional malaise: a systematic review and narrative synthesis.' *Journal of Translational Medicine 19* (1).

2. Stouten, B. (2005) 'Identification of ambiguities in the 1994 chronic fatigue syndrome research case definition and recommendations for resolution.' *BMC Health Services Research 13* (5).

3. Kluger, B.M., Krupp, L.B. & Enoka, R.M. (2013) 'Fatigue and fatigability in neurologic illnesses: proposal for a unified taxonomy.' *Neurology 80* (4).

4. Krupp, L. (2003) *Fatigue: The Most Common Complaints Series.* London: Butterworth-Heinemann.

5. Place, N. & Millet, G.Y. (2020) 'Quantification of neuromuscular fatigue: what do we do wrong and why?' *Sports Medicine 50* (3).

6. Carruthers, B.M., van de Sande, M.I., De Meirleir, K.L., Klimas, N.G., *et al.* (2011) 'Myalgic encephalomyelitis: International Consensus Criteria.' *Journal of Internal Medicine 270.*

7. Carruthers, B.M., Jain, A.K., De Meirleir, K.L., Peterson, D.L., *et al.* (2003) 'Myalgic encephalomyelitis/chronic fatigue syndrome.' *Journal of Chronic Fatigue Syndrome 11* (1).

8. Fukuda, K., Straus, S.E., Hickie, I., Sharpe, M C., Dobbins, J.G. & Komaroff, A.L. (1994) 'The chronic fatigue syndrome: a comprehensive approach to its definition and study.' *Annals of Internal Medicine 121.*

9. Sharpe, M.C., Archard, L.C. & Banatvala, J.E. (1991) 'A report – chronic fatigue syndrome: guidelines for research.' *Journal of the Royal Society of Medicine 84* (2).

10. Keech, A.C., Sandler, C.X., Vollmer-Conna, U., Cvejic, E., Lloyd, A.R. & Barry, B.K. (2015) 'Capturing the post-exertional exacerbation of fatigue following physical and cognitive challenge in patients with chronic fatigue syndrome.' *Journal of Psychosomatic Research 79* (6).

11. Jammes, Y. & Retornaz, F. (2020) 'Skeletal muscle weakness often occurs in patients with myalgic encephalomyelitis/chronic fatigue syndrome (ME/CFS).' *Journal of Experimental Neurology 1* (2).

12. Froyd, C., Millet, G.Y. & Noakes, T.D. (2013) 'The development of peripheral fatigue and short-term recovery during self-paced high-intensity exercise.' *Journal of Physiology 591.*

13. Wiles, C.M., Jones, D.A. & Edwards, R.H. (1981) 'Fatigue in human metabolic myopathy.' *Ciba Foundation Symposium 82.*

14. Davis, M.P. & Walsh, D. (2010) 'Mechanisms of fatigue.' *Journal of Supportive Oncology 8* (4).

15. Stackhouse, S.K., Stevens, J.E., Lee, S.C.K., Pearce, K.M., Snyder-Mackler, L. & Binder-Macleod, S.A. (2001) 'Maximum voluntary activation in nonfatigued and fatigued muscle of young and elderly individuals.' *Physical Therapy 81* (5).

16. Fraser, S.F., Li, J.L., Carey, M.F., Wang, X.N., *et al.* (2002) 'Fatigue depresses maximal in vitro skeletal muscle Na(+)-K(+)-ATPase activity in untrained and trained individuals.' *Journal of Applied Physiology [1985] 93* (5).
17. Juel, C. (2006) 'Muscle fatigue and reactive oxygen species.' *Journal of Physiology 576* (1).
18. Powers, S.K. & Jackson, M.J. (2008) 'Exercise-induced oxidative stress: cellular mechanisms and impact on muscle force production.' *Physiology Review 88* (4).
19. Dimauro, I., Mercatelli, N. & Caporossi, D. (2016) 'Exercise-induced ROS in heat shock proteins response.' *Free Radical Biology and Medicine 98.*
20. Pizzino, G., Irrera, N., Cucinotta, M., Pallio, G., *et al.* (2017) 'Oxidative stress: harms and benefits for human health.' *Oxidative Medicine and Cellular Longevity 2017.*
21. Urso, M.L. & Clarkson, P.M. (2003) 'Oxidative stress, exercise, and antioxidant supplementation.' *Toxicology 189* (1–2).
22. Nijs, J., Aelbrecht, S., Meeus, M. & Oosterwijck, J. (2010) 'Tired of being inactive: a systematic literature review of physical activity, physiological exercise capacity and muscle strength in patients with chronic fatigue syndrome.' *Disability and Rehabilitation 33* (17–18).
23. Sacco, P., Hope, P.A.J., Thickbroom, G.W., Byrnes, M.L. & Mastaglia, F.L. (1999) 'Corticomotor excitability and perception of effort during sustained exercise in the chronic fatigue syndrome.' *Clinical Neurophysiology 110* (11).
24. Kent-Braun, J.A., Sharma, K.R., Weiner, M.W., Massie, B. & Miller, R.G. (1993) 'Central basis of muscle fatigue in chronic fatigue syndrome.' *Neurology 43* (1).
25. Jäkel, B., Kedor, C. & Grabowski, P. (2021) 'Hand grip strength and fatigability: correlation with clinical parameters and diagnostic suitability in ME/CFS.' *Journal of Translational Medicine 19* (159).
26. Paul, L., Wood, L., Behan, W.M. & Maclaren, W.M. (1999) 'Demonstration of delayed recovery from fatiguing exercise in chronic fatigue syndrome.' *European Journal of Neurology 6* (1).
27. Tomas, C., Brown, A.E., Newton, J.L. & Elson, J.L. (2019) 'Mitochondrial complex activity in permeabilised cells of chronic fatigue syndrome patients using two cell types.' *PeerJ 7.*
28. Holden, S., Maksoud, R., Eaton-Fitch, N., Cabanas, H., Staines, D. & Marshall-Gradisnik, S. (2020) 'A systematic review of mitochondrial abnormalities in myalgic encephalomyelitis/chronic fatigue syndrome/systemic exertion intolerance disease.' *Journal of Translational Medicine 18* (1).
29. Fulle, S., Belia, S., Vecchiet, J., Morabito, C., Vecchiet, L. & Fanò, G. (2003) 'Modification of the functional capacity of sarcoplasmic reticulum membranes in patients suffering from chronic fatigue syndrome.' *Neuromuscular Disorders 13* (6).
30. Jammes, Y., Adjriou, N. & Kipson, N. (2020) 'Altered muscle membrane potential and redox status differentiates two subgroups of patients with chronic fatigue syndrome.' *Journal of Translational Medicine 18* (173).
31. Jammes, Y., Steinberg, J.G., Delliaux, S. & Brégeon, F. (2009) 'Chronic fatigue syndrome combines increased exercise-induced oxidative stress and reduced cytokine and Hsp responses.' *Journal of Internal Medicine 266* (2).
32. Brkic, S., Tomic, S., Maric, D., Novakov, M.A. & Turkulov, V. (2010) 'Lipid peroxidation is elevated in female patients with chronic fatigue syndrome.' *Medical Science Monitor 16* (12).
33. Kennedy, G., Spence, V.A., McLaren, M., Hill, A., Underwood, C. & Belch J.F. (2005) 'Oxidative stress levels are raised in chronic fatigue syndrome and are associated with clinical symptoms.' *Free Radical Biology and Medicine 39* (5).
34. Vecchiet, J., Cipollone, F., Falasca, K., Mezzetti, A., *et al.* (2003) 'Relationship between musculoskeletal symptoms and blood markers of oxidative stress in patients with chronic fatigue syndrome.' *Neuroscience Letters 335* (3).
35. Gibson, H., Carroll, N., Clague, J.E. & Edwards, R.H. (1993) 'Exercise performance and fatiguability in patients with chronic fatigue syndrome.' *Journal of Neurology, Neurosurgery, and Psychiatry 56* (9):

36. Gerwyn, M. & Maes, M. (2017) 'Mechanisms explaining muscle fatigue and muscle pain in patients with myalgic encephalomyelitis/chronic fatigue syndrome (ME/CFS): a review of recent findings.' *Current Rheumatology Reports 19* (1).

37. Sharples, S.A., Gould, J.A., Vandenberk, M.S. & Kalmar, J.M. (2016) 'Cortical mechanisms of central fatigue and sense of effort.' *PLOS ONE 11* (2).

38. Jammes, Y. & Retornaz, F. (2019) 'Understanding neuromuscular disorders in chronic fatigue syndrome.' *F1000Research 28* (8).

39. Berchicci, M., Menotti, F., Macaluso, A. & Di Russo, F. (2013) 'The neurophysiology of central and peripheral fatigue during sub-maximal lower limb isometric contractions.' *Frontiers of Human Neuroscience 7* (135).

40. Marcora, S. (2009) 'Perception of effort during exercise is independent of afferent feedback from skeletal muscles, heart, and lungs.' *Journal of Applied Physiology [1985] 106* (6).

41. Barhorst, E.E., Andrae, W.E., Rayne, T.J., Falvo, M.J., Cook, D.B. & Lindheimer, J.B. (2020) 'Elevated perceived exertion in people with myalgic encephalomyelitis/chronic fatigue syndrome and fibromyalgia: a meta-analysis.' *Medicine & Science in Sports & Exercise 52* (12).

42. Davis, J.M. & Bailey, S.P. (1997) 'Possible mechanisms of central nervous system fatigue during exercise.' *Medicine & Science in Sports & Exercise 29* (1).

43. Thakare, A.E., Mehrotra, R. & Singh, A. (2017) 'Effect of music tempo on exercise performance and heart rate among young adults.' *International Journal of Physiology, Pathophysiology and Pharmacology 9* (2).

44. Sheean, G.L., Murray, N.M., Rothwell, J.C., Miller, D.H. & Thompson, A.J. (1997) 'An electrophysiological study of the mechanism of fatigue in multiple sclerosis.' *Brain 120* (2).

45. Kent-Braun, J.A. & Miller, R.G. (2000) 'Central fatigue during isometric exercise in amyotrophic lateral sclerosis.' *Muscle Nerve 23* (6).

46. Menotti, F., Berchicci, M., Di Russo, F., Damiani, A., Vitelli, S. & Macaluso, A. (2014) 'The role of the prefrontal cortex in the development of muscle fatigue in Charcot-Marie-Tooth 1A patients.' *Neuromuscular Disorders 24* (6).

47. Garssen, M.P., Schillings, M.L., Van Doorn, P.A., Van Engelen, B.G. & Zwarts, M.J. (2007) 'Contribution of central and peripheral factors to residual fatigue in Guillain–Barré syndrome.' *Muscle Nerve 36* (1).

48. Siemionow, V., Fang, Y., Calabrese, L., Sahgal, V. & Yue, G.H. (2004) 'Altered central nervous system signal during motor performance in chronic fatigue syndrome.' *Clinical Neurophysiology 115* (10).

49. Schillings, M.L., Kalkman, J.S., van der Werf, S.P., van Engelen, B.G., Bleijenberg, G. & Zwarts, M.J. (2004) 'Diminished central activation during maximal voluntary contraction in chronic fatigue syndrome.' *Clinical Neurophysiology 115* (11).

50. Georgiades, E., Behan, W.M., Kilduff, L.P., Hadjicharalambous, M., *et al.* (2003) 'Chronic fatigue syndrome: new evidence for a central fatigue disorder.' *Clinical Science (London) 105* (2).

51. Davey, N.J., Puri, B.K., Catley, M., Main, J., Nowicky, A.V. & Zaman, R. (2003) 'Deficit in motor performance correlates with changed corticospinal excitability in patients with chronic fatigue syndrome.' *International Journal of Clinical Practice 57* (4).

52. de Lange, F.P., Kalkman, J.S., Bleijenberg, G., Hagoort, P., *et al.* (2004) 'Neural correlates of the chronic fatigue syndrome – an fMRI study.' *Brain 127* (9).

53. Rimmer, J.H., Schiller, W. & Chen, M.D. (2012) 'Effects of disability-associated low energy expenditure deconditioning syndrome.' *Exercise Sport Science Review 40* (1).

54. Bogdanis, G.C. (2012) 'Effects of physical activity and inactivity on muscle fatigue.' *Frontiers in Physiology 3* (142).

55. Gosker, H.R., van Mameren, H., van Dijk, P.J., Engelen, M.P., *et al.* (2002) 'Skeletal muscle fibre-type shifting and metabolic profile in patients with chronic obstructive pulmonary disease.' *European Respiratory Journal 19* (4).

56. Bloomfield, S.A. (1997) 'Changes in musculoskeletal structure and function with prolonged bed rest.' *Medicine & Science in Sports & Exercise 29* (2).
57. Marusic, U., Narici, M., Simunic, B., Pisot, R. & Ritzmann, R. (2021) 'Nonuniform loss of muscle strength and atrophy during bed rest: a systematic review.' *Journal of Applied Physiology [1985] 131* (1).
58. Wu, Y., Hu, X. & Chen, L. (2020) 'Chronic resistance exercise improves functioning and reduces toll-like receptor signaling in elderly patients with postoperative deconditioning.' *Journal of Manipulative and Physiological Therapeutics 43* (4).
59. Maher, J.L., McMillan, D.W. & Nash, M.S. (2017) 'Exercise and health-related risks of physical deconditioning after spinal cord injury.' *Topics in Spinal Cord Injury Rehabilitation 23* (3).
60. Ivey, F.M., Hafer-Macko, C.E. & Macko, R.F. (2008) 'Exercise training for cardio-metabolic adaptation after stroke.' *Journal of Cardiopulmonary Rehabilitation and Prevention 28* (1).
61. Pietrangelo, T., Toniolo, L., Paoli, A., Fulle, S., *et al.* 2009. 'Functional characterization of muscle fibres from patients with chronic fatigue syndrome: case-control study.' *International Journal of Immunopathology and Pharmacology 22* (2).
62. Nelson, M.J., Bahl, J.S., Buckley, J.D., Thomson, R.L. & Davison, K. (2019) 'Evidence of altered cardiac autonomic regulation in myalgic encephalomyelitis/chronic fatigue syndrome: a systematic review and meta-analysis.' *Medicine (Baltimore) 98* (43).
63. Cook, D.B., VanRiper, S., Dougherty, R.J., Lindheimer, J.B., Falvo, M.J. & Chen, Y. (2022) 'Cardiopulmonary, metabolic, and perceptual responses during exercise in myalgic encephalomyelitis/chronic fatigue syndrome (ME/CFS): a multi-site clinical assessment of ME/CFS (MCAM) sub-study.' *PLOS ONE 17* (3).
64. Cook, D.B., Nagelkirk, P.R., Poluri, A., Mores, J. & Natelson, B.H. (2006) 'The influence of aerobic fitness and fibromyalgia on cardiorespiratory and perceptual responses to exercise in patients with chronic fatigue syndrome.' *Arthritis & Rheumatology 54* (10).
65. Bazelmans, E., Bleijenberg, G., Van Der Meer, J.W. & Folgering, H. (2001) 'Is physical deconditioning a perpetuating factor in chronic fatigue syndrome? A controlled study on maximal exercise performance and relations with fatigue, impairment and physical activity.' *Psychological Medicine 31* (1).
66. Joseph, P., Arevalo, C., Oliveira, R.K.F., Faria-Urbina, M., *et al.* (2021) 'Insights from invasive cardiopulmonary exercise testing of patients with myalgic encephalomyelitis/chronic fatigue syndrome.' *Chest 160* (2).
67. van Campen, C.M.C., Rowe, P.C. & Visser, F.C. (2021) 'Deconditioning does not explain orthostatic intolerance in ME/CFS (myalgic encephalomyelitis/chronic fatigue syndrome).' *Journal of Translational Medicine 19* (193).
68. Davenport, T.E., Lehnen, M., Stevens, S.R., VanNess, J.M., Stevens, J. & Snell, C.R. (2019) 'Chronotropic intolerance: an overlooked determinant of symptoms and activity limitation in myalgic encephalomyelitis/chronic fatigue syndrome?' *Frontiers in Pediatrics 7* (82).
69. Davenport, T.E., Stevens, S.R., Stevens, J., Snell, C.R. & Van Ness, J.M. (2020) 'Properties of measurements obtained during cardiopulmonary exercise testing in individuals with myalgic encephalomyelitis/chronic fatigue syndrome.' *Work 66* (2).
70. Keller, B.A., Pryor, J.L. & Giloteaux, L. (2014) 'Inability of myalgic encephalomyelitis/chronic fatigue syndrome patients to reproduce VO_2peak indicates functional impairment.' *Journal of Translational Medicine 23* (12).
71. Larson, B., Davenport, T.E., Stevens, S., Stevens, J., Van Ness, M.J. & Snell, C. (2019) 'Reproducibility of measurements obtained during cardiopulmonary exercise testing in individuals with fatiguing health conditions: a case series.' *Cardiopulmonary Physical Therapy Journal 30* (4).
72. National Institute of Health and Care Excellence (2020) 'Guideline: myalgic encephalomyelitis (or encephalopathy)/chronic fatigue syndrome: diagnosis and

management; draft for consultation.' Accessed on 10/12/2022 at www.nice.org. uk/guidance/gid-ng10091/documents/draft-guideline.

73. Pesek, J.R., Jason, L.A. & Taylor, R.R. (2000) 'An empirical investigation of the envelope theory.' *Journal of Human Behavior in the Social Environment 3* (1).

74. Jason, L.A., Melrose, H., Lerman, A., Burroughs, V., *et al.* (1999) 'Managing chronic fatigue syndrome: overview and case study.' *American Association of Occupational Health Nurses Journal 47* (1).

75. Jason, L.A., Roesner, N., Porter, N., Parenti, B., Mortensen, J. & Till, L. (2010) 'Provision of social support to individuals with chronic fatigue syndrome.' *Journal of Clinical Psychology 66* (3).

76. Fragala, M.S., Cadore, E.L., Dorgo, S., Izquierdo, M., *et al.* (2019) 'Resistance training for older adults: position statement from the National Strength and Conditioning Association.' *Journal of Strength and Conditioning Research 33* (8).

77. Vogiatzis, I. (2011) 'Strategies of muscle training in very severe COPD patients.' *European Respiratory Journal 38* (4).

78. Cornish, A.K., Broadbent, S. & Cheema, B.S. (2011) 'Interval training for patients with coronary artery disease: a systematic review.' *European Journal of Applied Physiology 111* (4).

79. Chalder, T., Goldsmith, K.A., White, P., Sharpe, M. & Pickles, A. (2015) 'Rehabilitative therapies for chronic fatigue syndrome: a secondary mediation analysis of the PACE trial.' *The Lancet 2* (2).

80. White, P.D., Goldsmith, K.A., Johnson, A.L., Potts, L., Walwyn, R. & DeCesare, J.C. (2011) 'Comparison of adaptive pacing therapy, cognitive behaviour therapy, graded exercise therapy, and specialist medical care for chronic fatigue syndrome PACE): a randomised trial.' *The Lancet 377* (9768).

81. Clark, L., Pesola, F., Thomas, J.M., Vergara-Williamson, M., Beynon, M. & White, P.D. (2017) 'Guided graded exercise self-help plus specialist medical care versus specialist medical care alone for chronic fatigue syndrome (GETSET): a pragmatic randomised controlled trial.' *The Lancet 390* (10092).

82. Centers for Disease Control and Prevention (2022) 'Myalgic encephalomyelitis/ chronic fatigue syndrome.' Accessed on 10/12/2022 at www.cdc.gov/me-cfs/index. html.

83. National Institute for Health and Care Excellence (2021) 'Myalgic encephalomyelitis (or encephalopathy)/chronic fatigue syndrome: diagnosis and management.' Accessed on 2/12/2022 at www.nice.org.uk/guidance/ng206.

CHAPTER 8

Cognitive Dysfunction

PURPOSE OF THIS CHAPTER

Cognitive impairments are listed on most diagnostic criteria for ME/CFS (see chapter 1). While cognition is not an area of speciality for physiotherapists, it is still important to consider this symptom as a priority because:

- Memory and attentional problems will impact on how a person with ME/CFS can engage in a session and retain any advice provided.
- It is possible for a physiotherapist to cause or exacerbate cognitive symptoms, either through physical exertion or cognitive exertion (such as lengthy assessments).

This chapter details the nature of cognitive dysfunction found in people with ME/CFS and its potential pathophysiology, as well as the considerations that a physiotherapist should make when interacting with people with ME/CFS and planning interventions.

Cognition dysfunction in ME/CFS

The cognitive dysfunction associated with ME/CFS has a significant impact on a person's function and quality of life (1). Subjectively, cognitive dysfunction in ME/CFS is described as slow thinking, difficulty focusing, lack of concentration, forgetfulness and a haziness of thought process, often referred to colloquially as 'brain fog' (2).

Objectively, under research conditions, people with ME/CFS have demonstrated deficits in attention, memory and reaction time (1) (3), along with slow processing of information (4) and impaired performance with effortful tasks that require planning (5). No deficits have been found in fine motor speed, vocabulary, reasoning and global functioning in people with ME/CFS (3). The descriptor 'brain fog' could be considered a subjective experience of an objective cognitive dysfunction (2).

However, a systematic review and meta-analysis in 2022 (1) noted that many studies of cognitive function in people with ME/CFS have inconsistent findings, which could be due to methodological issues such as the lack of a control group or which criteria were used for participant inclusion, but also suggested that these discrepancies could reflect the varied nature of ME/CFS symptoms. Therefore not every person with ME/CFS may experience the same nature and severity of cognitive dysfunction.

Kim: 'I can concentrate for about forty-five minutes at a time, then I need to rest for thirty minutes. Being unable to talk, chat or engage with life has massively affected my relationship with my partner.'

Cognitive dysfunction can be one of the main symptoms of post exertional malaise (PEM), which is the addition of new symptoms, or exacerbation of current symptoms, after exertion. But it is also important to note that cognitive exertion can be a cause of PEM, and in fact trigger the same level of PEM symptoms compared to physical exertion (6). More discussion of PEM and the role of cognitive triggers can be found in chapter 6.

Causes of cognitive dysfunction in ME/CFS

A number of underlying physiological processes have been found in laboratory conditions that may explain the cognitive dysfunction found in people with ME/CFS.

Orthostatic intolerance

Cognitive dysfunction has been linked to postural orthostatic tachycardia syndrome (POTS), a form of orthostatic intolerance which is a common co-morbidity of people with ME/CFS and is discussed in chapters 2 and 12. When people with ME/CFS who have a diagnosis of POTS were tilted upright on a tilt table and given cognitive tests, their working memory, accuracy, reaction time and information processing deteriorated (7) (8) (9).

However, the cognitive impairments seen in people with ME/CFS are not restricted to those who are diagnosed with POTS (9). A leading theory to explain the cognitive deficits during a tilt test is the reduction in cerebral perfusion, which is the amount of blood flow to the brain (9). Cerebral blood flow can be measured using Doppler imaging and when people with ME/CFS were tilted against gravity, 90% showed an abnormal reduction in blood flow to the brain, irrespective of whether they had a POTS diagnosis or any change to their heart rate and blood pressure (9). The total reduction in blood flow was 28–29% in people with ME/CFS, in comparison to 7% in healthy controls. A tilt table test would be intolerable for those with severe ME/CFS, but another study found similar reductions in cerebral blood flow in people with severe ME/CFS simply by sitting upright (10). These studies are discussed further in chapter 12.

Physical exertion

Physical exertion has been shown to cause impairments in cognitive processing in people with ME/CFS (11) (12) both immediately following exercise and when tested 24 hours later. A potential reason for this is that during incremental increases in exercise, people with ME/CFS have been shown to have reduced oxygenation of the prefrontal cortex (13). It has not been established whether these effects are due solely to the physical exertion or are a further manifestation of the reduced blood flow linked to orthostatic intolerance due to the upright position maintained during the exercise testing.

Abnormalities in the brain

Several abnormalities have been found in the brains of people with ME/CFS (14). MRI studies have suggested there is an impaired nerve signal conduction through the brainstem in people with ME/CFS, which could cause cognitive dysfunction as well as problems with sleep and muscle tone (15). Neuroinflammatory processes are also suggested following abnormalities in temperature and metabolism found in whole brain imaging (16).

The hippocampus has a key role in cognition and memory. In neurodegenerative conditions such as Alzheimer's disease and multiple sclerosis, the volume of the hippocampus has been found to be reduced (17). However, when people with ME/CFS were scanned the hippocampus volume had actually increased, leading the researchers to suggest that there may be a neuroregulatory dysfunction and speculate that the increased volume may be to compensate for brain stem deficits (17).

Most studies on brain abnormalities in ME/CFS have small sample sizes so it is still difficult to generalize findings to the whole ME/CFS population, and it is not yet known whether the changes to the brain are causative or adaptive.

Mitochondrial dysfunction

While mitochondria are typically thought of as energy producers for cells, they also have a fundamental role in brain function (18). Dysfunction of mitochondria is seen in many disorders that exhibit cognitive dysfunction, including Alzheimer's disease and Parkinson's disease (18). Mitochondrial dysfunction has also been found in people with ME/CFS (19) (20) (21) and so could provide an explanation for cognitive dysfunction, although a specific mechanism has yet to be identified. More information on mitochondrial dysfunction is in chapter 6.

Mental health

The cognitive dysfunction in ME/CFS has been investigated as a link to mental health disorders (22), because the prevalence of depression and anxiety can be high in people with ME/CFS (23) and depression is linked closely with cognitive impairment (24).

> **Oliver:** 'Everything takes longer for my brain to compute. I can't concentrate intensely for as long as normal people.'

However, cognitive impairments found in people with ME/CFS often exist without any co-morbid mental health problems, so the link is unfounded (25) (26) (2).

Cognitive dysfunction caused by other symptoms of ME/CFS

Some of the other symptoms of ME/CFS could contribute to cognitive dysfunction, for example orthostatic intolerance, as discussed earlier in this chapter.

Other symptoms of ME/CFS have been linked to cognitive dysfunction in the general population such as fatigue (27), pain (28), sleep dysfunction (29) and food allergies (30). While the impact of these specific symptoms has not yet been explored on cognitive dysfunction in people with ME/CFS, it is important to recognize that some symptoms of ME/CFS may interact and influence each other.

Adaptation to physiotherapy practice
Communication
When working with a person with ME/CFS, a physiotherapist must consider that they may have cognitive dysfunction, and if required make the following adjustments to any interaction:

- Keep questions and instructions short and simple.
- Consider the position the person is in during any assessment in respect of orthostatic intolerances and cerebral blood perfusion. A prolonged upright position may exacerbate symptoms.
- A lengthy subjective assessment may challenge concentration and attention leading to cognitive exertion and PEM, so consider how to keep communication brief and maximize your contact time.
- Basic questions on past medical history, current regime, drug history etc. could be asked in advance, giving the person opportunity to build a response in their own time.
- Provide information and recommendations in written format after a session, rather than relying on attention and memory.

Chapter 14 provides more information on how to structure an assessment to account for cognitive dysfunction.

Assessment and monitoring
If assessing a person's typical daytime routine for potential triggers of PEM, be sure to include cognitive activities to identify possible cognitive exertion. Cognitive exertion may be from an obvious source such as working or studying, but typical leisure activities that may be thought of as restful, such as reading or watching television, can also be cognitively challenging and cause symptom flares.

As cognitive dysfunction can be a main symptom of PEM, a physiotherapist may need to consider how to measure and monitor this symptom in order to evaluate the tolerance of any intervention. See chapter 18 for more information on measuring cognition.

Medication
No pharmacological treatment for cognitive dysfunction in ME/CFS currently exists, but several medications or supplements may be used

to attempt to address some cognitive symptoms. These are listed in the Appendix.

Physiotherapy management of cognitive impairments
Energy management
Energy management involves managing activities to stay within the energy envelope. Ensure all cognitive activities are included in any plans and acknowledge that they may contribute equally to symptom exacerbation alongside physical exertion. Cognitive activities may include occupational tasks, reading, planning, medical appointments or social interactions.

It is important to note that energy management strategies, such as activity diaries, can also be cognitively exertional. Any change or addition to a management plan should be monitored and evaluated for signs of PEM. More information on energy management can be found in chapter 15.

Strategies and aids
Cognition specialists such as occupational therapists use a variety of strategies and aids to assist with cognitive dysfunction in all conditions. This can include (31):

- use of visual aids for orientation, such as prominent calendars and planners
- digital technology for tracking items that are easily misplaced
- recording notes and reminders, either in print or digitally via a voice recorder.

If a person's function and quality of life are being significantly affected by their cognitive dysfunction, consider referring them to an appropriate professional for further assessment and advice on aids and strategies.

What about exercise?
Exercise has been shown to improve both physical function and cognitive function in people with dementia (32) and those with mild cognitive impairments (33).

It has therefore been explored as an approach to treat the cognitive impairments found in people with ME/CFS. While some improvements have been demonstrated in objective cognitive performance (34) and visual attention (35), in contrast other studies have shown that people with ME/CFS have impaired cognitive processing following exertional exercise when compared to healthy controls (11) and in comparison to people diagnosed with depression, even when the baseline cognitive scores of the comparison groups were initially worse (36). However, all of these studies have significant methodological weaknesses including small sample sizes, large drop-out rates and being subject to the issues of diagnostic criteria discussed in chapter 1.

Currently there is not enough evidence to support the use of exercise to improve cognitive function in people with ME/CFS. Given physical exertion can cause PEM, which may involve further cognitive dysfunction, it is more likely that exercise may worsen cognitive symptoms and should therefore not be used as a management strategy for cognitive dysfunction.

SUMMARY

▸ People with ME/CFS may present with cognitive dysfunction, in particular reduced attention, memory and reaction time.

▸ Cognitive dysfunction may increase following physical or cognitive exertion.

▸ Cognitive exertion may cause symptom exacerbation in the form of PEM.

▸ Cognitive dysfunction may be linked to reduced blood flow to the brain when the body is in an upright position.

APPLICATION TO PRACTICE

▸ Modify communication style and methods to account for potential dysfunction in memory and attention.

▸ Understand that exertion may increase cognitive symptoms so any intervention should be closely monitored to ensure it does not exacerbate this symptom.

▸ Understand that cognitive activities may cause symptom exacerbation and should be considered carefully when helping patients with energy and activity planning.

▶ Utilize cognitive specialists when symptoms are impacting significantly on quality of life and function.

References

1. Aoun Sebaiti, M., Hainselin, M., Gounden, Y., Sirbuet, C.A., *et al.* (2022) 'Systematic review and meta-analysis of cognitive impairment in myalgic encephalomyelitis/chronic fatigue syndrome (ME/CFS).' *Scientific Reports 12* (2157).
2. Ocon, A. (2013) 'Caught in the thickness of brain fog: exploring the cognitive symptoms of chronic fatigue syndrome.' *Frontiers in Physiology 4* (63).
3. Cockshell, S.J. & Mathias, J.L. (2010) 'Cognitive functioning in chronic fatigue syndrome: a meta-analysis.' *Psychological Medicine 40* (8).
4. Cockshell, S.J. & Mathias, J.L. (2013) 'Cognitive deficits in chronic fatigue syndrome and their relationship to psychological status, symptomatology, and everyday functioning.' *Neuropsychology 27* (2).
5. Joyce, E., Blumenthal, S. & Wessely, S. (1996) 'Memory, attention, and executive function in chronic fatigue syndrome.' *Journal of Neurology, Neurosurgery and Psychiatry 60* (5).
6. Keech, A., Sandler, C.X., Vollmer-Conna, U., Cvejic, E., Lloyd, A.R. & Barry, B.K. (2015) 'Capturing the post-exertional exacerbation of fatigue following physical and cognitive challenge in patients with chronic fatigue syndrome.' *Journal of Psychosomatic Research 79* (6).
7. Ocon, A.J., Messer, Z.R., Medow, M.S. & Stewart, J.M. (2012) 'Increasing orthostatic stress impairs neurocognitive functioning in chronic fatigue syndrome with postural tachycardia syndrome.' *Clinical Science (London) 122* (5).
8. Stewart, J.M., Medow, M.S., Messer, Z.R., Baugham, I.L., Terilli, C. & Ocon, A.J. (2012) 'Postural neurocognitive and neuronal activated cerebral blood flow deficits in young chronic fatigue syndrome patients with postural tachycardia syndrome.' *American Journal of Physiology, Heart and Circulatory Physiology 302* (5).
9. van Campen, C.L.M.C, Rowe, P.C., Verheugt Freek, W.A. & Visser, F.C. (2020) 'Cognitive function declines following orthostatic stress in adults with myalgic encephalomyelitis/chronic fatigue syndrome ME/CFS.' *Frontiers in Neuroscience 14*.
10. Campen, C.M.V., Rowe, P.C. & Visser, F.C. (2020) 'Reductions in cerebral blood flow can be provoked by sitting in severe myalgic encephalomyelitis/chronic fatigue syndrome patients.' *Healthcare 8*.
11. LaManca, J.J., Sisto, S.A., DeLuca, J., Johnson, S.K., *et al.* (1998) 'Influence of exhaustive treadmill exercise on cognitive functioning in chronic fatigue syndrome.' *American Journal of Medicine 28* (105).
12. Mateo, L.J., Chu, L., Stevens, S., Stevens, J., *et al.* (2020) 'Post-exertional symptoms distinguish myalgic encephalomyelitis/chronic fatigue syndrome subjects from healthy controls.' *Work 66* (2).
13. Neary, P.J, Roberts, A.D, Leavins, N., Harrison, M.F., Croll, J.C. & Sexsmith, J.R. (2008) 'Prefrontal cortex oxygenation during incremental exercise in chronic fatigue syndrome.' *Clinical Physiology and Functional Imaging 28* (6).
14. Shan, Z.Y., Barnden, L.R. & Kwiatek, R.A. (2020) 'Neuroimaging characteristics of myalgic encephalomyelitis/chronic fatigue syndrome (ME/CFS): a systematic review.' *Journal of Translational Medicine 18* (335).
15. Barnden, L.R., Shan, Z.Y., Staines, D.R., Marshall-Gradisnik, S., *et al.* (2019) 'Intra brainstem connectivity is impaired in chronic fatigue syndrome.' *NeuroImage: Clinical 24* (102045).

16. Mueller, C., Lin, J.C., Sheriff, S., Maudsley, A.A. & Younger, J.W. (2020) 'Evidence of widespread metabolite abnormalities in myalgic encephalomyelitis/chronic fatigue syndrome: assessment with whole-brain magnetic resonance spectroscopy.' *Brain Imaging and Behavior 14* (2).
17. Thapaliya, K., Staines, D., Marshall-Gradisnik, S., Su, J. & Barnden, L. (2022) 'Volumetric differences in hippocampal subfields and associations with clinical measures in myalgic encephalomyelitis/chronic fatigue syndrome.' *Journal of Neuroscience Research 100* (7).
18. Khacho, M., Clark, A., Svoboda, D.S., MacLaurin, J.G., *et al.* (2017) 'Mitochondrial dysfunction underlies cognitive defects as a result of neural stem cell depletion and impaired neurogenesis.' *Human Molecular Genetics 26* (17).
19. Booth, N.E., Myhill, S. & McLaren-Howard, J. (2012) 'Mitochondrial dysfunction and the pathophysiology of myalgic encephalomyelitis/chronic fatigue syndrome (ME/CFS).' *International Journal of Clinical and Experimental Medicine 5* (3).
20. Tomas, C., Elson, J.L., Strassheim, V., Newton, J.L. & Walker, M. (2020) 'The effect of myalgic encephalomyelitis/chronic fatigue syndrome (ME/CFS) severity on cellular bioenergetic function.' *PLOS ONE 15* (4).
21. Holden, S., Maksoud, R., Eaton-Fitch, N., Cabanas, H., Staines, D. & Marshall-Gradisnik, S. (2020) 'A systematic review of mitochondrial abnormalities in myalgic encephalomyelitis/chronic fatigue syndrome/systemic exertion intolerance disease.' *Journal of Translational Medicine 18* (1).
22. Christley, Y., Duffy, T., Everall, I.P. & Martin, C.R. (2013) 'The neuropsychiatric and neuropsychological features of chronic fatigue syndrome: revisiting the enigma.' *Current Psychiatry Reports 15* (4).
23. Afari, N. & Buchwald, D. (2003) 'Chronic fatigue syndrome: a review.' *American Journal of Psychiatry 160* (2).
24. Pellegrino, L.D., Peters, M.E. & Lyketsos, C.G. (2013) 'Depression in cognitive impairment.' *Current Psychiatry Reports 15* (384).
25. Robinson, L.J., Gallagher, P., Watson, S., Pearce, R., *et al.* (2019) 'Impairments in cognitive performance in chronic fatigue syndrome are common, not related to co-morbid depression but do associate with autonomic dysfunction.' *PLOS ONE 14* (2).
26. DeLuca, J., Johnson, S.K., Ellis, S.P. & Natelson, B.H. (1997) 'Cognitive functioning is impaired in patients with chronic fatigue syndrome devoid of psychiatric disease.' *Journal of Neurology, Neurosurgery and Psychiatry 62* (2).
27. Abd-Elfattah, H.M., Abdelazeim, F.H. & Elshennawy, S. (2015) 'Physical and cognitive consequences of fatigue: a review.' *Journal of Advanced Research 6* (3).
28. Moriarty, O.T., McGuire, B.E. & Finn, D.P. (2011) 'The effect of pain on cognitive function: a review of clinical and preclinical research.' *Progress in Neurobiology 93* (3).
29. Pistacchi, M., Gioulis, M., Contin, F., Sanson, F. & Marsala, S.Z. (2014) 'Sleep disturbance and cognitive disorder: epidemiological analysis in a cohort of 263 patients.' *Neurological Science 35* (12).
30. Zhou, L., Chen, L., Li, X., Li, T., Dong, Z. & Wang, Y.T. (2019) 'Food allergy induces alteration in brain inflammatory status and cognitive impairments.' *Behavioural Brain Research 364.*
31. Stromsdorfer, S. (2022) 'Memory aids and strategies for patients with cognitive impairment.' My OT Spot. Accessed on 10/12/2022 at www.myotspot.com/memory-aids-cognitive-impairment.
32. Heyn, P., Abreu, B.C. & Ottenbacher, K.J. (2004) 'The effects of exercise training on elderly persons with cognitive impairment and dementia: a meta-analysis.' *Archives of Physical Medicine and Rehabilitation 85* (10).
33. Baker, L.D., Frank, L.L. & Foster-Schubert, K. (2010) 'Effects of aerobic exercise on mild cognitive impairment: a controlled trial.' *Archives of Neurology 67* (1).
34. Cvejic, E., Lloyd, A.R. & Vollmer-Conna, U. (2016) 'Neurocognitive improvements after best-practice intervention for chronic fatigue syndrome: Preliminary

evidence of divergence between objective indices and subjective perceptions.' *Comprehensive Psychiatry 66*.

35. Zalewski, P., Kujawski, S., Tudorowska, M., Morten, K. *et al.* (2020) 'The impact of a structured exercise programme upon cognitive function in chronic fatigue syndrome patients.' *Brain Science 10* (4).

36. Blackwood, S.K., MacHale, S.M., Power, M.J., Goodwin, G.M. & Lawrie, S.M. (1998) 'Effects of exercise on cognitive and motor function in chronic fatigue syndrome and depression.' *Journal of Neurology, Neurosurgery and Psychiatry 65* (4).

CHAPTER 9

Sleep Dysfunction

PURPOSE OF THIS CHAPTER

Sleep dysfunction is included in the list of symptoms that may be present in most diagnostic criteria for ME/CFS and it is essential for diagnosis according to the Canadian Clinical Criteria (1) and the Institute of Medicine (IOM)/National Academy of Medicine (NAM) criteria (2).

While sleep may not be a speciality of most physiotherapists, sleep dysfunction may have a major impact on a person's symptoms. For example, a qualitative study conducted 11 semi-structured interviews with people with ME/CFS and despite differing experiences each participant reported that sleep played a critical role in their general ME/CFS symptoms (3).

As a physiotherapist it is therefore important to consider sleep dysfunction when working with someone with ME/CFS because:

- the quality of their sleep may have an adverse effect on their other ME/CFS symptoms, such as cognitive dysfunction and pain
- the severity of ME/CFS symptoms may impact on the quality of sleep, so if an intervention exacerbates symptoms this may manifest in further sleep disruption.

This chapter provides an overview of known subjective and objective dysfunctions of sleep in people with ME/CFS and summarizes adaptations to practice and considerations to make when planning and monitoring any physiotherapy interventions.

Sleep dysfunction

Sleep can be dysfunctional in several ways (4) (5) (6):

- insomnia: difficulty falling asleep or maintaining sleep
- somnolence: excessive sleep and feeling drowsy
- disrupted sleep: frequent waking
- poor quality sleep: lack of restful sleep
- hypersomnia: excessive daytime sleepiness
- circadian rhythm sleep disorder: dysfunction of the circadian clock causing difficulties with sleep onset, frequent waking and daytime sleepiness.

While the exact purpose of sleep is yet to be determined, it is known to be important because deprivation of sleep in the general population results in deterioration of cognition, mood and performance (7).

Sleep dysfunction can be linked to a wide range of diseases, for example it is commonly found in relation to people with Parkinson's disease (8), gastrointestinal diseases (9), anxiety and depressive disorders (10) and Alzheimer's disease (11). It is still undetermined whether sleep dysfunction is a complication of these diseases or acts as a contributing factor.

Sleep dysfunction and ME/CFS

The general terminology for sleep dysfunction in ME/CFS is 'unrefreshing sleep' but symptoms of sleep disturbance may be reported as (12) (13):

- difficulty in initiating sleep
- frequent waking
- vivid dreams
- restless legs syndrome: overwhelming urge to move the legs, or unpleasant crawling sensations in the legs and feet
- sleep reversal: when sleep occurs during the day and wakefulness is at night
- excessive daytime sleepiness.

A strong association has been found between worsening sleep and an exacerbation of ME/CFS symptoms (14) although it is not clear whether sleep dysfunction in ME/CFS is a symptom of the disease, or becomes a contributing factor to the impairments suffered (7) (14).

Measuring sleep quality in people with ME/CFS

Polysomnography (PSG) is a method of objectively measuring sleep by looking at brain waves, oxygen levels, heart rate, breathing rate and movements of the eyes and limbs. A PSG usually takes place in a clinic, so the environment is different to a person's usual sleeping routine.

A review (15) in 2012 examined 15 papers using PSG to measure the sleep patterns of people with ME/CFS and found many variable and non-specific differences in sleep patterns between people with ME/CFS and healthy controls.

A later study (7) recruited 343 people with ME/CFS who were seen at a fatigue clinic and ran a single night of PSG to analyse their sleep after all medication was paused for several weeks prior to testing. The study identified 104 people with sleep apnoea or periodic limb movement disorder, which were deemed primary sleep disorders that would explain the person's fatigue symptoms. It is important to note that this study used the CDC (Fukuda) criteria for diagnosis of ME/CFS, which do not require post exertional malaise (PEM) as essential for diagnosis, and this may explain the high number of people with fatigue-like symptoms that could be attributed to other conditions. This highlights the issues around the use of different diagnostic criteria in research, which are discussed in more detail in chapter 1.

Oliver: 'I couldn't get to sleep until after 2am and would wake up feeling unrefreshed. Once I got my symptoms under control, my sleep improved.'

Of the remaining 239 people, 89.1% met criteria for at least one objective sleep problem. However, there was no single defining sleep pattern, which supported the earlier review's conclusion that based on available data there does not appear to be a single characteristic objective sleep disturbance for people with ME/CFS (15).

Cause of sleep dysfunction in people with ME/CFS

No single cause of sleep dysfunction has been identified in people with ME/CFS.

Sleep dysfunction may occur as a result of some of the key symptoms of ME/CFS, such as pain and autonomic dysfunction, or be linked to some of the numerous co-morbidities discussed in chapter 2 such as fibromyalgia, migraine or orthostatic intolerance. Other potential links include the following:

Heart rate variability and autonomic function

A measure of autonomic nervous system activity is heart rate variability (HRV), which is the variability in timing between successive heartbeats (16). A higher heart rate-variability is associated with better subjective and objective sleep quality (17). People with ME/CFS have been found to have a lower HRV compared to healthy controls (18) and have shown a low HRV during sleep (19) (20) (21). This suggests that there may be increased sympathetic nervous system activity throughout the night and has led some to suggest that this may be the cause of the 'unrefreshing sleep' experienced by people with ME/CFS (16). However, many studies have small sample sizes, struggle with issues around accurate diagnostic criteria, and the findings are correlational as opposed to causal (16), so no absolute conclusions can be drawn on current evidence. More information on HRV and autonomic nervous system function can be found in chapter 12.

> **Mo**: 'When I wake up in the morning it doesn't feel like I have slept at all.'

Mitochondrial dysfunction

Mitochondria have been associated with the regulation of circadian rhythm and the link between mitochondrial disorders and altered sleep patterns is under investigation (22) (23). Mitochondrial dysfunction has been found in people with ME/CFS (24); however the exact role that they play in relation to ME/CFS is yet to be established. Further discussion of mitochondrial dysfunction is in chapter 6.

Altered hypothalamic-pituitary-adrenal axis

One of the actions of the hypothalamic-pituitary-adrenal axis (HPA axis) is to modulate the sleep–wake cycle, and some studies have found that the HPA axis is underactive in people with ME/CFS (25). However, sleep deprivation can also cause a dysfunction of the HPA axis (26) so it is unclear as to what role any HPA axis dysfunction may play in people with ME/CFS. More discussion of the HPA axis is in chapter 13.

Pharmacological management of sleep dysfunction

There are pharmacological options for the management of sleep dysfunction in people with ME/CFS. For example melatonin, a hormone associated with the sleep–wake cycle, may be an effective treatment in people with ME/CFS (27) (28) although it may not be fully licensed for use in all countries (12). Sleep quality in people with ME/CFS may also be improved with low dose sedating tricyclic antidepressants such as amitriptyline, doxepin, desipramine, nortriptyline, clomipramine and imipramine (29).

Magnesium deficiency has been associated with sleep disorders (30) and for the general population magnesium supplements may improve the quality of sleep (30) although a systematic review found the evidence to be uncertain (31). People with ME/CFS have been found to have reduced levels of magnesium (32). A small clinical trial of 32 people with ME/CFS found intramuscular application of magnesium sulphate had a positive impact on energy levels and reduced pain in comparison to a placebo group, although there was no mention of its impact upon sleep (32).

Some people with ME/CFS have anecdotal success with cannabis or cannabinoids (13), which may have a therapeutic effect on insomnia (33). There have as yet been no clinical trials of this medication in relation to ME/CFS (13) and currently the evidence in general has mixed results with a need for further longitudinal research (33).

It is important to note that any pharmacological intervention may have side effects, particularly for people with ME/CFS who may have greater intolerance to certain medications.

Adaptation to practice
Timing of appointments

Considering the potential for dysfunctional sleep, it is important to check the best time of day for an appointment to ensure the person has had time to fully wake up, but equally that the exertion of an appointment does not further affect that night's sleep quality.

Physiotherapy management of sleep dysfunction
Assessment

Including sleep quality in an assessment can highlight additional symptoms that may be having a significant impact on quality of life. Further information on how to include sleep dysfunction questions in an assessment can be found in chapter 14.

There are screening tools available including questionnaires to look at sleepiness during the day and sleep practices at night, and these are discussed in more detail in chapter 18.

Referrals

People with ME/CFS may have co-morbid conditions, including sleep disorders. If a person is reporting significant sleep disturbance and has not been fully investigated for sleep disorders, then consider a referral to an appropriate specialist. Key symptoms of sleep apnoea include fatigue, difficulty concentrating, mood swings and morning headaches (34).

Given the number of pharmacological options that may improve sleep quality, if a person with ME/CFS reports sleep dysfunction as a primary symptom then they could be referred for a review of their medications.

Sleep hygiene

'Sleep hygiene' is a term that describes what are considered to be 'good sleeping habits'. However, a review (35) has highlighted that most recommendations for the general population have not been studied to evaluate their direct effects on sleep, and for those that have the evidence is often either based on extremes that are not generalizable to the wider population or drawn from studies that were not directly testing the impact of these practices on sleep. The review criticizes sleep hygiene recommendations for being too vague, inconsistent and lacking in real detail as to how they may be implemented.

Typical sleep hygiene recommendations include (36) (37):

- consistent bedtimes
- maintaining a low-stimulus sleep environment, considering light, noise and temperature
- reducing use of electronic equipment such as televisions and mobile phones before bed

- avoiding large meals, caffeine and alcohol before bed
- a pre-bedtime routine such as a warm shower or bath and meditation.

Although these recommendations are commonly used, there is no consensus on which are essential or specific parameters. There is some overlap between sleep hygiene practices and some cognitive behavioural therapy techniques (38), which have been shown to be effective for people diagnosed with chronic insomnia (39).

There is no research on the effectiveness of sleep hygiene practices on people with ME/CFS, so such generic, unevidenced advice should be given with caution. Some suggestions may be of use but any adjustments to sleep routines should be closely monitored for signs of further symptom exacerbation.

It is also important to consider that for people with ME/CFS the bedroom may be a space that is occupied for a larger amount of time compared to the general population, particularly for those with severe or very severe ME/CFS, so some typical sleep hygiene suggestions relating to environmental changes may be impractical.

What about exercise?

Exercise can be considered beneficial to sleep quality in many populations (40), for example exercise has been associated with moderate improvements in subjective and objective sleep quality in older adults (41) and people with mental illness (42). The generalizability of any evidence for exercise as a means to improve sleep is hampered by the many variables involved, for example type of exercise, time of day and the individual characteristics of the person (43).

There is no evidence that exercise improves sleep quality for people with ME/CFS, in fact it appears to be the opposite. People with ME/CFS have reported a deterioration in sleep quality following physical exertion as part of PEM, which is the hallmark feature of ME/CFS and discussed in chapter 6 (44) (45). Therefore exercise is more likely to cause further sleep dysfunction and should not be considered as a means to improve sleep quality.

If exercise is being used to treat an unrelated issue for a person with ME/CFS, then consider monitoring sleep quality to ensure the intervention is not causing further dysfunction.

SUMMARY

▸ People with ME/CFS may experience difficulties with sleep, but no single sleep dysfunction covers every person's experience.

▸ Quality of sleep may impact a person's ME/CFS symptoms – and the severity of their symptoms may impact on the quality of their sleep.

▸ No research has been carried out to determine the most effective treatments for sleep dysfunction for people with ME/CFS, and although some medications can be used successfully there may also be side effects to consider.

APPLICATION TO PRACTICE

▸ Include questions about sleep quality in a general assessment to gain further understanding of how ME/CFS symptoms impact on all aspects of a person's life, as well as to identify possible avenues for onward referral.

▸ Consider using sleep quality as an outcome measure to determine tolerance or success of an intervention.

▸ There are many pharmacological options that may improve sleep quality, so refer for medical review if appropriate.

▸ Generic advice on 'sleep hygiene' practices could be given but with caution, as there is no evidence base for their effectiveness in ME/CFS. Any adjustments to routine should be monitored for their impact on overall symptoms and PEM.

References

1. Carruthers, B.M., Jain, A.K., De Meirleir, K L., Peterson, D.L., *et al.* (2003) 'Myalgic encephalomyelitis/chronic fatigue syndrome.' *Journal of Chronic Fatigue Syndrome 11* (1).

2. Centers for Disease Control and Prevention (2021) *IOM 2015 Diagnostic Criteria.* Accessed on 10/12/2022 at www.cdc.gov/me-cfs/healthcare-providers/diagnosis/iom-2015-diagnostic-criteria.html.

3. Gotts, Z.M., Newton, J.L., Ellis, J.G. & Deary, V. (2016) 'The experience of sleep in chronic fatigue syndrome: a qualitative interview study with patients.' *British Journal of Health Psychology 21* (1).

4. Devine, E.B., Hakim, Z. & Green, J. (2005) 'A systematic review of patient-reported outcome instruments measuring sleep dysfunction in adults.' *Pharmacoeconomics 23* (9).

5. Dauvilliers, Y. & Buguet, A. (2005) 'Hypersomnia.' *Dialogues in Clinical Neuroscience 7* (4).

6. Zee, P.C., Attarian, H. & Videnovic, A. (2013) 'Circadian rhythm abnormalities.' *Continuum (Minneap Minn) 19* (1 Sleep Disorders).
7. Gotts, Z.M., Deary, V., Newton, J., Van der Dussen, D., De Roy, P. & Ellis, J.G. (2013) 'Are there sleep-specific phenotypes in patients with chronic fatigue syndrome? A cross-sectional polysomnography analysis.' *BMJ Open 3* (6).
8. Comella, C.L. (2007) 'Sleep disorders in Parkinson's disease: an overview.' *Movement Disorders 22.*
9. Khanijow, V., Prakash, P., Emsellem, H.A., Borum, M.L. & Doman, D.B. (2015) 'Sleep dysfunction and gastrointestinal diseases.' *Gastroenterology & Hepatology (NY) 11* (12).
10. Becker, P.M. (2006) 'Treatment of sleep dysfunction and psychiatric disorders.' *Current Treatment Options in Neurology 8.*
11. Uddin, M.S.C., Tewari, D, Mamun, A.A., Kabir, M.T., *et al.* (2020) 'Circadian and sleep dysfunction in Alzheimer's disease.' *Ageing Research Reviews 60.*
12. Shepherd, C. & Chaudhuri, A. (2019) *ME/CFS/PVFS: An Exploration of the Key Clinical Issues.* Gawcott: The ME Association.
13. Rowe, P.C., Underhill, R.A., Friedman, K.J., Gurwitt, A., *et al.* (2017) 'Myalgic encephalomyelitis/chronic fatigue syndrome diagnosis and management in young people: a primer.' *Frontiers in Pediatrics 5* (121).
14. Morriss, R.K., Wearden, A.J. & Battersby, L. (1997) 'The relation of sleep difficulties to fatigue, mood and disability in chronic fatigue syndrome.' *Journal of Psychosomatic Research 42* (6).
15. Jackson, M.L. & Bruck, D. (2012) 'Sleep abnormalities in chronic fatigue syndrome/myalgic encephalomyelitis: a review.' *Journal of Clinical Sleep Medicine 8* (6).
16. Fatt, S.J., Beilharz, J.E., Joubert, M., Wilson, C., *et al.* (2020) 'Parasympathetic activity is reduced during slow-wave sleep, but not resting wakefulness, in patients with chronic fatigue syndrome.' *Journal of Clinical Sleep Medicine 16* (1).
17. Werner, G.G., Ford, B.Q., Mauss, I.B., Schabus, M., Blechert, J. & Wilhelm, F.H. (2015) 'High cardiac vagal control is related to better subjective and objective sleep quality.' *Biological Psychology 106.*
18. Nelson, M.J., Bahl, J.S., Buckley, J.D., Thomson, R.L. & Davison, K. (2019) 'Evidence of altered cardiac autonomic regulation in myalgic encephalomyelitis/chronic fatigue syndrome: a systematic review and meta-analysis.' *Medicine (Baltimore) 98* (43).
19. Boneva, R.S., Decker, M.J., Maloney, E.M., Lin, J.M., *et al.* (2007) 'Higher heart rate and reduced heart rate variability persist during sleep in chronic fatigue syndrome: a population-based study.' *Autonomic Neuroscience: Basic and Clinical 137* (1–2).
20. Rahman, K., Burton, A., Galbraith, S., Lloyd, A. & Vollmer-Conna, U. (2011) 'Sleep-wake behavior in chronic fatigue syndrome.' *Sleep 34* (5).
21. Burton, A.R., Rahman, K., Kadota, Y., Lloyd, A. & Vollmer-Conna, U. (2010) 'Reduced heart rate variability predicts poor sleep quality in a case-control study of chronic fatigue syndrome.' *Experimental Brain Research 204* (1).
22. Sardon Puig, L., Valera-Alberni, M., Cantó, C. & Pillon, N.J. (2018) 'Circadian rhythms and mitochondria: connecting the dots.' *Frontiers in Genetics 8* (9).
23. Aguilar-López, B.A., Moreno-Altamirano, M.M.B., Dockrell, H.M., Duchen, M.R. & Sánchez-García, F.J. (2020) 'Mitochondria: an integrative hub coordinating circadian rhythms, metabolism, the microbiome, and immunity.' *Frontiers in Cell and Developmental Biology 7* (8).
24. Holden, S., Maksoud, R., Eaton-Fitch, N., Cabanas, H., Staines, D. & Marshall-Gradisnik, S. (2020) 'A systematic review of mitochondrial abnormalities in myalgic encephalomyelitis/chronic fatigue syndrome/systemic exertion intolerance disease.' *Journal of Translational Medicine 18* (1).
25. Tanriverdi, F., Karaca, Z., Unluhizarci, K. & Kelestimur, F. (2007) 'The hypothalamo-pituitary-adrenal axis in chronic fatigue syndrome and fibromyalgia syndrome.' *Stress 10* (1).

26. Hirotsu, C., Tufik, S. & Andersen, M.L. (2015) 'Interactions between sleep, stress, and metabolism: from physiological to pathological conditions.' *Sleep Science 8* (3).

27. van Heukelom, R.O., Prins, J.B., Smits, M.G. & Bleijenberg, G. (2006) 'Influence of melatonin on fatigue severity in patients with chronic fatigue syndrome and late melatonin secretion.' *European Journal of Neurology 13* (1).

28. Castro-Marrero, J., Zaragozá, M.C., López-Vílchez, I., Galmés, J.L., *et al.* (2021) 'Effect of melatonin plus zinc supplementation on fatigue perception in myalgic encephalomyelitis/chronic fatigue syndrome: a randomized, double-blind, placebo-controlled trial.' *Antioxidants (Basel) 10* (7).

29. Castro-Marrero, J., Sáez-Francàs, N., Santillo, D. & Alegre, J. (2017) 'Treatment and management of chronic fatigue syndrome/myalgic encephalomyelitis: all roads lead to Rome.' *British Journal of Pharmacology 174* (5).

30. Nielsen, F.H. (2015) 'Relation between Magnesium Deficiency and Sleep Disorders and Associated Pathological Changes.' In R.R. Watson (ed.) *Modulation of Sleep by Obesity, Diabetes, Age, and Diet.* San Diego, CA: Academic Press.

31. Arab, A., Rafie, N., Amani, R. & Shirani, F. (2023) 'The role of magnesium in sleep health: a systematic review of available literature.' *Biological Trace Element Research 201* (1).

32. Cox, I.M., Campbell, M.J. & Dowson, D. (1991) 'Red blood cell magnesium and chronic fatigue syndrome.' *Lancet 337* (8744).

33. Babson, K.A., Sottile, J. & Morabito, D. (2017) 'Cannabis, cannabinoids, and sleep: a review of the literature.' *Current Psychiatry Reports 19* (23).

34. NHS (2019) 'Sleep apnoea.' Accessed on 10/12/2022 at www.nhs.uk/conditions/sleep-apnoea/.

35. Irish, L.A., Kline, C.E., Gunn, H.E., Buysse, D.J. & Hall, M.H. (2015) 'The role of sleep hygiene in promoting public health: a review of empirical evidence.' *Sleep Medicine Reviews 22.*

36. American Sleep Association (2022) 'Get better sleep.' Accessed on 10/12/2022 at www.sleepassociation.org/about-sleep/get-better-sleep.

37. Centers for Disease Control and Prevention (2016) 'Sleep and sleep disorders.' Accessed on 10/12/2022 at www.cdc.gov/sleep/about_sleep/sleep_hygiene.html.

38. Stepanski, E.J. & Wyatt, J.K. (2003) 'Use of sleep hygiene in the treatment of insomnia.' *Sleep Medicine Review 7* (3).

39. Trauer, J.M., Qian, M.Y., Doyle, J.S., Rajaratnam, S.M.W. & Cunnington, D. (2015) 'Cognitive behavioral therapy for chronic insomnia: a systematic review and meta-analysis.' *Annals of Internal Medicine 163.*

40. Chennaoui, M., Arnal, P.J., Sauvet, F. & Léger, D. (2015) 'Sleep and exercise: a reciprocal issue?' *Sleep Medicine Reviews 20.*

41. King, A.C., Pruitt, L.A., Woo, S., Castro, C.M., *et al.* (2008) 'Effects of moderate-intensity exercise on polysomnographic and subjective sleep quality in older adults with mild to moderate sleep complaints.' *Journal of Gerontology: Biological Sciences 63* (9).

42. Lederman, O., Ward, P.B., Firth, J., Maloney, C., *et al.* (2019) 'Does exercise improve sleep quality in individuals with mental illness? A systematic review and meta-analysis.' *Journal of Psychiatric Research 109.*

43. Driver, H.S. & Taylor, S.R. (2000) 'Exercise and sleep.' *Sleep Medical Review 4* (4).

44. Chu, L., Valencia, I.J., Garvert, D.W. & Montoya, J.G. (2018) 'Deconstructing post-exertional malaise in myalgic encephalomyelitis/chronic fatigue syndrome: a patient-centered, cross-sectional survey.' *PLOS ONE 12* (6).

45. Holtzman, C.S., Bhatia, S., Cotler, J. & Jason, L.A. (2019) 'Assessment of post-exertional malaise (PEM) in patients with myalgic encephalomyelitis (ME) and chronic fatigue syndrome (CFS): a patient-driven survey.' *Diagnostics (Basel) 9* (1).

CHAPTER 10

Pain

PURPOSE OF THIS CHAPTER

Pain is a common symptom in people with ME/CFS (1) but while it is clinically significant, there is no agreed definition of chronic pain specifically in relation to ME/CFS (2). The presence of pain is linked to a reduced quality of life and functional status in people with ME/CFS (3) so a physiotherapist should treat pain in this population as seriously as they would address pain arising from any other condition (4). Additionally, a physiotherapist needs to recognize when pain is a symptom independent of ME/CFS and always ensure that other causes or sources of pain are considered.

This chapter discusses the known pathophysiology of pain in ME/CFS and the common co-morbidities of ME/CFS that may also be a cause of pain, and details pain management options that are appropriate for people with ME/CFS.

What is pain
The International Association for the Study of Pain defines pain as 'an unpleasant sensory and emotional experience associated with, or resembling that associated with, actual or potential tissue damage' (5). Pain is a personal experience that may be influenced by biological, psychological and social factors (6).

Pain in ME/CFS
Pain is a common feature of ME/CFS and included on almost every diagnostic criteria, although only marked as essential for diagnosis in one (Canadian Clinical Criteria (7)). Pain in relation to ME/CFS is

not linked to a single part of the body and tends to be described as widespread (8), arising from muscles, joints or nerves; however not every person with ME/CFS may experience pain as part of their core ME/CFS symptoms, and the nature of any pain will vary between individuals. Pain can also be a symptom of post exertional malaise (PEM) (9), which is the exacerbation of current symptoms or addition of new symptoms caused by exertion, discussed in chapter 6.

An analysis of case definitions of ME/CFS suggests that pain is not necessarily an independent characteristic but could be a manifestation of other symptoms of ME/CFS (10). Additionally, a number of co-morbidities linked to ME/CFS can also cause pain, and it can therefore be very difficult to determine the primary cause of this symptom.

Pathophysiology of pain in ME/CFS

Hyperalgesia is an increased sensitivity to pain measured using pressure pain threshold testing, which can closely reflect clinical presentations (11). Using this technique, some people with ME/CFS have been found to have significantly lower pressure pain thresholds in comparison to healthy controls (12) and people with chronic lower back pain (13). While pain thresholds are much lower in muscles, they appear to be normal in the skin and subcutis in people with ME/CFS (14). As well as lowered pain thresholds, some people with ME/CFS have been found to have slower pain inhibitory responses, which are controlled by areas of the brain and central nervous system (15).

The cause of decreased pain thresholds in some people with ME/CFS is still to be determined. One theory was hypocortisolism, which is a reduction in the action of the adrenal gland, but no evidence has been found to support this (15). Research has also looked at muscle composition with varying results. One study showed the type and quantity of enzymes involved in energy production of a muscle were found to be normal in people who reported pain with ME/CFS (16), but another study took muscle biopsies from specific painful points and found abnormalities in structure, enzyme activity and mitochondrial DNA (14).

Pain is a complex topic in which to conduct robust research and most studies feature small sample sizes along with the problem of diagnostic discrepancies in ME/CFS discussed in chapter 1.

Pain in association with co-morbidities of ME/CFS

A number of co-morbidities of ME/CFS may be a cause of the pain experienced.

Pain associated with fibromyalgia

Fibromyalgia is characterized by chronic widespread pain (17) but has several overlapping features with ME/CFS (18). Key symptoms of fibromyalgia are widespread muscle pain, fatigue, morning stiffness, non-restorative sleep and cognitive dysfunction (19). Fibromyalgia can be diagnosed irrespective of other co-morbidities that may cause similar symptoms (20) and as such it can co-exist with ME/CFS (21). The presence of fibromyalgia can significantly increase the frequency and severity of PEM (21).

ME/CFS and fibromyalgia are diagnostically different conditions (22) so fibromyalgia cannot be the sole contributor of pain symptoms in people with ME/CFS. Further information on fibromyalgia can be found in chapter 2.

Pain associated with hypermobility

Joint hypermobility describes any joint that is mobile beyond the normal range of motion, and this appears to be common in people with ME/CFS (23). A retrospective cross-sectional study (24) of people in a specialist ME/CFS clinic in Sweden examined the prevalence of hypermobility. Out of 229 people diagnosed with severe ME/CFS, general joint hypermobility was identified in 115 (50%), with 20% already having an established diagnosis of hypermobile Ehlers–Danlos syndrome (EDS). Other studies have not found as high a prevalence, with evidence of hypermobility found in 25% (25) or 20% (26) of people with ME/CFS compared to 4% in the general population (26). More information on hypermobility can be found in chapter 2.

Pain is prevalent in hypermobility conditions. Chronic pain is the dominating symptom of joint hypermobility syndrome (27). In EDS the severity of pain is strongly correlated with the scale of hypermobility (28) and in Marfan syndrome back pain due to scoliosis is three times more frequent than in the general population (29). As a higher proportion of people with ME/CFS also have hypermobility, it could be considered as a potential source of the pain experienced by people with ME/CFS. However, so far no statistically significant correlations have been found in people with ME/CFS between the presence of hypermobility, self-reported pain and activity limitations (25) and there seems to be no association between musculoskeletal pain and joint hypermobility (26).

Therefore hypermobility alone is unlikely to be the sole reason for pain experienced by people with ME/CFS (22), but physiotherapists should have an awareness of the potential of hypermobile joints when working with people with ME/CFS.

Pain associated with orthostatic intolerance

A specific pattern of pain in the neck and shoulders is given the term 'coat-hanger pain' (30) and this can be associated with orthostatic intolerance, which is an intolerance to an upright position. A potential cause of coat-hanger pain is through orthostatic hypotension, which is a decrease in blood pressure on standing and may lead to reduced blood flow and ischaemia to the upper back and neck muscles resulting in pain (31). Neck and shoulder pain is also commonly reported in postural orthostatic tachycardia syndrome (POTS) (32). However, no direct association has been found between coat-hanger pain and orthostatic intolerance, with inter-individual and intra-individual variability (30). More information on orthostatic intolerance is in chapter 12.

Pain associated with temporomandibular disorders (TMDs)

Temporomandibular disorders involve pain in the temporomandibular joint (TMJ) and associated structures such as the jaw, teeth, ear, temples and cheeks (33). Temporomandibular disorders are considered to be a co-morbidity of ME/CFS (34) and can be treated effectively with physiotherapy interventions (35). Temporomandibular disorders are discussed further in chapter 2.

Pain associated with migraines and headaches

Migraines are a common co-morbidity of ME/CFS (34). A cross-sectional study of 143,000 people with ME/CFS in England found 76% reported headaches and 39.2% reported migraines, in comparison to 32.8% and 21.3% respectively in healthy controls (36). Pharmacological management of migraines and headaches is feasible for people with ME/CFS (37) so if not yet addressed a person presenting with migraine or headache symptoms should be referred for medical review. Further information regarding migraine is in chapter 2.

Pain associated with irritable bowel syndrome

Abdominal pain along with other symptoms such as changes to bowel movements can be associated with irritable bowel syndrome, which is discussed in chapter 3. There may be a number of other causes of abdominal pain so it is important that a thorough medical review takes place if this symptom is occurring.

Central sensitization, 'catastrophizing' and kinesiophobia

Central sensitization, where repeated noxious stimulation leads to neuroplastic changes in the central nervous system, has been used as a potential explanation of the widespread pain in people with ME/CFS (38). The resultant sensitization can cause exaggerated perceptions of noxious stimuli, nociceptive responses to non-noxious stimuli and the generation of widespread, unspecified locations of pain (39).

Oliver: 'I get pain in my leg muscles as part of PEM if I overdo things. Massage helps when they are very sore.'

Central sensitization has been explored in depth in relation to fibromyalgia but not ME/CFS (38) and while there may be an overlap between the two conditions there is still a clear distinction (see Fibromyalgia section in this chapter). Central sensitization in people with ME/CFS is suggested by the presence of hyperalgesia, lack of obvious peripheral tissue damage and lowered pain thresholds following exercise, which are all indicative of a dysfunctional nociceptive system (38). However, currently there is no direct evidence supporting central sensitization specifically in people with ME/CFS (40).

Another pain phenomenon, 'catastrophizing', has been suggested as a contributing factor to chronic pain in ME/CFS (22). Catastrophizing in chronic pain conditions is a way of thinking about a pain experience, characterized by rumination, magnification and helplessness (41). However, there is very little evidence that catastrophizing is demonstrated in ME/CFS (42) and therefore it is unlikely to be a contributing factor to pain in ME/CFS.

The concept of 'fear avoidance' and 'kinesiophobia' (an irrational fear of movement) has been associated with chronic pain states and a related increase in disability (43) and this has also been explored in people with ME/CFS who experience pain. However, no correlation has been found between a person's exercise capacity and activity limitations and the presence of kinesiophobia in ME/CFS (44).

Adaptation to practice
Assessment and referrals

If pain is reported by a person with ME/ CFS it is important to carry out a thorough assessment. Examples of outcome measures for pain can be found in chapter 18. While pain is a common symptom of ME/CFS, it could also be in relation to a co-morbidity or a completely unrelated issue, so it is important not to immediately attribute every symptom of pain to ME/CFS.

Mo: 'My pain is in my whole body and medication will only take the edge off.'

Analgesics, whether over-the-counter (aspirin, paracetamol, ibuprofen) or prescribed, can have varying benefits in relation to pain relief. People with ME/CFS may have sensitivities to some medications so an appropriate medical practitioner should be considered if the person wishes to explore analgesic options. The Appendix lists some common medications used for people with ME/CFS.

Physiotherapy management of pain

There are many non-pharmacological approaches to pain management but there is no single over riding treatment recommendation for pain management in ME/CFS. For example, one study interviewed people with ME/CFS who had chronic pain, and of the 45 people interviewed there were 19 different approaches tried, all with varying results (45).

Massage therapy

Massage therapy may improve pain, as well as depression and anxiety, in people with ME/CFS (46) and some types of massage may improve physical symptoms (47); however, it is not clear whether any effects can be sustained in the long term and the quality of evidence is poor (48). While massage has reduced pain for some people with ME/CFS it has also caused an increase in pain for others (45).

If a physiotherapist is considering using massage as part of pain management it is important to remember that people with ME/CFS have lower pressure pain thresholds (49) and therefore the intensity of massage should be moderated accordingly. People with ME/CFS may also have sensory intolerances to smell (see chapter 11) so any lubricating medium with strong scents should be avoided.

Any treatment should be constantly monitored for signs of new symptoms, or exacerbation of current symptoms, both during the intervention and in the period following the intervention, considering the delayed nature of PEM.

Acupuncture

Acupuncture has been reported in qualitative data to provide pain relief in some people with ME/CFS (45). A favourable response compared to sham acupuncture has been found but most studies have low methodological quality (50) and there have been recorded drop-out rates from trials of up to 35% (48) which suggests it may not be tolerated by all.

Any use of acupuncture should be constantly monitored for tolerance both during and in the period following the intervention, considering the delayed nature of PEM.

Spinal mobilizations

Mobilization of the spine in the general population is considered to create a hypoalgesic effect (51); however very few studies have been carried out in relation to ME/CFS (52). A small qualitative study reported no improvements with spinal mobilizations in people with ME/CFS (45).

Consideration of the lower pressure pain thresholds in people with ME/CFS (49) and the potential for hypermobility should add caution to any treatment requiring larger amplitudes of pressure.

Pain education

Education about pain and central sensitization can have a positive effect on pain in people with chronic pain conditions (53) and could be considered as an intervention for people with ME/CFS who experience chronic pain (22). Pain physiology education was shown to improve pain physiology knowledge and reduce catastrophizing in people with ME/CFS immediately after a 30-minute session, but no long-term effects or reduction in pain symptoms have been recorded (54).

General pain education is not specific to ME/CFS and the timing and delivery method of any information should be carefully considered given the potential cognitive impairments of some people with ME/CFS, in particular attention and memory. Additionally, there is the risk of causing cognitive fatigue with in-depth educational sessions, which may lead to PEM and symptom exacerbation, including the potential for causing further pain. Chapter 8 discusses cognitive dysfunction in more detail and provides methods of adapting communication to limit the impact of an intervention.

Heat
Use of basic techniques such as warm baths, heat pads, electric blankets and hot water bottles have been the most reported methods of easing pain in people with ME/CFS (45) although with regards to baths the energy expenditure required to dry the body afterwards can make the intervention counter-productive. Heat may increase vasodilation and lead to improved blood flow, which could help with any circulatory impairments.

Transcutaneous electrical stimulation
Transcutaneous electrical stimulation (TENS) is a non-invasive pain relief method using a mild electrical current. A comprehensive appraisal of reviews and meta-analysis on use of TENS for acute and chronic pain in the general population concluded that there was sufficient data showing benefits of TENS, insufficient data showing no benefit, but also many studies that were inconclusive (55). Currently there has been no research on the benefits of TENS specifically for people with ME/CFS so, as with any intervention, there should be careful monitoring of symptom response if TENS is trialled.

Ana: 'I am in constant pain. Acupuncture was helpful at first, but getting to the appointments was too exhausting.'

What about exercise?
In the general population exercise can have a beneficial effect on pain, causing 'exercise-induced hypoalgesia' (56). A single bout of resistance exercise can raise pain thresholds and lower pain ratings in a healthy population (57), and for people with chronic low back pain aerobic exercise has been found to reduce pressure pain perception (58) and increase pain thresholds (13). Isometric exercises, where muscles are contracted without movement of joints, can reduce pain during recovery from lower limb fracture (59) and tendinopathy (60) although this is not consistently found in research (61).

While exercise may reduce pain in the general population, for some people with ME/CFS exercise appears to cause further pain (45) and it has been shown to lower pressure pain thresholds (13) (49) (62). This decreased pain threshold may be associated with PEM (62) which is triggered by exertion. In an international survey of over 1500 people with ME/CFS (63) 87.9% reported worsening muscle pain, 73% joint pain and 63% nerve pain after physical and cognitive exertion. More information about PEM can be found in chapter 6.

Exercise can cause pain in the general population in the form of delayed onset muscle soreness (DOMS), which typically peaks between 24 and 48 hours after exercise and subsides within 96 hours (64). While DOMS may also be experienced by people with ME/CFS, the impact of exercise on pain has been found to be more prevalent and more severe. One study found that 82% of people with ME/CFS reported muscle or joint pain, and 53% reported general pain following maximal exercise tests, compared to 40% and 10% respectively in matched sedentary controls. The researchers noted that the pain in healthy controls may be indicative of DOMS and the participants quickly returned to their baseline levels of health, whereas there was a substantial difference in the severity and duration of post exertional symptoms in people with ME/CFS (65).

The origin of a lowered pain threshold after exercise may be due to a central dysfunction (49), for example one theory (66) considers that the hypoalgesia effect of exercise is produced by several areas of the brain, and blood flow to the brain is known to decrease in people with ME/CFS when upright (see chapter 12). Therefore the reduced blood flow may impact on the capability of the brain to create the hypoalgesia affect in people with ME/CFS (66).

Other findings suggest there may be peripheral factors contributing to increased pain, for example enhanced gene expression for receptors detecting muscle metabolites have been found following moderate exercise in people with ME/CFS (67).

While exercise may have benefits in reducing pain in the general population, there do not appear to be the same benefits for people with ME/CFS and in fact the introduction of exercise may increase pain for this population. The primary focus of any intervention for a person with ME/CFS should always be avoiding PEM, so any approach designed to manage pain in ME/CFS must be regularly monitored and evaluated for signs of symptom exacerbation.

SUMMARY

▸ People with ME/CFS may experience pain in muscles and joints, as part of PEM and in relation to other co-morbidities.

▸ Exertion can further reduce the pressure pain threshold for some people with ME/CFS and may trigger PEM, which can increase pain symptoms.

APPLICATION TO PRACTICE

▸ Pain negatively affects quality of life and therefore pain management should be addressed as a priority.

▸ Pain may be a symptom independent of ME/CFS and therefore it is important to ensure that other causes or sources of pain are considered.

▸ Pain management techniques such as massage therapy and acupuncture could be considered but treatment should always be individualized and regularly monitored for adverse effects.

▸ Exercise is more likely to cause pain than relieve it in people with ME/CFS.

References

1. Jason, L.A., Richman, J.A., Rademaker, A.W., Jordan, K.M., *et al.* (1999) 'A community-based study of chronic fatigue syndrome.' *Archives of Internal Medicine 159* (18).
2. Meeus, M., Nijs, J. & Meirleir, K.D. (2007) 'Chronic musculoskeletal pain in patients with the chronic fatigue syndrome: a systematic review.' *European Journal of Pain 11* (4).
3. Strand, E.B., Mengshoel, A.M., Sandvik, L., Helland, I.B., Abraham, S. & Nes, L.S. (2019) 'Pain is associated with reduced quality of life and functional status in patients with myalgic encephalomyelitis/chronic fatigue syndrome.' *Scandinavian Journal of Pain 19* (1).
4. Marshall, R., Paul, L., McFadyen, A.K., Rafferty, D. & Wood, L. (2010) 'Pain characteristics of people with chronic fatigue syndrome.' *Journal of Musculoskeletal Pain 18* (2).
5. Raja, S.N., Carr, D.B., Cohen, M., Finnerup, N.B., *et al.* (2020) 'The revised International Association for the Study of Pain definition of pain: concepts, challenges, and compromises.' *Pain 161* (9).
6. International Association for the Study of Pain (1994) 'Pain terms and definitions.' Accessed on 10/12/2022 at www.iasp-pain.org/resources/terminology.
7. Carruthers, B.M., Jain, A.K., De Meirleir, K.L., Peterson, D.L., *et al.* (2003) 'Myalgic encephalomyelitis/chronic fatigue syndrome.' *Journal of Chronic Fatigue Syndrome 11* (1).

8. Bateman, L., Bested, A.C., Bonilla, H.F., Chheda, B.V., *et al.* (2021) 'Myalgic encephalomyelitis/chronic fatigue syndrome: essentials of diagnosis and management.' *Mayo Clinic Proceedings 96* (11).

9. Chu, L., Valencia, I.J., Garvert, D.W. & Montoya, J.G. (2018) 'Deconstructing post-exertional malaise in myalgic encephalomyelitis/chronic fatigue syndrome: a patient-centered, cross-sectional survey.' *PLOS ONE 13* (6).

10. Conroy, K.E., Islam, M.F. & Jason, L.A. (2022) 'Evaluating case diagnostic criteria for myalgic encephalomyelitis/chronic fatigue syndrome (ME/CFS): toward an empirical case definition.' *Disability and Rehabilitation.* Epub ahead of print.

11. Geisser, M.E., Gracely, R.H., Giesecke, T., Petzke, F.W., Williams, D.A. & Clauw, D.J. (2007) 'The association between experimental and clinical pain measures among persons with fibromyalgia and chronic fatigue syndrome.' *European Journal of Pain 11* (2).

12. Meeus, M., Nijs, J., Huybrechts, S. & Truijen, S. (2010) 'Evidence for generalized hyperalgesia in chronic fatigue syndrome: a case control study.' *Clinical Rheumatology 29* (4).

13. Meeus, M., Roussel, N.A., Truijen, S. & Nijs, J. (2010) 'Reduced pressure pain thresholds in response to exercise in chronic fatigue syndrome but not in chronic low back pain: an experimental study.' *Journal of Rehabilitative Medicine 42* (9).

14. Vecchiet, L., Montanari, G., Pizzigallo, E., Iezzi, S., *et al.* (1996) 'Sensory characterization of somatic parietal tissues in humans with chronic fatigue syndrome.' *Neuroscience Letters 208* (2).

15. Meeus, M., Nijs, J., Van de Wauwer, N., Toeback, L. & Truijen, S. (2008) 'Diffuse noxious inhibitory control is delayed in chronic fatigue syndrome: an experimental study.' *Pain 139* (2).

16. Byrne, E. & Trounce, I. (1987) 'Chronic fatigue and myalgia syndrome: mitochondrial and glycolytic studies in skeletal muscle.' *Journal of Neurology, Neurosurgery and Psychiatry 50* (6).

17. Bazzichi, L., Giacomelli, C., Consensi, A., Giorgi, V., *et al.* (2020) 'One year in review 2020: fibromyalgia.' *Clinical and Experimental Rheumatology 123* (1).

18. Clauw, D.J. & Chrousos, G.P. (1997) 'Chronic pain and fatigue syndromes: overlapping clinical and neuroendocrine features and potential pathogenic mechanisms.' *Neuroimmunomodulation 4* (3).

19. Häuser, W., Zimmer, C., Felde, E. & Köllner, V. (2008) 'What are the key symptoms of fibromyalgia? Results of a survey of the German Fibromyalgia Association.' *Schmerz (Pain) 22* (2).

20. Wolfe, F., Clauw, D.J., Fitzcharles, M.A., Goldenberg, D.L., *et al.* (2016) '2016 revisions to the 2010/2011 fibromyalgia diagnostic criteria.' *Seminars in Arthritis and Rheumatology 46* (3).

21. McManimen, S.L. & Jason, L.A. (2017) 'Post-exertional malaise in patients with ME and CFS with comorbid fibromyalgia.' *SRL Neurological Neurosurgery 3* (1).

22. Nijs, J., Crombez, G., Meeus, M., Knoop, H., *et al.* (2012) 'Pain in patients with chronic fatigue syndrome: time for specific pain treatment?' *Pain Physician 15* (5).

23. Nijs, J. (2005) 'Generalized joint hypermobility: an issue in fibromyalgia and chronic fatigue syndrome?' *Journal of Bodywork and Movement Therapies 9* (4).

24. Bragée, B., Michos, A., Drum, B., Fahlgren, M., Szulkin, R. & Bertilson, B.C. (2020) 'Signs of intracranial hypertension, hypermobility, and craniocervical obstructions in patients with myalgic encephalomyelitis/chronic fatigue syndrome.' *Frontier of Neurology 28* (11).

25. Nijs, J., De Meirleir, K. & Truyen S. (2004) 'Hypermobility in patients with chronic fatigue syndrome: preliminary observations.' *Journal of Musculoskeletal Pain 12* (1).

26. Nijs, J., Aerts, A. & De Meirleir, K. (2006) 'Generalized joint hypermobility is more common in chronic fatigue syndrome than in healthy control subjects.' *Journal of Manipulative Physiological Therapeutics 29* (1).

27. Grahame, R. (2009) 'Joint hypermobility syndrome pain.' *Current Science 13.*

28. Voermans, N.C., Knoop, H., Bleijenberg, G. & van Engelen, B.G. (2010) 'Pain in Ehlers–Danlos syndrome is common, severe, and associated with functional impairment.' *Journal of Pain and Symptom Management 40* (3).

29. Dean, J. (2007) 'Marfan syndrome: clinical diagnosis and management.' *European Journal of Human Genetics 15.*

30. Khurana, R.K. (2012) 'Coat-hanger ache in orthostatic hypotension.' *Cephalalgia 32* (10).

31. Wieling, W. & Schatz, I.J. (2009) 'The consensus statement on the definition of orthostatic hypotension: a revisit after 13 years.' *Journal of Hypertension 27* (5).

32. Henry, A.H., Samy, A.H., Ashangari, C. & Suleman, A. (2015) 'Frequency of symptoms in postural orthostatic tachycardia syndrome (POTS).' *Autonomic Neuroscience 192.*

33. National Institute for Health and Care Excellence (2021) 'Temporomandibular disorders (TMDs).' Accessed on 10/12/2022 at https://cks.nice.org.uk/topics/temporomandibular-disorders-tmds.

34. Carruthers, B.M., van de Sande, M.I., De Meirleir, K.L., Klimas, N.G., *et al.* (2011) 'Myalgic encephalomyelitis: International Consensus Criteria.' *Journal of Internal Medicine 270.*

35. Paço, M., Peleteiro, B., Duarte, J. & Pinho, T. (2016) 'The effectiveness of physiotherapy in the management of temporomandibular disorders: a systematic review and meta-analysis.' *Journal of Oral & Facial Pain and Headache 30* (3).

36. Nacul, L.C., Lacerda, E.M., Pheby, D., Campion, P., *et al.* (2011) 'Prevalence of myalgic encephalomyelitis/chronic fatigue syndrome (ME/CFS) in three regions of England: a repeated cross-sectional study in primary care.' *BMC Medical 28* (9).

37. Shepherd, C. & Chaudhuri, A. (2019) *ME/CFS/PVFS: An Exploration of the Key Clinical Issues.* Gawcott: The ME Association.

38. Meeus, M. & Nijs, J. (2007) 'Central sensitization: a biopsychosocial explanation for chronic widespread pain in patients with fibromyalgia and chronic fatigue syndrome.' *Clinical Rheumatology 26* (4).

39. Li, J., Simone, D.A. & Larson, A.A. (1999) 'Windup leads to characteristics of central sensitization.' *Pain 79* (1).

40. Nijs, J., Meeus, M. & De Meirleir, K. (2006) 'Chronic musculoskeletal pain in chronic fatigue syndrome: recent developments and therapeutic implications.' *Manual Therapies 11* (3).

41. Sullivan, M.J.L., Bishop, S.R. & Pivik, J. (1995) 'The pain catastrophizing scale: development and validation.' *Psychological Assessment 7.*

42. Nijs, J., Van de Putte, K., Louckx. F., Truijen, S. & De Meirleir, K. (2008) 'Exercise performance and chronic pain in chronic fatigue syndrome: the role of pain catastrophizing.' *Pain Medicine 9* (8).

43. Luque-Suarez, A., Martinez-Calderon, J. & Falla, D. (2019) 'Role of kinesiophobia on pain, disability and quality of life in people suffering from chronic musculoskeletal pain: a systematic review.' *British Journal of Sports Medicine 53.*

44. Nijs, J., Vanherberghen, K., Duquet, W. & De Meirleir, K. (2004) 'Chronic fatigue syndrome: lack of association between pain-related fear of movement and exercise capacity and disability.' *Physical Therapy 84* (8).

45. Marshall, R., Paul, L. & Wood, L. (2011) 'The search for pain relief in people with chronic fatigue syndrome: a descriptive study.' *Physiotherapy Theory and Practice 27* (5).

46. Field, T., Sunshine, W., Hernandez-Reif, M., Quintino, O., *et al.* (2011) 'Massage therapy effects on depression and somatic symptoms in chronic fatigue syndrome.' *Journal of Chronic Fatigue Syndrome 3.*

47. Wang, J.H., Chai, T.Q., Lin, G.H. & Luo, L. (2009) 'Effects of the intelligent-turtle massage on the physical symptoms and immune functions in patients with chronic fatigue syndrome.' *Journal of Traditional Chinese Medicine 29* (1).

48. Porter, N.S., Jason, L.A., Boulton, A., Bothne, N. & Coleman, B. (2010) 'Alternative medical interventions used in the treatment and management of myalgic

encephalomyelitis/chronic fatigue syndrome and fibromyalgia.' *Journal of Alternative and Complementary Medicine 16* (3).

49. Whiteside, A., Hansen, S. & Chaudhuri, A. (2004) 'Exercise lowers pain threshold in chronic fatigue syndrome.' *Pain 109.*

50. Zhang, Q., Gong, J., Dong, H., Xu, S., Wang, W. & Huang, G. (2019) 'Acupuncture for chronic fatigue syndrome: a systematic review and meta-analysis.' *Acupuncture Medicine 37* (4).

51. Krouwel, O., Hebron, C. & Willett, E. (2010) 'An investigation into the potential hypoalgesic effects of different amplitudes of PA mobilisations on the lumbar spine as measured by pressure pain thresholds (PPT).' *Manual Therapy 15* (1).

52. Yee, C.W. & Chellappan, D.K. (2013) 'Are the current complementary and alternative therapies available for the treatment of low back pain and chronic fatigue syndrome reliable clinically? A review of the literature.' *Journal of Evidence-Based Complementary & Alternative Medicine 18* (3).

53. Louw, A., Diener, I., Butler, D.S. & Puentedura, E.J. (2011) 'The effect of neuroscience education on pain, disability, anxiety, and stress in chronic musculoskeletal pain.' *Archives of Physical Medicine and Rehabilitation 92* (12).

54. Meeus, M., Nijs, J., Van Oosterwijck, J., Van Alsenoy, V. & Truijen, S. (2010) 'Pain physiology education improves pain beliefs in patients with chronic fatigue syndrome compared with pacing and self-management education: a double-blind randomized controlled trial.' *Archives of Physical Medicine and Rehabilitation 91* (8).

55. Paley, C.A., Wittkopf, P.G., Jones, G. & Johnson, M.I. (2021) 'Does TENS reduce the intensity of acute and chronic pain? A comprehensive appraisal of the characteristics and outcomes of 169 reviews and 49 meta-analyses.' *Medicina (Kaunas) 57* (10).

56. Wewege, M.A. & Jones, M.D. (2021) 'Exercise-induced hypoalgesia in healthy individuals and people with chronic musculoskeletal pain: a systematic review and meta-analysis.' *Journal of Pain 22* (1).

57. Koltyn, K.F. & Arbogast, R.W. (1998) 'Perception of pain after resistance exercise.' *British Journal of Sports Medicine 32* (1).

58. Hoffman, M.D., Shepanski, M.A., Mackenzie, S.P. & Clifford, P.S. (2005) 'Experimentally induced pain perception is acutely reduced by aerobic exercise in people with chronic low back pain.' *Journal of Rehabilitation Research and Development 42* (2).

59. Khosrojerdi, H., Tajabadi, A., Amadani, M., Akrami, R. & Tadayonfar, M. (2018) 'The effect of isometric exercise on pain severity and muscle strength of patients with lower limb fractures: a randomized clinical trial study.' *MEDSURG Nursing: The Journal of Adult Health 7* (1).

60. Rio, E., Kidgell, D., Purdam, C., Gaida, J., *et al.* (2015) 'Isometric exercise induces analgesia and reduces inhibition in patellar tendinopathy.' *British Journal of Sports Medicine 49* (19).

61. van der Vlist, A.C., van Veldhoven, P.L.J., van Oosterom, R.F., Verhaar, J.A.N. & de Vos, R.J. (2020) 'Isometric exercises do not provide immediate pain relief in Achilles tendinopathy: a quasi-randomized clinical trial.' *Scandinavian Journal of Medicine & Science in Sports 30* (9).

62. Van Oosterwijck, J., Nijs, J., Meeus, M., Lefever, I., *et al.* (2010) 'Pain inhibition and postexertional malaise in myalgic encephalomyelitis/chronic fatigue syndrome: an experimental study.' *Journal of Internal Medicine 268* (3).

63. Holtzman, C.S., Bhatia, S., Cotler, J. & Jason, L.A. (2019) 'Assessment of post-exertional malaise (PEM) in patients with myalgic encephalomyelitis (ME) and chronic fatigue syndrome (CFS): a patient-driven survey.' *Diagnostics (Basel) 9* (1).

64. Connolly, D.A., Sayers, S.P. & McHugh, M.P. (2003) 'Treatment and prevention of delayed onset muscle soreness.' *Journal of Strength & Conditioning Research 17* (1).

65. Mateo, L.J., Chu, L., Stevens, S., Stevens, J., *et al.* (2020) 'Post-exertional symptoms distinguish myalgic encephalomyelitis/chronic fatigue syndrome subjects from healthy controls.' *Work 66* (2).

66. Nijs, J. & Ickmans, K. (2013) 'Postural orthostatic tachycardia syndrome as a clinically important subgroup of chronic fatigue syndrome: further evidence for central nervous system dysfunctioning.' *Journal of Internal Medicine 273* (5).

67. Light, A.R., White, A.T., Hughen, R.W. & Light, K.C. (2009) 'Moderate exercise increases expression for sensory, adrenergic, and immune genes in chronic fatigue syndrome patients but not in normal subjects.' *Pain 10* (10).

CHAPTER 11

Neurological Impairments

PURPOSE OF THIS CHAPTER

Neurological impairments are included in two of the major diagnostic criteria for ME/CFS and are listed as motor impairments and sensory disturbances.

As a physiotherapist it is important to understand the potential neurological impairments in people with ME/CFS because:

- typical exercise-based neurological rehabilitation may be a trigger for post exertional malaise (PEM)
- sensory disturbances may be aggravated by any interaction and therefore adaptations to practice may be required.

This chapter details the nature of neurological impairments for people with ME/CFS and what considerations should be made to adapt practice and management.

Neurological dysfunction in ME/CFS

The World Health Organization lists 'myalgic encephalomyelitis' as a disorder of the nervous system under code G93.3, alongside post viral fatigue syndrome. Symptoms of neurological dysfunction in ME/CFS, as described in diagnostic criteria, cover motor and sensory impairments.

It has not been established whether the origins of the neurological symptoms of ME/CFS are from damage of the nervous system. Abnormalities in brain scans of people with ME/CFS have been identified and a systematic review (1) of all reported brain imaging to 2018 found frequent and consistent abnormalities in the brains of people with ME/CFS compared to healthy controls, including:

- recruitment of additional brain regions for cognitive tasks
- structural anomalies in the brain stem
- indication of local neuroinflammation in the brain stem
- reduced serotonin transporters.

Despite these findings, studies often feature small sample sizes or use diagnostic criteria that may not truly represent the population, as discussed in chapter 1, and it is difficult to conclude the implications for diagnosis and treatment. While neurological inflammation is suspected, the technology to investigate these processes is only recently becoming available (2).

Kim: 'I cannot cope for long with things like loud noises, lively restaurants or public events with music and people talking.'

Motor impairments in people with ME/CFS

Common motor impairments linked to ME/CFS are muscle weakness, ataxia and fasciculations (3). It is important to be aware that these are also signs and symptoms of other neurological conditions, so if indicated a thorough neurological screen should be carried out, or onward referral made to an appropriate specialist for review to rule out other causes.

Muscle weakness

People with ME/CFS have muscles that are weaker and quicker to fatigue in comparison to the general population (4). It is not clear however whether the muscle weakness experienced by people with ME/CFS is caused by a neurological pathology (5). Other explanations for the mechanisms behind this weakness include impaired metabolic processes, peripheral fatigue, central fatigue or deconditioning, and these are explored in detail in chapters 6 and 7. Muscle weakness can also be a symptom of PEM, for example 87.3% of 1500 people with ME/CFS reported that physical or cognitive exertion caused muscle weakness (6).

While reduced muscle strength is reported in research, there is no reported record of muscle atrophy being commonly found in people with ME/CFS. Significant atrophy without obvious causation should be investigated further to rule out other conditions or causes.

One implication of muscle weakness is reduced strength in lower limbs leading to impaired muscle pump and subsequent intolerance to an upright position. Further explanation of such orthostatic intolerance can be found in chapter 12.

Ataxia/balance problems

Ataxia is an impaired co-ordination of voluntary movement (7). One review (3) reports that people with ME/CFS often describe clumsiness and difficulty with balance. Ataxia was reported to be exacerbated by physical or cognitive exertion by 77.6% of 1500 people with ME/CFS in an international survey (6). A small study found 29% of participants with ME/CFS presented with unstable tandem gait and impairments in the ability to stand with eyes closed, without sway, and stand on one leg, which they suggested could be truncal ataxia (8). However, it is unclear whether true axial or truncal ataxia is present in the ME/CFS population as there is limited evidence and this presentation could be explained by a number of other symptoms such as muscle weakness and fatigue.

Fasciculations

A fasciculation is a spontaneous discharge of a motor unit in a muscle, observed as localized muscle twitches (9). Fasciculations are listed as a possible symptom of ME/CFS but can also be seen in a range of disorders such as peripheral neuropathy, motor neurone disease and hyper-excitability of the peripheral nerves, as well as occurring spontaneously in the general population (9). 'Muscle twitches' were reported by 68.1% of 1500 people with ME/CFS in an international survey exploring symptoms that were made worse by physical or cognitive exertion (6).

Sensory disturbances

People with ME/CFS can be hypersensitive to sensory stimulation, including light, noise, touch, smell and temperature (3) (10) and are described as being in a 'sensory overload' (11). One study (12) explored self-reported symptoms in over 400 people with ME/CFS and found over half reported moderate to severe sensory disturbances, which were linked to significantly reduced scores for physical functioning, general health, social functioning and higher levels of unemployment.

Sensory overload was reported as a trigger for PEM in over 80% of 1500 people with ME/CFS in an international survey (6). Sensory symptoms may also be one of the symptoms exacerbated by triggers of PEM.

People with severe or very severe ME/CFS may have extremely debilitating sensory disturbances, and these are discussed in more detail in chapter 3.

Visual disturbances

Visual disturbances in some people with ME/CFS include photosensitivity, difficulty focusing, poor depth perception, inaccurate eye movements, discomfort with visual patterns, eye pain, visual migraine, reduced tear secretion and impaired visual attention (13) (14) (15) (11) (16) with the suggestion that the severity of visual symptoms are in line with the severity of ME/CFS symptoms (11).

Tear production and contraction of the ciliary muscle in the eye are both controlled by the parasympathetic nervous system (17). As a significant number of people with ME/CFS have a dysfunction of the autonomic nervous system, this could explain the reduced tear production and eyesight problems. More information regarding autonomic dysfunction can be found in chapter 12.

Ana: 'I am hypersensitive to light and noise, so I am unable to cope with visitors as even the movement of a person in my room exacerbates my symptoms.'

Visual disturbances can affect the ability to carry out activities of daily living, including driving (18). Corrective lenses and prisms could be considered for some visual dysfunction (11), so if visual symptoms are reported then a referral to an appropriate eye specialist should be considered.

Touch sensitivity

Some people with ME/CFS may be hypersensitive to touch. One explanation for this is that some people with ME/CFS have been found to have significantly lower pressure pain thresholds compared to the general population (19). Further information regarding pain processing in people with ME/CFS can be found in chapter 10.

Adaptation to practice

Whether seeing a person with ME/CFS as an outpatient, inpatient or in their own home, check with the person which adjustments to the environment and your approach may help in order to minimize sensory overload, for example (10):

- Dim lights/closed blinds and curtains.
- Keep background noise to a minimum.
- Consider the volume of your own voice and the speed of speech.
- Avoid perfume or air fresheners.
- Consider the lowered pressure pain threshold if applying a hands-on intervention.
- Avoid prolonged sessions to reduce the time exposed to sensory stimulation.
- With virtual appointments, consider whether a video call or phone call is most tolerable in respect of the person's vision and hearing sensitivities.

More in-depth adaptations to practice in relation to sensory stimulation can be found in chapter 14.

Physiotherapy management of neurological impairments
Motor impairments
Assessment
A physiotherapy assessment of someone with ME/CFS should include a neurological component, checking for any red flags or signs and symptoms that may indicate a differential diagnosis. If there are neurological symptoms that have not been adequately investigated then a referral to a specialist for further assessment may be indicated.

What about exercise?
In other neurological conditions muscle weakness and ataxia are typically treated with a motor relearning and strengthening approach (20). However, the underlying cause of muscle weakness in ME/CFS is not necessarily linked to a neurological pathology, and therefore may not respond in the same way to neurological rehabilitation.

For example, multiple sclerosis (MS) is a degenerative neurological condition that causes muscle weakness and fatigue. People with MS have been shown to benefit from intensive exercise programmes without a negative impact on their fatigue symptoms (21) (22). In comparison, people with ME/CFS show a decline in performance on repeated exercise, with further weakness and reduced muscular control, suggesting that the muscle weakness has a bioenergetic cause (23) (24) (4).

If a person with ME/CFS also has a neurological co-morbidity involving motor weakness, then any rehabilitation programme should be designed to avoid PEM, on the understanding that muscles are quicker to fatigue and take longer to recover. More information regarding how to approach exercise for a person with ME/CFS can be found in chapter 17.

Sensory disturbances
Desensitization therapy

Hypersensitivity to touch could be addressed using desensitization therapy, which aims to normalize sensations that are causing pain by exposing the affected area to sensation (25). Prolonged exposure to sensation is thought to desensitize peripheral nerves, for example vibration applied to the skin has been shown to decrease perception of sensation and decrease neuronal firing (26). Desensitization therapy involves applying sensory stimulation, for example gently rubbing skin with cotton wool or applying pressure to an unaffected area and then to the sensitized area for a sustained period of time, repeated daily. Desensitization therapy has been shown to help reduce pain in peripheral neuropathies caused by diabetes (25) and is recommended in the treatment of hypersensitivity at the surgical site of amputations (27).

> **Faith**: 'If I have to be in an environment with multiple sound sources, then I need to use ear plugs or noise cancelling headphones.'

However, there is no standardized protocol for desensitization therapy and no research in relation to its use with ME/CFS. If hypersensitivity to touch is causing significant issues then it may be worth considering desensitization work with a cautious approach and regular monitoring of symptom exacerbation, both during and in a period of up to 48 hours afterwards to ensure it has not caused PEM.

Pharmacological treatment

Hypersensitivities may cause severe pain, in which case medications such as gabapentin and low dose amitriptyline may be beneficial (28); however there may be unwanted side effects. If pain is a significant factor and pharmacological options have not yet been explored, then refer to a medical specialist to address this symptom.

SUMMARY

▸ People with ME/CFS may present with neurological impairments in the form of motor impairments and sensory disturbances.

▸ It is not clear whether these impairments are caused by a neurological pathology or are a symptom of another component of ME/CFS.

APPLICATION TO PRACTICE

▸ Avoid applying traditional neuro-rehabilitation approaches to motor impairments in ME/CFS as these may be ineffective and cause further symptom exacerbation.

▸ If sensory disturbances are present, adapt every aspect of an interaction to minimize sensory stimulation.

▸ Utilize other specialities to assist in the case of visual disturbances and pain management.

▸ Be alert for signs of other neurological conditions that may be co-morbid and refer to specialists for further investigations where appropriate.

References

1. Shan, Z.Y., Barnden, L.R. & Kwiatek, R.A. (2020) 'Neuroimaging characteristics of myalgic encephalomyelitis/chronic fatigue syndrome (ME/CFS): a systematic review.' *Journal of Translational Medicine 18* (335).

2. Johnson, C. (2018) 'Brain on fire: widespread neuroinflammation found in chronic fatigue syndrome (ME/CFS).' Healthrising. Accessed on 11/12/2022 at www.health-rising.org/blog/2018/09/24/brain-fire-neuroinflammation-found-chronic-fatigue-syndrome-me-cfs.

3. Bested, A.C. & Marshall, L.M. (2015) 'Review of myalgic encephalomyelitis/chronic fatigue syndrome: an evidence-based approach to diagnosis and management by clinicians.' *Reviews on Environmental Health 30* (4).

4. Nijs, J., Aelbrecht, S., Meeus, M., Van Oosterwijck, J., Zinzen, E. & Clarys, P. (2011) 'Tired of being inactive: a systematic literature review of physical activity, physiological exercise capacity and muscle strength in patients with chronic fatigue syndrome.' *Disability Rehabilitation 33* (17–18).

5. Wirth, K.J., Scheibenbogen, C. & Paul, F. (2021) 'An attempt to explain the neurological symptoms of myalgic encephalomyelitis/chronic fatigue syndrome.' *Journal of Translational Medicine 19* (471).

6. Holtzman, C.S., Bhatia, S., Cotler, J. & Jason, L.A. (2019) 'Assessment of post-exertional malaise (PEM) in patients with myalgic encephalomyelitis (ME) and chronic fatigue syndrome (CFS): a patient-driven survey.' *Diagnostics (Basel) 9* (1).

7. Ashizawa, T. & Xia, G. (2016) 'Ataxia.' *Continuum (Minneap Minn) 22* (4 Movement Disorders).

8. Miwa, K. & Inoue, Y. (2017) 'Truncal ataxia or disequilibrium is an unrecognised cause of orthostatic intolerance in patients with myalgic encephalomyelitis.' *International Journal of Clinical Practice 71* (6).
9. Mills, K.R. (2010) 'Characteristics of fasciculations in amyotrophic lateral sclerosis and the benign fasciculation syndrome.' *Brain 133* (11).
10. Carruthers, B.M., van de Sande, M.I., De Meirleir, K.L., Klimas, N.G., *et al.* (2011) 'Myalgic encephalomyelitis: International Consensus Criteria.' *Journal of Internal Medicine 270.*
11. Vedelago, L.J. (1997) 'Visual dysfunction in chronic fatigue syndrome – behavioural optometric assessment and management.' *Journal of Behavioral Optometry 8* (6).
12. Eaton-Fitch, N., Johnston, S.C. & Zalewski, P. (2020) 'Health-related quality of life in patients with myalgic encephalomyelitis/chronic fatigue syndrome: an Australian cross-sectional study.' *Quality of Life Research 29.*
13. Caffery, B.E., Josephson, J.E. & Samek, M.J. (1994) 'The ocular signs and symptoms of chronic fatigue syndrome.' *Journal of the American Optometric Association 65* (3).
14. Ahmed, N.S., Gottlob, I., Proudlock, F.A. & Hutchinson, C.V. (2018) 'Restricted spatial windows of visibility in myalgic encephalomyelitis (ME).' *Vision (Basel) 2* (1).
15. Wilson, R.L., Paterson, K.B., McGowan, V. & Hutchinson, C.V. (2018) 'Visual aspects of reading performance in myalgic encephalomyelitis (ME).' *Frontiers in Psychology 9* (1).
16. Wilson, R.L., Paterson, K.B. & Hutchinson, C.V. (2015) 'Increased vulnerability to pattern-related visual stress in myalgic encephalomyelitis.' *Perception 44* (12).
17. Wehrwein, E.A., Orer, H.S. & Barman, S.M. (2016) 'Overview of the anatomy, physiology, and pharmacology of the autonomic nervous system.' *Comprehensive Physiology 6* (3).
18. Potaznick, W. & Kozol, N. (1992) 'Ocular manifestations of chronic fatigue and immune dysfunction syndrome.' *Optometry and Vision Science 69* (10).
19. Meeus, M., Nijs, J., Huybrechts, S. & Truijen, S. (2010) 'Evidence for generalized hyperalgesia in chronic fatigue syndrome: a case control study.' *Clinical Rheumatology 29* (4).
20. Zonta, M.B., Diaferia, G., Pedroso, J.L. & Teive, H.A.G. (2017) 'Rehabilitation of ataxia.' In H. Chien & O. Barsottini (eds) *Movement Disorders Rehabilitation.* Cham: Springer.
21. Jonsdottir, J., Gervasoni, E., Bowman, T., Bertoni, R., *et al.* (2018) 'Intensive multimodal training to improve gait resistance, mobility, balance and cognitive function in persons with multiple sclerosis: a pilot randomized controlled trial.' *Frontiers in Neurology 28* (9).
22. Mark, V.W., Taub, E., Uswatte, G., Bashir, K., *et al.* (2013) 'Constraint-induced movement therapy for the lower extremities in multiple sclerosis: case series with 4-year follow-up.' *Archives of Physical Medicine and Rehabilitation 94* (4).
23. Davenport, T.E., Lehnen, M., Stevens, S.R., VanNess, J.M., Stevens, J. & Snell, C.R. (2019) 'Chronotropic intolerance: an overlooked determinant of symptoms and activity limitation in myalgic encephalomyelitis/chronic fatigue syndrome?' *Frontiers in Pediatrics 7* (82).
24. Davenport, T.E., Stevens, S.R., Stevens, J., Snell, C.R. & Van Ness, J.M. (2020) 'Properties of measurements obtained during cardiopulmonary exercise testing in individuals with myalgic encephalomyelitis/chronic fatigue syndrome.' *Work 66* (2).
25. Battesha, H.H.M., Ahmed, G.M., Amer, H.A., Gohary, A.M.E. & Ragab, W.M. (2018) 'Effect of core stability exercises and desensitisation therapy on limit of stability in diabetic peripheral neuropathy patients.' *International Journal of Therapy and Rehabilitation 25* (3).
26. Graczyk, E.L., Delhaye, B.P., Schiefer, M.A., Bensmaia, S.J. & Tyler, D.J. (2018) 'Sensory adaptation to electrical stimulation of the somatosensory nerves.' *Journal of Neural Engineering 15* (4).

27. Inverarity, L. (2021) 'Desentization exercises after limb amputation.' VeryWell Health. Accessed on 11/12/2022 at www.verywellhealth.com/desensitization-exercises-2696171.
28. Shepherd, C. & Chaudhuri, A. (2019) *ME/CFS/PVFS: An Exploration of the Key Clinical Issues*. Gawcott: The ME Association.

CHAPTER 12

Autonomic Dysfunction

PURPOSE OF THIS CHAPTER

Autonomic dysfunction is included in three of the various diagnostic criteria for ME/CFS (the International Consensus Criteria, the Canadian Clinical Criteria and the Institute of Medicine (IOM)/National Academy of Medicine (NAM) Criteria), although it is not classed as essential for diagnosis in any of the criteria.

It is important for any physiotherapist working with someone with ME/CFS to be aware of the potential for autonomic dysfunction because:

- A physiotherapist could use their assessment skills to identify disorders of the autonomic system, which will be vital information for onward referral or treatment planning.
- Orthostatic intolerance will dictate positional choices for any assessment and treatment.
- A physiotherapy intervention may benefit some symptoms of autonomic dysfunction, but it may also be detrimental. Knowledge of the best approach is key in any speciality.

This chapter has split the components of autonomic dysfunction into three sections: a dysfunctional balance between the sympathetic and parasympathetic systems, orthostatic intolerance and dysfunctional breathing.

The autonomic nervous system

The autonomic nervous system (ANS) is responsible for the regulation of bodily systems such as blood pressure, heart rate, respiration, thermoregulation and bladder and bowel function (1). The ANS transmits impulses from the central nervous system to the smooth muscle of peripheral organs, causing contraction and relaxation as required (for example to regulate the heart rate) and can cause constriction and dilation of blood vessels, as well as glandular secretions (2). The ANS is not consciously controlled and is therefore also known as the involuntary nervous system (3).

The primary function of the ANS is to maintain the homeostasis of cells, tissues and organs throughout the body (3). When external or internal demands change, for example physical activity, encountering a threat or an inflammatory response to infection, the ANS makes adjustments to functions like cardiac output, blood flow and respiratory rate to meet demands and restore homeostasis (3).

Components of the autonomic nervous system

The autonomic nervous system (ANS) is composed of three subsystems (3).

The sympathetic nervous system

Commonly known as 'fight or flight', while the sympathetic nervous system is most associated with physiological responses to threats, it also continues to function in rest states, for example maintaining tone in the arterial walls or bladder.

The parasympathetic nervous system

Commonly known as 'rest and digest', with a role in conserving energy, the digestive process and removal of waste products from the body. In addition to the concept of restful states the parasympathetic system also causes active states such as contraction of muscles in the eye, tear production and control of sexual organs.

Enteric nervous system

The enteric nervous system works alongside the sympathetic and parasympathetic nervous systems to control digestion. Dysfunction of this system may be linked to irritable bowel syndrome, which is a common co-morbidity of ME/CFS discussed in chapter 2.

Many organs, such as the heart, bronchi, stomach and bladder, are innervated by more than one sub-system of the ANS, often with the sympathetic and parasympathetic systems acting as physiological agonists and antagonists (3). Other parts of the body may only be controlled by one part of the system.

Autonomic dysfunction

Dysfunction of the ANS can occur as a result of many different diseases, and such dysfunction can be known as 'dysautonomia' (1). Many drugs and medications can also affect the ANS (3).

Failure or dysfunction of the ANS can be across multiple regions, known as generalized autonomic failure, which can be seen in diseases such as multiple system atrophy, diabetic autonomic neuropathy and autoimmune autonomic ganglionopathy (1). Dysfunction can also occur in specific functions of the ANS, which is known as selective autonomic failure (1).

Symptoms of autonomic dysfunction can include orthostatic intolerance, light-headedness, extreme pallor, nausea, temperature dysregulation, irritable bowel syndrome, bladder dysfunction, palpitations with or without cardiac arrhythmias, and exertional dyspnoea (4). 'Orthostatic intolerance' is an umbrella term, covering conditions such as orthostatic hypotension (OH), postural orthostatic tachycardia syndrome (POTS) and neurally mediated hypotension (NMH), which are discussed later in this chapter.

A disruption in the balance between the sympathetic and parasympathetic nervous systems can be identified by an elevated resting heart rate (5). It may also be measured by assessing heart rate variability (HRV), which looks at the variability of the interval between consecutive heart beats (6). HRV has been shown by some to have good reliability in measuring autonomic function (7), where a low heart rate variability indicates an imbalance in the autonomic nervous system (6). However, others have suggested that HRV is not a valid measure of cardiac autonomic function (8) (9) (10).

Autonomic dysfunction and ME/CFS

Symptoms of autonomic dysfunction in ME/CFS are listed in diagnostic criteria as (11) (12):

- orthostatic intolerance

- palpitations, with or without arrhythmias
- light-headedness
- laboured breathing
- exertional dyspnoea (breathlessness)
- nausea
- bladder or bowel dysfunction.

Some people with ME/CFS have been shown to have altered cardiac regulation compared to healthy controls, including a higher resting heart rate, lower maximal peak heart rate, higher heart rate responses to head-up tilt tests and a lower heart rate at submaximal exercise threshold (5). These results indicate increased activity of the sympathetic nervous system in the modulation of cardiac function.

Heart rate variability (HRV) has been used to measure autonomic function in people with ME/CFS, with a low variability suggesting a dysfunction in the autonomic nervous system (7). HRV is lower in people with ME/CFS compared to healthy controls (13) (5) which persists during sleep (14). This suggests there could be an imbalance between the sympathetic and parasympathetic nervous systems, which could provide explanation for some of the physical and cognitive symptoms experienced by people with ME/CFS (15). However, a low HRV can also be associated with POTS (16) (discussed later in this chapter), and is not exclusively controlled by the autonomic nervous system (17).

Additionally, brain imaging of people with ME/CFS has found potential nerve conduction deficits within the brainstem and midbrain, which are areas that have a key role in the autonomic nervous system (18).

Adaptation to practice
Assessment and referrals
An assessment of someone with ME/CFS should include questions around the symptoms of autonomic dysfunction to highlight whether they are impacting on their quality of life. An objective measure such as heart rate variability could be considered. More information on assessment can be found in chapter 14.

Several medications may be used for autonomic dysfunction including midodrine, which can be used to treat hypotension (19). If symptoms of autonomic dysfunction are having a significant impact and the person has not been medically reviewed for this, then consider a referral to an appropriate practitioner.

Physiotherapy management of autonomic dysfunction
Vagus nerve stimulation

The vagus nerve is the tenth cranial nerve and the main neural component of the parasympathetic nervous system (20). The idea of improving the balance within the autonomic nervous system by using stimulation of the vagus nerve to trigger the parasympathetic system has been widely researched (21).

Direct stimulation of the vagus nerve is a method that has been explored to treat a wide range of conditions, currently including epilepsy, depression, anxiety, pain and migraines (20).

Vagus nerve stimulation has been explored in a small study of 31 people with ME/CFS in a randomized placebo-controlled trial using intranasal mechanical stimulation, which is a device inserted up the nose (22). Stimulation was twice a week for 20 minutes and results were reported as an average 30% reduction in subjectively reported overall symptoms after eight weeks, in comparison to a placebo.

Transcutaneous auricular vagus nerve stimulation (taVNS) involves stimulation of the vagus nerve via electrodes applied to part of the ear. One study of taVNS included 11 people with ME/CFS and found a significant reduction in reported daytime sleepiness, abnormal fatigue, anxiety and depression (23), although this study had no control group so it is difficult to determine if the results were due to the placebo effect.

While results of these studies show promising effects of vagus nerve stimulation, larger-scale trials are required to determine safe and effective treatment parameters.

Non-invasive methods of vagus nerve stimulation

There are many methods of stimulating the vagus nerve and parasympathetic nervous system (21) although very few of these methods have been directly researched in relation to people with ME/CFS. A systematic review of 'mind–body interventions' for ME/CFS (24) found 12 studies, seven of which were randomized controlled trials and the remainder single-arm trials. While subjective fatigue, anxiety and quality of life measures were improved in some studies, the review noted that none of the studies measured post exertional malaise (PEM), the hallmark feature of ME/CFS, and most studies used diagnostic criteria that did not include PEM. The review concluded that while practices such as mindfulness, cognitive behavioural therapy and yoga may improve fatigue severity and anxiety in people with ME/CFS, these results could be biased due to poor reporting, small sample sizes and diagnostic issues.

There are a range of methods below to stimulate the vagus nerve in healthy populations and for other chronic diseases. Many are inexpensive and simple techniques that could be considered for people with ME/CFS who are exhibiting autonomic nervous system dysfunction; however none of the methods have been robustly studied in people with ME/CFS so there should be careful monitoring for signs of PEM.

- A variety of massage techniques have been shown to increase heart rate variability, suggesting an influence over the parasympathetic nervous system (21). If considering massage it is important to consider the potential for reduced pressure–pain threshold in people with ME/CFS. Massage is discussed in more detail in chapter 10.
- Slow breathing exercises featuring prolonged exhalation have been shown to lower blood pressure and heart rate (25).
- 'OM' chanting can reduce activity in the limbic system, echoing the outcome of vagus nerve stimulation (26).
- Music therapy (27) and listening to Mozart (28) have been shown to affect parasympathetic activity.
- Exposure to positive emotions, social connections (29) and even laughter (30) has been shown to increase vagal tone.
- The practice of mindfulness can enhance parasympathetic influences on heart rate (31).
- Immersing the face in cold water after exercise can lead to greater reactivation of the parasympathetic nervous system (32).
- High fish intake or omega-3 fatty acid supplementation can increase parasympathetic nervous system activity (33).

What about exercise?

For healthy populations and people with other chronic diseases exercise has been linked with improving heart rate variability and vagal tone (21). The type of exercise required to stimulate the parasympathetic nervous system does not appear to be limited, with research finding results from strenuous exercise (34), stretching (35) and resistance training (36), as well as various forms of yoga (37).

Unfortunately, exercise has been found to have the opposite effect in people with ME/CFS, causing a reduced reactivation of the parasympathetic nervous system in a case-control study (38). Equally, the potential for physical exertion to cause PEM would likely negate any intended symptom improvement. Chapter 17 discusses safe exercise prescription for people with ME/CFS in more detail.

Orthostatic intolerance

When the body adopts an upright posture there is a sudden gravitational redistribution of blood volume towards the lower extremities (39). Maintaining adequate blood flow to the upper body, particularly the brain, requires a rapid cardiovascular response, and this relies on adequate blood volume, intact skeletal and respiratory muscle pumps, and the regulation of blood pressure and heart rate by the autonomic nervous system (40).

> **Kim**: 'I developed orthostatic intolerance symptoms after a secondary infection with COVID-19. I would have to lie down after sitting or standing for any period of time. The right medication has made a huge difference to my symptoms.'

'Orthostatic intolerance' is the umbrella term for conditions that feature an intolerance to being in an upright position (39). Mild orthostatic intolerance is characterized by light-headedness and may be experienced by anyone simply by standing up too quickly, or episodically in the form of fainting, known as postural vasovagal syncope (40).

Chronic intolerances such as orthostatic hypotension (OH) or postural orthostatic tachycardia syndrome (POTS) are longstanding and have a significant impact on a person's quality of life (40). General symptoms of orthostatic intolerances include dizziness, weakness, fatigue, cognitive disturbance and, in extreme situations, loss of consciousness (39). Pain in the neck and shoulders, termed 'coat-hanger pain', can also be associated with orthostatic intolerances (41) and is discussed in chapter 10.

Orthostatic hypotension (OH) describes a sustained objective drop in blood pressure (at least 20 mm Hg in systolic or 10 mm Hg in diastolic) within three minutes of standing up (39). The occurrence of OH has been linked with increasing age and in people with chronic diseases such as hypertension and diabetes, as well as neurodegenerative diseases like Parkinson's disease (39). When the drop in blood pressure is caused by a change in the autonomic nervous system the condition is called 'neurally mediated hypotension' (NMH) (42).

Postural orthostatic tachycardia syndrome (POTS) features a marked increase in heart rate on standing with diagnostic criteria in adults stipulating an increase of over 30 beats per minute or above 120 beats per minute within the first ten minutes of standing (43). POTS can also be present in children and adolescents, with a slightly altered criteria of over 40 beats per minute or a maximum heart rate of over 130 beats per minute (44). POTS is more commonly seen in the younger population (15–40 years) and predominantly in women (80%) (43). POTS is discussed in more detail in chapter 2.

Symptoms of orthostatic intolerance in the general population may also be present without there being measurable changes to heart rate or blood pressure (45). A number of studies have explored this further by looking at cerebral blood flow, which is the rate of delivery of arterial blood to the brain. A reduction in cerebral blood flow when upright could explain the dizziness, weakness and occasional loss of consciousness that is indicative of orthostatic intolerances. Cerebral blood flow can be measured using Doppler imaging of the carotid and vertebral arteries while gradually tilting a participant upright on a tilt-table (46). Autoregulation of cerebral blood flow when adopting an upright position in people with POTS appears to be less effective than the general population (47).

Some people may present with symptoms of orthostatic intolerance but show no changes to blood pressure or heart rate when tested in upright positions, yet this population have consistently been found to have a comparable drop in cerebral blood flow (46) (48) (49) suggesting orthostatic intolerance can exist without changes to heart rate or blood pressure, and may be due solely to reduced cerebral blood flow.

Orthostatic intolerance and ME/CFS

The exact occurrence of orthostatic intolerance in people with ME/CFS is difficult to determine as research in this area is contradictory, with the prevalence of POTS in people with ME/CFS ranging from 19% to 70% (50). One study estimates that POTS may occur twice as frequently in people with ME/CFS compared to healthy controls (50), while another of 179 people with ME/CFS found only 13% presented with POTS, who appeared to form a distinct subgroup who were younger, demonstrated less reported fatigue and depression, and had significantly more orthostatic symptoms (51). The inability to form a consensus is due in part to the issues around which diagnostic criteria for ME/CFS is used to select participants, discussed in chapter 1, and many studies are small scale with varying assessment modalities for orthostatic intolerance (4).

A reduction in cerebral blood flow when upright has been found consistently in people with ME/CFS. In healthy people cerebral blood flow reduces by up to 6% when they are tilted fully upright (52). In people with ME/CFS cerebral blood flow was found to be reduced by 19–26% at mid-tilt position and 24–29% at a 70-degree tilt (53). This finding was replicated in people with severe ME/CFS with a 27% reduction after just a 20-degree tilt (54) and a 24.5% reduction by simply sitting upright (55).

In replication of other studies, cerebral blood flow was comparably reduced in people with ME/CFS who had no changes to heart rate or blood pressure during a tilt-table test (53). The abnormalities in cerebral blood flow have also been observed up to five minutes after the tilt-test was complete, even though the body was supine and cardiac function had returned to baseline levels (56).

Adaptation to practice
Assessment and referral
Assessment of people with ME/CFS should include questions around symptom behaviour when the person is upright. If POTS is suspected, the active stand or NASA lean are both valid diagnostic tests (57) and are discussed in chapter 18. While a physiotherapist may be able to carry out either of these tests quite easily, their interpretation of results should be used as a screening tool as opposed to a diagnostic aid, and a person with suspected POTS should be referred for a medical review with an appropriate clinician (45).

A physiotherapist should consider that orthostatic intolerance cannot be ruled out in the absence of altered heart rate or blood pressure, given the potential for reduced cerebral perfusion as detailed earlier in this chapter, so it is therefore important to take note of symptoms reported by the person as well as using objective measures.

If a person has not had their orthostatic intolerance medically reviewed then a referral would be appropriate as pharmacological therapies can be beneficial for POTS (44). Drug treatment may be aimed at reducing tachycardia (for example beta blockers), increasing blood pressure (for example midorine) or boosting blood volume (fludrocortisone or desmopressin) (19).

Position

As some people with ME/CFS may have reduced blood blow to their brain in an upright position, consider the positioning of a person during assessment and any treatment intervention. Discuss which position is most comfortable to them and be prepared to adapt your environment to accommodate accordingly.

Physiotherapy management of orthostatic intolerance

Very few non-pharmacological interventions for orthostatic intolerance have been validated in large clinical trials (58), let alone including people with ME/CFS.

Compression garments

Venous return may be improved using compression garments such as stockings or abdominal binders (59). Heart rate and reported symptoms can be reduced using compression of either the legs or abdomen, with blood pressure and stroke volume better maintained with compression of both areas combined (60). An inflatable abdominal compression device has been shown to improve POTS symptoms; however the true physiological effects are still uncertain and studies have not yet translated to outside of a clinic environment (58).

Mo: 'When I was standing upright in the shower to wash my hair, I felt like my legs were going to collapse and I needed my wife to support me. I now have to use a shower stool.'

It is important to note that people with ME/CFS, particularly those with more severe ME/CFS, can have sensory intolerances that may be triggered by compression (see chapter 10). Additionally, a degree of physical exertion is required to put on and take off compression garments. Such sensory and physical exertion may be enough to trigger PEM and therefore may make wearing compression garments counter-productive, so any exploration of these items must be done with care.

Cervical collars

A small study (61) of ten people with POTS found reduced orthostatic intolerance symptoms when using a Q-collar. The theory was that the collar helped to increase blood flow to the brain. This study did not stipulate whether the participants also had a diagnosis of ME/CFS. While some people with ME/CFS have anecdotally reported an improvement in their general symptoms using a collar (62) there is currently no further evidence on whether cervical collars would be effective for managing orthostatic intolerance in this population.

Orthostatic tilt training

One suggested method of addressing orthostatic intolerance is tilt training, by spending time in progressively more upright postures using a tilt table (63). A small study compared tilt training to a sham intervention with people diagnosed with ME/CFS and found reductions in orthostatic intolerance after four weeks which were maintained at six-month follow up (63). However, the intervention did not improve fatigue levels, which made other researchers question the clinical importance of the treatment effect (64) and participants were selected using a diagnostic criteria that does not require PEM, therefore its application to all people with ME/CFS is questionable.

Saline

One of the factors required for an adequate response to adopting an upright position is sufficient blood volume. In adults with ME/CFS who also had clinical signs of orthostatic intolerance, a significantly lower blood volume was found, both in comparison to the expected value and to people with ME/CFS who did not have intolerances (65).

To combat low blood volume, one strategy explored in research is the use of saline infusions via an intravenous line. In people with POTS intermittent saline infusions have been found to significantly reduce symptoms (66) and one small study found even rapidly drinking 500ml of water improved working memory when in an upright position (67).

A single ME/CFS case study (68) has been reported where a person received a saline infusion via a central line once a day for 678 days. Cardiopulmonary exercise testing was used to monitor objective responses and found improved metabolic responses during exertion, as well as reduced recovery time following the testing, a reduction in total number of reported symptoms and an improvement in subjective cognitive dysfunction ('brain fog'). Larger-scale studies need to be carried out before this treatment can be considered, especially as there are risks of infection with a central line and the as-yet-undefined appropriate dosage or duration of saline infusions.

Salt and hydration

Due to low blood volume contributing to POTS symptoms, a high salt and fluid intake is recommended (19) although high levels of salt can be dangerous for some people so medical guidance is recommended.

What about exercise?

Strength training for the lower limbs and core is recommended to help improve muscle pump and increase venous return in upright positions (69) much in the same way that compression garments may improve symptoms. Isometric exercises for the lower limbs in supine could be at a tolerable level for some people with ME/CFS, but when considering the introduction of any exercise it is imperative to develop a means to monitor for PEM. Key considerations for any exercise programme are discussed in chapter 17.

Aerobic exercise has been investigated as a potential treatment for POTS. A group of researchers (69) recommend aerobic reconditioning in a recumbent position as treatment for POTS, for example rowing, swimming or a recumbent bike, linking the intervention to complete remission from POTS in people who completed a three-month training programme. However, in a research setting 76% of participants were able to complete the programme but in the community this dropped to just 41%. Numerous reasons were given for lack of adherence, including 'mitochondrial disorders' and that training was considered 'too difficult' by some participants. There was no mention of whether any participants had a concurrent diagnosis of ME/CFS, but aerobic training could involve enough physical exertion to trigger PEM for people with ME/CFS, which may even cause a further increase of orthostatic intolerance symptoms. Therefore any aerobic exercise, regardless of the position it is in, is unlikely to be suitable for someone with ME/CFS and there is no evidence that recumbent aerobic training is tolerated or beneficial to people with ME/CFS.

Orthostatic intolerance has also been linked to deconditioning from prolonged bedrest (45). One study found 90% of people diagnosed with POTS had a reduced VO_2 max that suggests deconditioning (70).

However, this link is inconsistent, as another study (71) used cardio-pulmonary exercise testing in people with POTS to demonstrate that although peak oxygen uptake and heart rate were significantly reduced, most people demonstrated an exercise capacity considered 'normal' and that any impairment may be due to a dysfunctional breathing pattern rather than cardiovascular deconditioning.

Given people with ME/CFS have reduced activity levels, sometimes to the point of being confined to bed, it would be logical to conclude that deconditioning may occur and therefore could be the cause of orthostatic intolerance symptoms. To test this hypothesis, one study (72) explored the reduction in cerebral blood flow during a tilt test on groups of people with ME/CFS who had no, mild or severe deconditioning, as measured with cardiopulmonary exercise testing. The study found that every participant with ME/CFS had significant reduction in cerebral blood flow, regardless of the level of their deconditioning.

There is an important distinction between orthostatic intolerance symptoms that have been caused by deconditioning, and deconditioning that has been caused by inactivity as a result of orthostatic intolerance (45). Regardless, the typical treatment for deconditioning involves incremental increases in exercise, which will inevitably trigger PEM in people with ME/CFS and is therefore an inappropriate treatment method. Further discussion of deconditioning and ME/CFS can be found in chapter 6.

Dysfunctional breathing and autonomic dysfunction

One of the systems regulated by the autonomic nervous system (ANS) is respiration (1).

'Dysfunctional breathing' or 'breathing pattern disorder' (BPD) are terms used to describe a dysfunctional breathing pattern that is symptomatic (73). The causes of dysfunctional breathing patterns are wide ranging and include physiological, psychological and biomechanical components (73). Symptoms of dysfunctional breathing can include:

- dyspnoea (breathlessness)
- frequent yawning or sighing
- air hunger (unable to get a deep enough breath)
- dizziness
- chest pain

- altered vision
- general fatigue
- nausea
- difficulty concentrating.

Assessment of breathing includes an observational and hands-on assessment of breathing technique, as well as subjective outcome measures (see chapter 18) and pulse oximetry (73).

Dysfunctional breathing and ME/CFS

Breathlessness is a symptom included under autonomic dysfunction on two of the diagnostic criteria for ME/CFS. Breathlessness is also a prevalent symptom of POTS (74).

Very little research has been carried out to date on breathing disorders in people with ME/CFS. A small pilot study (75) assessed 20 people with ME/CFS for breathing patterns and found 5 people (25%) with a breathing pattern disorder, but no differences in respiratory muscle strength or pulmonary function. Breathing disorders are clearly an area that require further research for people with ME/CFS before any conclusions can be drawn.

Adaptation to practice
Assessment

Given the benefits of optimizing breathing rate for any population group, physiotherapists should consider the assessment of breathing pattern for every person they work with, including people with ME/CFS (73). A brief assessment can involve questions about breathing symptoms and observation of the person during an interaction for any obvious signs of dysfunction, and if indicated consider a more detailed assessment.

Further information on including breathing pattern in assessment of someone with ME/CFS can be found in chapter 14.

Physiotherapy management for dysfunctional breathing
Breathing retraining

Breathing retraining involves teaching breathing control with the aim to achieve nasal breathing, use of the diaphragm and establish a normal respiratory rate with an appropriate inspiratory/expiratory ratio (74). A retrospective observational cohort study of 66 people diagnosed with POTS who had been referred for respiratory physiotherapy due to symptoms of breathlessness found that breathing retraining resulted in significant improvements in breathing pattern and symptom burden (74).

Ana: 'My digestive system, bladder and bowel are all affected by ME/CFS. This leads to incontinence, vomiting, and periods of constipation or diarrhoea.'

Very little research has been conducted on breathing retraining for people with ME/CFS. A small pilot study (75) found that breathing retraining resulted in a decreased respiratory rate and increased tidal volume in people with ME/CFS, but included no information with regards to the impact on ME/CFS symptoms or long-term carry over.

If a breathing disorder is suspected but breathing retraining is outside of the scope of practice, a physiotherapist should consider referring to respiratory specialists for treatment. If a respiratory specialist is unfamiliar with ME/CFS specifically, they should be provided with information regarding PEM so that they are aware to monitor for this in relation to their treatment.

SUMMARY

▸ People with ME/CFS may have a dysfunction of the autonomic nervous system resulting in a dominant sympathetic nervous system.

▸ People with ME/CFS may have an orthostatic intolerance, which involves symptoms such as dizziness, light-headedness, cognitive dysfunction and fatigue when in an upright position.

▸ Orthostatic intolerance may also be present without changes to heart rate and blood pressure, and is due to a reduced cerebral blood flow.

▸ While deconditioning may be linked to orthostatic intolerances, it is not a primary cause and typical exercise-based rehabilitation approaches will be ineffective due to their impact on PEM.

▶ People with ME/CFS may have a dysfunctional breathing pattern due to changes in their autonomic nervous system.

APPLICATION TO PRACTICE

▶ Include autonomic dysfunction, orthostatic intolerance and dysfunctional breathing in assessments as they will impact on symptoms and influence management decisions.
▶ There are many non-invasive techniques to stimulate the parasympathetic nervous system, though none have been verified for use specifically with ME/CFS.
▶ Treatment options for orthostatic intolerances are more limited in people with ME/CFS due to PEM. Consider low level strengthening exercises for legs and core, and compression garments or positional advice to improve venous return.
▶ Breathing retraining could be considered if a breathing pattern disorder is indicated.

References

1. Low, P.A., Tomalia, V.A. & Park, K.J. (2013) 'Autonomic function tests: some clinical applications.' *Journal of Clinical Neurology 9* (1).
2. Van Cauwenbergh, D., Nijs, J., Kos, D., Van Weijnen, L., Struyf, F. & Meeus, M. (2014) 'Malfunctioning of the autonomic nervous system in patients with chronic fatigue syndrome: a systematic literature review.' *European Journal of Clinical Investigation 44* (5).
3. Wehrwein, E.A., Orer, H.S. & Barman, S.M. (2016) 'Overview of the anatomy, physiology, and pharmacology of the autonomic nervous system.' In R. Terjung (ed.) *Comprehensive Physiology*. London: Wiley Online Library.
4. Newton, J.L., Okonkwo, O., Sutcliffe, K., Seth, A., Shin, J. & Jones, D.E.J. (2007) 'Symptoms of autonomic dysfunction in chronic fatigue syndrome.' *QJM: An International Journal of Medicine 100* (8).
5. Nelson, M.J., Bahl, J.S., Buckley, J.D., Thomson, R.L. & Davison, K. (2019) 'Evidence of altered cardiac autonomic regulation in myalgic encephalomyelitis/ chronic fatigue syndrome: a systematic review and meta-analysis.' *Medicine (Baltimore) 98* (43).
6. Tracy, L.M., Ioannou, L., Baker, K.S., Gibson, S.J., Georgiou-Karistianis, N. & Giummarra, M. (2016) 'Meta-analytic evidence for decreased heart rate variability in chronic pain implicating parasympathetic nervous system dysregulation.' *PAIN 157* (1).
7. Bertsch, K., Hagemann, D., Naumann, E., Schächinger, H. & Schulz, A. (2012) 'Stability of heart rate variability indices reflecting parasympathetic activity.' *Psychophysiology 49* (5).
8. Rahman, F., Pechnik, S., Gross, D., Sewell, L. & Goldstein, D.S. (2011) 'Low frequency power of heart rate variability reflects baroreflex function, not cardiac sympathetic innervation.' *Clinical Autonomic Research 21* (3).

9. Hopf, H.B., Skyschally, A., Heusch, G. & Peters, J. (1995) 'Low-frequency spectral power of heart rate variability is not a specific marker of cardiac sympathetic modulation.' *Anesthesiology 82* (3).

10. Thomas, B.L., Claassen, N., Becker, P. & Viljoen, M. (2019) 'Validity of commonly used heart rate variability markers of autonomic nervous system function.' *Neuropsychobiology 78* (1).

11. Carruthers, B.M., van de Sande, M.I., De Meirleir, K.L., Klimas, N.G., *et al.* (2011) 'Myalgic encephalomyelitis: International Consensus Criteria.' *Journal of Internal Medicine 270.*

12. Carruthers, B.M., Jain, A.K., De Meirleir, K.L., Peterson, D.L., *et al.* (2003) 'Myalgic encephalomyelitis/chronic fatigue syndrome.' *Journal of Chronic Fatigue Syndrome 11* (1).

13. Stewart, J. (2000) 'Autonomic nervous system dysfunction in adolescents with postural orthostatic tachycardia syndrome and chronic fatigue syndrome is characterized by attenuated vagal baroreflex and potentiated sympathetic vasomotion.' *Pediatric Research 48.*

14. Boneva, R.S., Decker, M.J., Maloney, E.M., Lin, J.M., *et al.* (2007) 'Higher heart rate and reduced heart rate variability persist during sleep in chronic fatigue syndrome: a population-based study.' *Autonomic Neuroscience 137.*

15. Gandasegui, I.M., Laka, L.A., Gargiulo, P.-Á., Gómez-Esteban, J.-C. & Sánchez, J.-V.L. (2021) 'Myalgic encephalomyelitis/chronic fatigue syndrome: a neurological entity?' *Medicina 57.*

16. Swai, J., Hu, Z., Zhao, X., Rugambwa, T. & Ming, G. (2019) 'Heart rate and heart rate variability comparison between postural orthostatic tachycardia syndrome versus healthy participants: a systematic review and meta-analysis.' *BMC Cardiovascular Disorders 19* (1).

17. Stauss, H.M. (2003) 'Heart rate variability.' *American Journal of Physiology – Regulatory, Integrative and Comparative Physiology 285* (5).

18. Barnden, L.R., Kwiatek, R., Crouch, B., Burnet, R. & Del Fante, P. (2016) 'Autonomic correlations with MRI are abnormal in the brainstem vasomotor centre in chronic fatigue syndrome.' *NeuroImage: Clinical 31* (11).

19. Shepherd, C. & Chaudhuri, A. (2019) *ME/CFS/PVFS: An Exploration of the Key Clinical Issues.* Gawcott: The ME Association.

20. Farmer, A.D., Strzelczyk, A., Finisguerra, A., Gourine, A.V., *et al.* (2021) 'International consensus based review and recommendations for minimum reporting standards in research on transcutaneous vagus nerve stimulation (version 2020).' *Frontiers in Human Neuroscience 14* (409).

21. Yuen, A.W.C. & Sander, J.W. (2017) 'Can natural ways to stimulate the vagus nerve improve seizure control?' *Epilepsy & Behavior 67.*

22. Rodriguez, L., Pou, C., Tadepally, L., Jingdian, Z., *et al.* (2020) 'Achieving symptom relief in patients with myalgic encephalomyelitis by targeting the neuro-immune interface and inducing disease tolerance.' Preprint.

23. Traianos, E., Dibnah, B., Lendrem, D., Clark, Y., *et al.* (2021) 'The effects of non-invasive vagus nerve stimulation on immunological responses and patient reported outcome measures of fatigue in patients with chronic fatigue syndrome, fibromyalgia, and rheumatoid arthritis.' *Annals of the Rheumatic Diseases 80.*

24. Khanpour Ardestani, S., Karkhaneh, M., Stein, E., Punja, S., *et al.* (2021) 'Systematic review of mind-body interventions to treat myalgic encephalomyelitis/chronic fatigue syndrome.' *Medicina 57.*

25. Pramanik, T., Sharma, H.O., Mishra, S., Mishra, A., Prajapati, R. & Singh, S. (2009) 'Immediate effect of slow pace bhastrika pranayama on blood pressure and heart rate.' *Journal of Alternative and Complementary Medicine 15* (3).

26. Kalyani, B.G, Venkatasubramanian, G., Arasappa, R., Rao, N.P., *et al.* (2011) 'Neurohemodynamic correlates of "OM" chanting: a pilot functional magnetic resonance imaging study.' *International Journal of Yoga 4* (1).

A PHYSIOTHERAPIST'S GUIDE TO UNDERSTANDING AND MANAGING ME/CFS

27. Chuang, C.Y., Han, W.R., Li, P.C. & Young, S.T. (2010) 'Effects of music therapy on subjective sensations and heart rate variability in treated cancer survivors: a pilot study.' *Complementary Therapy Medicine 18*.
28. Lin, L.C. & Yang, R.C. (2015) 'Mozart's music in children with epilepsy.' *Translational Pediatrics 4*.
29. Kok, B.E., Coffey, K.A., Cohn, M.A., Catalino, L.I., *et al.* (2013) 'How positive emotions build physical health: perceived positive social connections account for the upward spiral between positive emotions and vagal tone.' *Psychology Science 24* (7).
30. Dolgoff-Kaspar, R., Baldwin, A., Johnson, M.S., Edling, N. & Sethi, G.K. (2012) 'Effect of laughter yoga on mood and heart rate variability in patients awaiting organ transplantation: a pilot study.' *Alternative Therapies in Health and Medicine 18*.
31. Mankus, A.M., Aldao, A., Kerns, C., Mayville, E.W. & Mennin, D.S. (2013) 'Mindfulness and heart rate variability in individuals with high and low generalized anxiety symptoms.' *Behaviour Research and Therapy 51* (7).
32. Al, H.H., Laursen, P.B., Ahmaidi, S. & Buchheit, M. (2010) 'Influence of cold water face immersion on post-exercise parasympathetic reactivation.' *European Journal of Applied Physiology 108*.
33. Mozaffarian, D., Stein, P.K., Prineas, R.J. & Siscovick, D.S. (2008) 'Dietary fish and omega-3 fatty acid consumption and heart rate variability in US adults.' *Circulation 117*.
34. Soares-Miranda, L., Sandercock, G., Valente, H., Vale, S., Santos, R. & Mota, J. (2009) 'Vigorous physical activity and vagal modulation in young adults.' *European Journal of Preventive Cardiology 16*.
35. Farinatti, P.T., Brandao, C., Soares, P.P. & Duarte, A.F. (2011) 'Acute effects of stretching exercise on the heart rate variability in subjects with low flexibility levels.' *Journal of Strength and Conditioning Research 25*.
36. Caruso, F.R., Arena, R., Phillips, S.A., Bonjorno, J.C., Jr., *et al.* (2015) 'Resistance exercise training improves heart rate variability and muscle performance: a randomized controlled trial in coronary artery disease patients.' *European Journal of Physical and Rehabilitation Medicine 51*.
37. Vinay, A.V., Venkatesh, D. & Ambarish, V. (2016) 'Impact of short-term practice of yoga on heart rate variability.' *International Journal of Yoga 9*.
38. Van Oosterwijck, J., Marusic, U., De Wandele, I., Paul, L., *et al.* (2017) 'The role of autonomic function in exercise-induced endogenous analgesia: a case-control study in myalgic encephalomyelitis/chronic fatigue syndrome and healthy people.' *Pain Physician 20* (3).
39. Freeman, R., Wieling, W., Axelrod, F.B., Benditt, D.G., *et al.* (2011) 'Consensus statement on the definition of orthostatic hypotension, neurally mediated syncope and the postural tachycardia syndrome.' *Clinical Autonomic Research 21* (2).
40. Stewart, J.M. (2013) 'Common syndromes of orthostatic intolerance.' *Pediatrics 131* (5).
41. Wieling, W. & Schatz, I.J. (2009) 'The consensus statement on the definition of orthostatic hypotension: a revisit after 13 years.' *Journal of Hypertension 27* (5).
42. Rowe, P.C., Bou-Holaigah, I., Kan, J.S. & Calkins, H. (1995) 'Is neurally mediated hypotension an unrecognised cause of chronic fatigue?' *The Lancet 345* (8950).
43. Fedorowski, A. (2019) 'Postural orthostatic tachycardia syndrome: clinical presentation, aetiology and management.' *Journal of Internal Medicine 285* (4).
44. Chen, G., Du, J., Jin, H. & Huang, Y. (2020) 'Postural tachycardia syndrome in children and adolescents: pathophysiology and clinical management.' *Frontiers in Pediatrics 20* (8).
45. Bourne, K.M., Lloyd, M.G. & Raj, S.R. (2021) 'Diagnostic Criteria for Postural Tachycardia Syndrome: Consideration of the Clinical Features Differentiating PoTS from Other Disorders of Orthostatic Intolerance.' In N. Gall, L. Kavi & M.D. Lobo (eds) *Postural Tachycardia Syndrome*. Cham: Springer International.

46. Shin, K.J., Kim, S.E., Park, K.M., Park, J., *et al.* (2016) 'Cerebral hemodynamics in orthostatic intolerance with normal head-up tilt test.' *Acta Neurologica Scandinavica 134.*

47. Ocon, A.J., Medow, M.S., Taneja, I., Clarke, D. & Stewart, J.M. (2009) 'Decreased upright cerebral blood flow and cerebral autoregulation in normocapnic postural tachycardia syndrome.' *American Journal of Physiology: Heart and Circulatory Physiology 297* (2).

48. Novak, P. (2018) 'Hypocapnic cerebral hypoperfusion: a biomarker of orthostatic intolerance.' *PLOS ONE 13* (9).

49. Park, J., Kim, H.-T., Park, K.M., Ha, S.Y., *et al.* (2017) 'Orthostatic dizziness in Parkinson's disease is attributed to cerebral hypoperfusion: a transcranial Doppler study.' *Journal of Clinical Ultrasound 45.*

50. Freeman, R. (2002) 'The chronic fatigue syndrome is a disease of the autonomic nervous system. Sometimes.' *Clinical Autonomic Research 12* (4).

51. Lewis, I., Pairman, J., Spickett, G. & Newton, J.L. (2013) 'Clinical characteristics of a novel subgroup of chronic fatigue syndrome patients with postural orthostatic tachycardia syndrome.' *Journal of Internal Medicine 273* (5).

52. van Campen, C.L.M.C., Verheugt, F.W.A. & Visser, F.C. (2018) 'Cerebral blood flow changes during tilt table testing in healthy volunteers, as assessed by Doppler imaging of the carotid and vertebral arteries.' *Clinical Neurophysiology Practice 23* (3).

53. van Campen, C.L.M.C., Verheugt, F.W.A., Rowe, P.C. & Visser, F.C. (2020) 'Cerebral blood flow is reduced in ME/CFS during head-up tilt testing even in the absence of hypotension or tachycardia: a quantitative, controlled study using Doppler echography.' *Clinical Neurophysiology Practice 8* (5).

54. van Campen, C.L.M.C., Rowe, P.C. & Visser, F.C. (2020) 'Cerebral blood flow is reduced in severe myalgic encephalomyelitis/chronic fatigue syndrome patients during mild orthostatic stress testing: an exploratory study at 20 degrees of head-up tilt testing.' *Healthcare 8* (169).

55. van Campen, C.L.M.C., Rowe, PC. & Visser, F.C. (2020) 'Reductions in cerebral blood flow can be provoked by sitting in severe myalgic encephalomyelitis/chronic fatigue syndrome patients.' *Healthcare (Basel) 8* (4).

56. van Campen, C.L.M.C., Rowe, P.C. & Visser, F.C. (2021) 'Cerebral blood flow remains reduced after tilt testing in myalgic encephalomyelitis/chronic fatigue syndrome patients.' *Clinical Neurophysiology Practice 6.*

57. Plash, W.B., Diedrich, A., Biaggioni, I., Garland, E.M, *et al.* (2013) 'Diagnosing postural tachycardia syndrome: comparison of tilt testing compared with standing haemodynamics.' *Clinical Science (London) 124* (2).

58. Miller, A.J. & Bourne, K.M. (2020) 'Abdominal compression as a treatment for postural tachycardia syndrome.' *Journal of the American Heart Association 9* (14).

59. Mar, P.L. & Raj, S.R. (2020) 'Postural orthostatic tachycardia syndrome: mechanisms and new therapies.' *Annual Review of Medicine 27* (71).

60. Bourne, K.M., Sheldon, R.S., Hall, J., Lloyd, M., *et al.* (2021) 'Compression garment reduces orthostatic tachycardia and symptoms in patients with postural orthostatic tachycardia syndrome.' *Journal of the American College of Cardiology 77* (3).

61. Nardone, M., Guzman, J., Harvey, P.J., Floras, J.S. & Edgell, H. (2020) 'Effect of a neck compression collar on cardiorespiratory and cerebrovascular function in postural orthostatic tachycardia syndrome (POTS).' *Journal of Applied Physiology 128* (4).

62. Johnson, C. (2019) 'Could craniocervical instability be causing ME/CFS, fibromyalgia & POTS? Pt I – The spinal series.' Health Rising. Accessed on 10/12/2022 at www.healthrising.org/blog/2019/02/27/brainstem-compression-chronic-fatigue-syndrome-me-cfs-fibromyalgia-pots-craniocervical-instability.

63. Sutcliffe, K., Gray, J., Tan, M.P., Pairman, J., *et al.* (2010) 'Home orthostatic training in chronic fatigue syndrome – a randomized, placebo-controlled feasibility study.' *European Journal of Clinical Investigation 40.*

64. Nijs, J. & Ickmans, K. (2013) 'Postural orthostatic tachycardia syndrome as a clinically important subgroup of chronic fatigue syndrome: further evidence for central nervous system dysfunctioning.' *Journal of Internal Medicine 273* (5).

65. van Campen, C.L M.C., Rowe, P.C. & Visser, F.C. (2018) 'Blood volume status in ME/CFS correlates with the presence or absence of orthostatic symptoms: preliminary results.' *Frontiers in Pediatrics 6.*

66. Ruzieh, M., Baugh, A., Dasa, O., Parker, R.L., *et al.* (2017) 'Effects of intermittent intravenous saline infusions in patients with medication-refractory postural tachycardia syndrome.' *Journal of Interventional Cardiac Electrophysiology 48* (3).

67. Rodriguez, B., Zimmermann, R., Gutbrod, K., Heinemann, D. & Z'Graggen, W.J. (2019) 'Orthostatic cognitive dysfunction in postural tachycardia syndrome after rapid water drinking.' *Frontiers in Neuroscience 13.*

68. Davenport, T.E., Ward, M.K., Stevens, S.R., Stevens, J., Snell, C.R. & VanNess, J.M. (2020) 'Cardiopulmonary responses to exercise in an individual with myalgic encephalomyelitis/chronic fatigue syndrome during long-term treatment with intravenous saline: a case study.' *Work 66* (2).

69. Fu, Q. & Levine, B.D. (2018) 'Exercise and non-pharmacological treatment of POTS.' *Autonomic Neuroscience 215.*

70. Parsaik, A., Allison, T.G., Singer, W., Sletten, D.M., *et al.* (2012) 'Deconditioning in patients with orthostatic intolerance.' *Neurology 79* (14).

71. Loughnan, A., Gall, N. & James, S. (2021) 'Observational case series describing features of cardiopulmonary exercise testing in postural tachycardia syndrome (PoTS).' *Autonomic Neuroscience 231.*

72. van Campen, C.L.M.C., Rowe, P.C. & Visser, F.C. (2021) 'Deconditioning does not explain orthostatic intolerance in ME/CFS (myalgic encephalomyelitis/chronic fatigue syndrome).' *Journal of Translational Medicine 19.*

73. Cliftonsmith, T. & Rowley, J. (2011) 'Breathing pattern disorders and physiotherapy: inspiration for our profession.' *Physical Therapy Reviews 16.*

74. Reilly, C.C., Floyd, S.V., Lee, K., Warwick, G., *et al.* (2020) 'Breathlessness and dysfunctional breathing in patients with postural orthostatic tachycardia syndrome (POTS): the impact of a physiotherapy intervention.' *Autonomic Neuroscience 223.*

75. Nijs, J., Adriaens, J., Schuermans, D., Buyl, R. & Vincken, W. (2008) 'Breathing retraining in patients with chronic fatigue syndrome: a pilot study.' *Physiotherapy Theory Practice 24* (2).

CHAPTER 13

Immune and Neuroendocrine Dysfunction

PURPOSE OF THIS CHAPTER

The impact and influence of the immune and neuroendocrine systems in relation to ME/CFS is arguably the most detailed area of current research, but they are also the systems that will have the least benefit from physiotherapy management strategies.

However, a physiotherapist should have an awareness of symptoms related to immune and neuroendocrine dysfunction because they could be linked to post exertional malaise (PEM), which is the exacerbation of current symptoms or addition of new symptoms caused by exertion.

This chapter provides a brief summary of current findings in the immune and neuroendocrine systems of people with ME/CFS and highlights which symptoms should be of particular note for a physiotherapist.

Immune and neuroendocrine dysfunction in ME/CFS

A key role of the immune system is to defend the body against infection.

Symptoms of immune system dysfunction feature on several diagnostic criteria for ME/CFS (1) (2) (3), although they are not essential for diagnosis. Immune system symptoms described for diagnosis of ME/CFS are:

- flu-like symptoms
- susceptibility to viral infections
- sensitivities to food

- tender or swollen lymph nodes
- recurrent sore throat
- recurrent flu-like symptoms, e.g. general malaise.

An altered immunological state has been found in people with ME/CFS, particularly those with more severe symptoms (4). It is not yet clear whether such changes to the immune system are the cause of ME/CFS, a reflection of ongoing or recent infection, or an indication that a person with ME/CFS will be more susceptible to future infections (4) (5).

'Neuroendocrine' describes the interaction between the nervous system and the endocrine system. The endocrine system involves the secretion of hormones into the circulatory system to regulate metabolic processes such as the growth and development of skeletal tissues. Overall, the neuroendocrine system allows the body to respond to change and maintain homeostasis (6) including a role in thermoregulation (7).

Neuroendocrine symptoms feature on several diagnostic criteria for ME/CFS (8) (1) (2), although they are not essential for diagnosis. Neuroendocrine symptoms included for diagnosis of ME/CFS are:

- chills or night sweats
- loss of thermostatic stability
- intolerance to heat or cold.

Several areas of the immune and neuroendocrine systems have been explored in research and shown to have dysfunction in people with ME/CFS. Summaries are provided in this chapter, and physiotherapists with a specialist interest in these areas are encouraged to read the source materials.

Increased immune activity

Increased immune activity has been associated with ME/CFS (5) (9), therefore some research has looked at the potential benefits of using immunological treatments. For example, some treatments for cancer, autoimmune diseases and inflammatory diseases that suppress the immune system have been trialled on people with ME/CFS. While some benefits were reported they were not found in all participants, and others suffered serious adverse events (10) (11). There is currently no clear evidence as to the effectiveness of immunological treatments for people with ME/CFS (9).

Mast cell activation disease

Mast cells are a type of white blood cell which are involved in the immune system (12). When activated in response to infection or environmental threats, mast cells travel to peripheral tissues where they release mediators (12) and in healthy people their activity is common and necessary (13). There are more than 200 mediators, including chemicals such as histamine and cytokines which are commonly involved in allergic reactions, but mast cells respond to both allergic and nonallergic triggers (12).

Ana: 'The effects of ME/CFS are systemic and it is almost impossible to separate the immune symptoms from neuroendocrine symptoms that I experience, such as fever, sweating, swollen glands, joint and muscle pain, profound fatigue, temperature dysregulation and skin rashes.'

Mast cells may become overproduced or overactive (13), and this dysfunction is known as mast cell activation disease (12), an umbrella term that includes mast cell activation syndrome (MCAS), a common co-morbidity of ME/CFS which is discussed in more detail in chapter 2.

The role that mast cells play in ME/CFS has been investigated, with one small study (14) comparing 18 people with ME/CFS to 13 healthy controls and finding significantly increased numbers of mast cells in people with ME/CFS, with numbers increasing alongside the severity of ME/CFS symptoms. However, this area of research remains in its infancy and warrants further investigation before conclusions can be drawn.

Gut health and immune response

People with ME/CFS have been found to have an imbalance of gut microbiota and increased microbial translocation (15). One study found there were increased levels of antibodies for common gut bacteria in people with ME/CFS compared to healthy controls, and that the level of antibodies correlated with the severity of their reported fatigue as well as other symptoms such as muscle tension and cognitive dysfunction (16).

A small study (17) looked at the blood and stool samples of ten people with ME/CFS and ten healthy controls, which were taken at rest and at intervals following a maximal exercise test. The microbiomes in stool samples differed between groups at baseline, and in people with ME/CFS there was an increase in six out of nine of the major bacteria, immediately following exercise and up to 72 hours after the exertion, that were not observed in healthy controls. Clearance of bacteria from blood was also delayed in people with ME/CFS, suggesting gut permeability may be occurring during PEM. An increased permeability of the gastrointestinal barrier could lead to an immune response or increased inflammation (5).

Potential management strategies for gut health are included in the section on irritable bowel syndrome in chapter 2.

The hypothalamic-pituitary-adrenal axis

The hypothalamic-pituitary-adrenal axis ('HPA axis') is the term used to describe the interaction between the hypothalamus (below the thalamus in the brain), the pituitary gland (located just above the brain-stem), and the adrenal glands (on top of the kidneys) (18). The HPA axis serves to maintain homeostasis as it coordinates neural, endocrine and immune responses (19).

Hormones involved in the HPA axis include glucocorticoids such as cortisol, which are essential for metabolic and homeostatic processes (20). These hormones also modulate immune and inflammatory pro-cesses (21) and their effects have been utilized in drug development primarily as anti-inflammatories (20).

Some studies have found that the HPA axis is underactive in people with ME/CFS (22), with a number of deficiencies found in relation to reduced or altered cortisol levels and a blunted responsiveness of the whole system (23). Lower levels of cortisol (24) (22) and another hormone involved in the HPA axis (25) have been found in people with ME/CFS compared to healthy controls. However, the exact mechanism causing low cortisol levels is yet to be fully understood (24) and these findings are not universal in people with ME/CFS (26). Excessively low cortisol levels can be caused by a disorder of the adrenal glands called Addison's disease, where early symptoms include fatigue and muscle weakness as well as loss of appetite and increased thirst (27). Addison's disease can be a differential diagnosis for ME/CFS (9).

Oliver: 'I used to get a cold and sore throat really often, but this has settled down since I've been on antivirals.'

While the HPA axis can modulate the sleep–wake cycle, sleep

deprivation can also cause a dysfunction of the HPA axis (28) and, given sleep dysfunction is a key symptom of ME/CFS (see chapter 9), it is possible that changes to the HPA axis are secondary complications as opposed to primary causes of ME/CFS.

Pharmacological interventions to address lower levels of cortisol have been investigated in several studies that looked at the use of a synthetic preparation of cortisol called hydrocortisone. The reported effectiveness of hydrocortisone differed between 'moderate', 'mild', 'slight' and 'not effective at all' (29), but how studies measure 'effectiveness' in a condition as complex as ME/CFS is notable. For example, in a randomized, double-blind placebo-controlled study of hydrocortisone (30) the main outcome measure was a general 'wellness scale', and while there was a greater improvement in scores for the participants taking hydrocortisone compared to those taking a placebo, there were no statistically significant changes to any other self-rating scales used. At present there is not enough evidence to support the routine use of corticosteroids such as hydrocortisone for ME/CFS (22).

Thermoregulation

People with ME/CFS have reported problems with thermoregulation, for example feeling unusually hot or cold and sudden changes to skin colour (31). A small study of 15 young people with ME/CFS found that those with ME/CFS showed abnormal thermoregulatory responses during a skin cooling procedure in comparison to healthy controls (31).

Kim: 'Every viral illness has hit me badly and requires two weeks or more to recover from. I am intolerant to excessive heat, which makes my orthostatic intolerance symptoms even worse.'

Immune and neuroendocrine symptoms in PEM

PEM is the hallmark characteristic of ME/CFS and involves an addition of symptoms or exacerbation of current symptoms in response to exertion (32). More information regarding PEM can be found in chapter 6.

An international survey of over 1500 people with ME/CFS (33) captured symptoms that were exacerbated by physical or cognitive exertion. In relation to immune and neuroendocrine systems, the following symptoms were reported:

- flu-like symptoms (86.6%)

- sore throat (70.9%)
- night sweats and chills (67.7%)
- tender lymph nodes (62.9%).

A physiotherapist should ask about the prevalence of these types of symptoms during an assessment of anyone with ME/CFS as this information may help them to identify PEM. More information regarding assessment can be found in chapter 14.

Adaptation to practice
Assessment and referrals

- For in-person interactions, strict infection control procedures should be followed considering the potential for immune system dysfunction.
- Check before an appointment what temperatures are most comfortable for each individual and make the necessary adjustments to the environment.
- Include questions on immune and neuroendocrine symptoms in assessments of people with ME/CFS to build a picture of all possible indicators of PEM.
- Consider referrals for medical review if persistent viral infection symptoms are present.

SUMMARY

▶ The immune and neuroendocrine systems may play a role in the ongoing physiological processes of ME/CFS.
▶ People with ME/CFS may have dysfunction of their immune and neuroendocrine systems.

APPLICATION TO PRACTICE

▶ Immune and neuroendocrine symptoms may occur as part of an individual's experience of PEM. The severity and behaviour of these symptoms may help a physiotherapist to identify and avoid triggers of PEM.

References

1. Carruthers, B.M., van de Sande, M.I., De Meirleir, K.L., Klimas, N.G., *et al.* (2011) 'Myalgic encephalomyelitis: International Consensus Criteria.' *Journal of Internal Medicine 270.*

2. Carruthers, B.M., Jain, A.K., De Meirleir, K.L., Peterson, D.L., *et al.* (2003) 'Myalgic encephalomyelitis/chronic fatigue syndrome.' *Journal of Chronic Fatigue Syndrome 11* (1).

3. Fukuda, K., Straus, S.E., Hickie, I., Sharpe, M.C., Dobbins, J.G., Komaroff, A.L. (1994) 'The chronic fatigue syndrome: a comprehensive approach to its definition and study.' *Annals of Internal Medicine 121* (12).

4. Cliff, J.M., King, E.C., Lee, J.S., Sepúlveda, N., *et al.* (2019) 'Cellular immune function in myalgic encephalomyelitis/chronic fatigue syndrome (ME/CFS).' *Frontiers in Immunology 10* (796).

5. Klimas, N.G. & Koneru, A.O. (2007) 'Chronic fatigue syndrome: inflammation, immune function, and neuroendocrine interactions.' *Current Rheumatology Reports 9* (6).

6. Levine, J.E. (2012) 'An Introduction to Neuroendocrine Systems.' In G. Fink, D.W. Pfaff & J.E. Levine (eds) *Handbook of Neuroendocrinology.* London: Academic Press.

7. Gale, C.C. (1973) 'Neuroendocrine aspects of thermoregulation.' *Annual Review of Physiology 35.*

8. Centers for Disease Control and Prevention (2021) *IOM 2015 Diagnostic Criteria.* Centers for Disease Control and Prevention. Accessed on 2/12/2022 at www.cdc.gov/me-cfs/healthcare-providers/diagnosis/iom-2015-diagnostic-criteria.html.

9. Shepherd, C. & Chaudhuri, A. (2019) *ME/CFS/PVFS: An Exploration of the Key Clinical Issues.* Gawcott: The ME Association.

10. Rekeland, I.G., Fosså, A., Lande, A., Ktoridou-Valen, I, *et al.* (2020) 'Intravenous cyclophosphamide in myalgic encephalomyelitis/chronic fatigue syndrome. An open-label phase II study.' *Front Med (Lausanne) 7* (162).

11. Fluge, Ø., Rekeland, I.G., Lien, K., Thürmer, H, *et al.* (2019) 'B-lymphocyte depletion in patients with myalgic encephalomyelitis/chronic fatigue syndrome: a randomized, double-blind, placebo-controlled trial.' *Annals of Internal Medicine 170* (9).

12. Selleck, B. & Selleck, C. (2021) 'A primer on mast cell activation disease for the nurse practitioner.' *Journal for Nurse Practitioners 17* (7).

13. Akin, C. (2017) 'Mast cell activation syndromes.' *Journal of Allergy and Clinical Immunology 140* (2).

14. Nguyen, T., Johnston, S., Chacko, A., Gibson, D., *et al.* (2017) 'Novel characterisation of mast cell phenotypes from peripheral blood mononuclear cells in chronic fatigue syndrome/myalgic encephalomyelitis patients.' *Asian Pacific Journal of Allergy and Immunology 35* (2).

15. Giloteaux, L., Goodrich, J.K., Walters, W.A., Levine, S.M., Ley, R.E. & Hanson, M.R. (2016) 'Reduced diversity and altered composition of the gut microbiome in individuals with myalgic encephalomyelitis/chronic fatigue syndrome.' *Microbiome 4* (30).

16. Maes, M., Mihaylova, I. & Leunis, J.C. (2007) 'Increased serum IgA and IgM against LPS of enterobacteria in chronic fatigue syndrome (CFS): indication for the involvement of gram-negative enterobacteria in the etiology of CFS and for the presence of an increased gut-intestinal permeability.' *Journal of Affective Disorders 99* (1–3).

17. Shukla, S.K., Cook, D., Meyer, J., Vernon, S.D., *et al.* (2015) 'Changes in gut and plasma microbiome following exercise challenge in myalgic encephalomyelitis/chronic fatigue syndrome (ME/CFS).' *PLOS ONE 10* (12).

18. Chrousos, G.P. (2009) 'Stress and disorders of the stress system.' *Nature Reviews Endocrinology 5* (7).

19. Fulford, A.J. & Harbuz, M.S. (2005) 'An introduction to the HPA axis.' In T. Steckler, N.H. Kalin, & J.M.H.M. Reul (eds) *Techniques in the Behavioral and Neural Sciences.* London: Elsevier.

20. Akalestou, E., Genser, L. & Rutter, G.A. (2020) 'Glucocorticoid metabolism in obesity and following weight loss.' *Frontiers in Endocrinology (Lausanne) 20* (11).

21. Cruz-Topete, D. & Cidlowski, J.A. (2015) 'One hormone, two actions: anti- and pro-inflammatory effects of glucocorticoids.' *Neuroimmunomodulation 22* (1–2).

22. Tanriverdi, F., Karaca, Z., Unluhizarci, K. & Kelestimur, F. (2007) 'The hypothalamo-pituitary-adrenal axis in chronic fatigue syndrome and fibromyalgia syndrome.' *Stress 10* (1).

23. Papadopoulos, A. & Cleare, A. (2012) 'Hypothalamic–pituitary–adrenal axis dysfunction in chronic fatigue syndrome.' *Nature Reviews Endocrinology 8.*

24. Demitrack, M.A., Dale, J.K., Straus, S.E., Laue, L., *et al.* (1991) 'Evidence for impaired activation of the hypothalamic-pituitary-adrenal axis in patients with chronic fatigue syndrome.' *Journal of Clinical Endocrinology & Metabolism 73* (6).

25. Gaab, J., Engert, V., Heitz, V., Schad, T., Schürmeyer, T.H. & Ehlert, U. (2004) 'Associations between neuroendocrine responses to the Insulin Tolerance Test and patient characteristics in chronic fatigue syndrome.' *Journal of Psychosomatic Research 56* (4).

26. Papanicolaou, D.A., Amsterdam, J.D., Levine, S., McCann, S.M., *et al.* (2004) 'Neuroendocrine aspects of chronic fatigue syndrome.' *Neuroimmunomodulation 11* (2).

27. NHS (2021) 'Addison's disease.' Accessed on 2/12/2022 at www.nhs.uk/conditions/addisons-disease.

28. Hirotsu, C., Tufik, S. & Andersen, M.L. (2015) 'Interactions between sleep, stress, and metabolism: from physiological to pathological conditions.' *Sleep Science 8* (3).

29. Collatz, A., Johnston, S.C., Staines, D.R. & Marshall-Gradisnik, S.M. (2016) 'A systematic review of drug therapies for chronic fatigue syndrome/myalgic encephalomyelitis.' *Clinical Therapy 38* (6).

30. McKenzie, R., O'Fallon, A., Dale, J., Demitrack, M., *et al.* (1998) 'Low-dose hydrocortisone for treatment of chronic fatigue syndrome: a randomized controlled trial.' *JAMA 280* (12).

31. Wyller, V.B., Godang, K., Mørkrid, L., Saul, J.P., Thaulow, E. & Walløe, L. (2007) 'Abnormal thermoregulatory responses in adolescents with chronic fatigue syndrome: relation to clinical symptoms.' *Pediatrics 120* (1).

32. Bateman, L., Bested, A.C., Bonilla, H.F., Chheda, B.V., *et al.* (2021) 'Myalgic encephalomyelitis/chronic fatigue syndrome: essentials of diagnosis and management.' *Mayo Clinic Proceedings 96* (11).

33. Holtzman, C.S., Bhatia, S., Cotler, J. & Jason, L.A. (2019) 'Assessment of post-exertional malaise (PEM) in patients with myalgic encephalomyelitis (ME) and chronic fatigue syndrome (CFS): a patient-driven survey.' *Diagnostics (Basel) 9* (1).

PHYSIOTHERAPY ASSESSMENT and MANAGEMENT of ME/CFS

CHAPTER 14

Assessment

PURPOSE OF THIS CHAPTER

People with ME/CFS can experience additional symptoms or an exacerbation of current symptoms after physical, cognitive, sensory and emotional exertion (post exertional malaise, PEM). Irrespective of the problem being addressed, any physiotherapy assessment of a person with ME/CFS must seek to understand the severity of their ME/CFS symptoms and identified triggers. This will enable the physiotherapist to monitor and evaluate the impact of their intervention to ensure they avoid causing PEM. A physiotherapist must also recognize that the assessment process itself may trigger PEM and be able to adapt their assessments accordingly.

There are a variety of reasons why someone with ME/CFS may seek physiotherapy input:

- for support and management after a recent diagnosis of ME/CFS
- to address specific symptoms in relation to ME/CFS
- to address a problem relating to a co-morbidity of ME/CFS
- to have assessment and treatment of a problem completely unrelated to ME/CFS.

This chapter provides guidance on how to adapt every aspect of an assessment to minimize the potential for PEM. An outline of a general assessment of someone with ME/CFS is also provided, although as every assessment should be individualized there is no single recommended process.

The recommendations in this chapter are based on the knowledge and understanding of the physiological processes that influence the symptoms of ME/CFS along with best practice, clinical experience and feedback from people with ME/CFS.

Adaptations to the assessment approach

There are many factors to consider before carrying out an assessment of someone with ME/CFS in order to minimize the potential for symptom exacerbation and maximize the person's comfort and tolerance of the interaction.

You: the physiotherapist

You will have an impact on the person with ME/CFS and therefore create the potential to increase their symptoms, because people with ME/CFS may have sensitivities to sensory stimulation (see chapter 11) and cognitive exertion (see chapter 8). You can minimize your sensory stimulus and therefore improve the person's tolerance and experience of the assessment by considering the following.

- Scent: avoid strong smelling deodorant, perfumes, aftershave, body spray, washing powders, hair sprays, shampoos and cigarette smoke. While infection control is important, be aware that alcohol gels and soaps can also be heavily scented.
- Communication: consider lowering the volume of your voice, but ensure the person is still able to hear you. Also consider how fast you talk, the number of questions you use and whether they are open or closed, and the length of your sentences. Establish the person's preferred method of communication (e.g. written or verbal).
- Appearance: avoid bright colours and patterned materials to minimize visual stimulus.
- Body awareness: personal space is an important consideration that should be established with each person. Minimize gesticulation and body movement to reduce visual stimulus.

Location

Some people with ME/CFS may not be able to leave their home and most will incur significant exertion by simply attending a clinic appointment. Where possible, an appointment in the home environment is recommended.

If the appointment is in a clinic, provide clear information as to the location and parking facilities so that the person can plan in advance and find the location easily.

Virtual appointments by video or telephone calls have the benefit of the person being able to stay at home; however, consideration of cognitive and sensory exertion is important. You can reduce the sensory load by turning off cameras and minimizing the duration of the appointment.

Some people with ME/CFS will be admitted to hospital, either due to the severity of their ME/CFS symptoms or for an unrelated matter. A hospital ward environment can be extremely challenging to people with ME/CFS due to the sensory stimulation, risk of hospital-acquired harms and altered routine. Any physiotherapist involved in the care of people with ME/CFS in a hospital setting should make every effort to adapt the environment and advocate for the person to ensure other staff are aware of these issues. More information regarding hospital admissions is included in chapter 3.

Time of assessment

People with ME/CFS have fluctuating symptoms and/or sleep patterns, so the time of assessment should be arranged with the person in advance, with the understanding that symptoms can be unpredictable and there may be some flexibility required.

Environment

Consider potential environmental triggers such as lighting, temperature, smell (e.g. air fresheners) and noise (e.g. background music). If seeing a person with ME/CFS in a clinic, try to make the environment as comfortable as possible with limited sensory stimulation. Be aware that some people with ME/CFS may choose to wear noise cancelling ear defenders and/or sunglasses or eye masks to reduce levels of stimulation.

If using a shared clinic space ensure other staff members are also aware of the adaptations required and the reasons behind it.

Assessment duration

Consider offering time for the person to rest during the appointment, which may mean increasing the length of appointment time or splitting the appointment into several shorter interactions.

Positioning

Consider the position of the person during the interaction and the support of any seating used. Ascertain whether the person is physically able to manage an upright posture. Discuss with the person which position is most comfortable to maintain with less chance of symptom exacerbation, for example having feet elevated or being in supine.

Further suggestions for adapting interactions, particularly for those with severe or very severe ME/CFS, can be found in chapter 3.

Assessment preparation

People with ME/CFS can experience cognitive impairments, which are discussed in chapter 8. There is potential to cause cognitive fatigue from a lengthy assessment, therefore consider ways to obtain subjective information beforehand by contacting the person or asking their carer. Forms and/or questionnaires can be used to gather information in advance; however, open questions can be more cognitively challenging to complete so the design or selection of the pre-assessment documents should be carefully considered, and ensure plenty of time is provided for the person to complete them so they are able to pace themselves leading up to the appointment.

Establishing the nature of the person's PEM should be a priority of pre-assessment information gathering as this will determine how much the person may be able to tolerate and how the in-person assessment will be structured. Outcome measures and screening tools are discussed further in chapter 18.

Information such as medication, past medical history and details of their daily routine is also easy to obtain beforehand in order to save time in the assessment.

Assessment structure

The first step in an assessment of any person with ME/CFS is to establish why they are seeking support from a physiotherapist and what their priorities are for treatment. For people with ME/CFS this is of particular importance as you will be time-limited, so their priorities should form the focus of the assessment.

This chapter provides information on how to carry out a detailed assessment of someone with ME/CFS. It is for the physiotherapist to use their clinical judgement and the person's priorities to determine which areas of assessment are applicable and in which order you complete the assessment. Given the potential level of detail involved, a full assessment may have to happen over more than one appointment to avoid symptom exacerbation.

Consent

Ensure the person is able to provide informed consent by explaining the potential effects of the assessment and any intervention in terms of symptom exacerbation.

Be aware that some people with ME/CFS may not be able to give verbal consent so alternative methods of gaining consent may be required. This is especially relevant for those with severe and very severe ME/CFS (see chapter 3).

Present condition

Ask the person why they are seeking physiotherapy support and identify their main problems or priorities. This may or may not be linked to their ME/CFS diagnosis.

Further prompts in relation to specific ME/CFS symptoms are listed later in this chapter and should be considered irrespective of the initial presenting condition as they may influence how you adapt your assessment and treatment.

History of present condition

Establish whether the person has had a formal diagnosis of ME/CFS, who gave this diagnosis and when, and whether the cause of onset is known. A brief timeline of the person's history with ME/CFS is useful, bearing in mind some people may have had this condition for years or even decades. Establish also whether there are patterns of relapse and remission, and how this relates to their present state.

Has the person had any medical investigations in the past and what were the results? This is information that can be gathered in the pre-assessment period.

Past medical history and co-morbidities

People with ME/CFS may have other co-morbidities that might impact upon their symptoms. Establish if they are already under the care of any other medical professionals or teams.

Some co-morbidities may influence how any management or treatment may be delivered. Chapter 2 provides more detail on select co-morbidities and what should be considered.

Past experience of physiotherapy

Ask the person what physiotherapy treatment they have previously had and determine:

- what approach has been helpful
- whether any approach has caused symptom exacerbation
- how they feel physiotherapy might help them in this instance.

It is important to validate the person's experience and consider they may not have had a positive experience of physiotherapy and health-care in the past.

Medication

Establish what medication the person is on, taking note of any that may affect heart rate (for example beta blockers) as this may influence any objective measures or management strategies that involve the heart rate as a marker. Some medications may also have an impact on the autonomic nervous system. A list of common medications and supplements can be found in the Appendix.

Hydration and nutrition

Dietary intake and sensitivities may impact on symptoms including sleep and rest quality, for example alcohol or caffeine intake. Information regarding fluid and salt intake may be of particular interest if orthostatic intolerances are suspected or already diagnosed. Consider whether the person would benefit from a referral to a dietician for expert advice in this area.

Gastrointestinal symptoms such as bloating, cramps or changes to the frequency or nature of stools may be indicative of irritable bowel syndrome, which is a common co-morbidity of ME/CFS (see chapter 2). Abdominal discomfort and fatigue can also be symptoms of other serious conditions such as ovarian cancer or inflammatory bowel disease, so any unexplained gastrointestinal symptoms should be referred for a medical review.

Social history

A typical social history includes information on employment, family and hobbies. When working with people with ME/CFS it is also helpful to build a greater understanding about the person's physical and emotional environment to identify areas of support, potential stressors and key priorities for energy.

- Social support: find out who is in their social network, for example family, carers and friends. Are any relationships affected by their condition? It is helpful to determine whether there are people who can support any physiotherapy intervention, or whether they may be any challenges.
- Employment (if applicable): requirements, routine, adaptations and support available.
- Education (if applicable): requirements, routine, adaptations and support available.
- Relaxation/enjoyment/hobbies: are there activities that provide respite or are of great importance to the person? Would an additional intervention mean they lose the ability to carry out these activities and potentially have a negative effect on their quality of life? Are there important activities that the person is currently unable to manage?

Home environment

Understanding the home environment helps to build a picture of how the person currently manages and may raise key areas that could be addressed with aids and adaptations.

- bed type: profiling, size, mattress type
- distance between key points (bedroom, bathroom, kitchen)
- steps, stairs and access
- aids and adaptations already in use: e.g. perching stools, rails, shower chair, mobility aids
- specific activities or access to parts of the home that are impacted by symptoms.

Activities of daily living

Discussing normal activities of daily living can lead to a greater understanding of how much energy is currently being expended, how great an impact their symptoms are having on everyday life and identify areas where aids or modifications could provide benefit.

- Washing: how often do they shower/bathe, and how does this affect their symptoms?
- Dressing: are any items of clothing difficult, and do they need assistance?
- Preparing meals: how much can they manage in the kitchen environment, and what activities do they find most difficult?
- Housework: which tasks are difficult/impossible, and which tasks are essential?
- Assistance: are they receiving assistance for any activities of daily living? Is support available?
- Household admin: who is responsible for general administration tasks such as managing finance, household bills etc.?

Daily routine

One of the most important parts of the subjective assessment is to find out about the person's daily routine in fine detail. Create a timeline of a typical day and work with the person to list the physical and cognitive tasks, as well as periods of rest. A daily routine diary can be time consuming to complete so it is helpful to gather an outline of this information in the pre-assessment process, but it is beneficial to discuss the routine in more detail in the context of their symptoms during the assessment.

An overview of a person's daily routine will help you to build a picture of current activity levels throughout the day, as well as potentially identify triggers of PEM.

Subjective symptoms of ME/CFS

Regardless of the reason for a physiotherapy assessment, it is important to understand a person's main ME/CFS symptoms and how they impact on their daily living and potential ability to tolerate any intervention. For example, when treating a person with ME/CFS who has had a knee replacement, the physiotherapist must know whether they could tolerate a typical rehabilitation programme or if this will need to be adapted to take into account their PEM, pain, orthostatic intolerance, muscle fatiguability and current energy management requirements.

Establish the person's key ME/CFS symptoms, what triggers them, whether anything eases them and how severe they are. There are a number of screening tools and outcome measures that can be used to capture symptom severity and progression but given the number of potential symptoms and the cognitive load required to complete each measure it is important to carefully select these. How to determine which tool is most appropriate for each person is discussed in chapter 18.

Table 14.1 is a list of the main symptoms of ME/CFS and what should be considered when carrying out a subjective assessment.

Table 14.1 Subjective assessment of ME/CFS symptoms

Post exertional malaise	An addition of symptoms or exacerbation of current symptoms following exertion (see chapter 6)
	A person may not identify their symptoms using this terminology. They may describe a pattern of symptoms which could include fatigue, pain and cognitive dysfunction ('brain fog') that are made worse by exertion, which may be physical, cognitive, sensory, emotional, social, or undefined
	Mapping out a typical daily or weekly schedule may help to identify patterns of PEM
	Potential outcome measures for PEM are discussed in chapter 18
Fatigue	'Fatigue' is a vague term that may mean different things to different people (see chapter 7)
	Look for how fatigue impacts upon the person's quality of life in terms of how they are managing their activities of daily living, and whether they are able to work, socialize, exercise or continue with hobbies
	Fatigue may present as physical or cognitive (or both)
	There are outcome measures for fatigue that capture the general extent to which fatigue impacts on quality of life and function, and these are detailed in chapter 18
Cognitive dysfunction	Does the person report difficulty with cognitive tasks such as: • memory • attention • concentration • planning and problem solving • word finding difficulties? If so, how does this impact on their ability to function? Have their cognitive problems been assessed and investigated by an appropriate medical specialist?

cont.

Sleep dysfunction	Ascertain whether there are any symptoms impacting on sleep quality: pain, racing mind, restless legs, breathing difficulties, anxiety, depression, urinary frequency, sleep–wake cycle issues. See chapter 9 for more information
	Establish their current sleep routine/pattern: what time do they go to bed, what is their routine at bedtime, how many hours do they sleep and what position do they sleep in (e.g. elevated head/legs)? Is their sleep pattern fixed or changeable? Do they find it easy to get to sleep? Do they wake often?
	What is the sleep environment like? Is there any sensory stimulation from light, sound, screens or other environmental factors?
	Does their symptom severity impact on their sleep quality or vice versa? Do they feel refreshed after sleep?
	Do they suffer from sleep apnoea, insomnia or other sleep disorders? Have they been formerly assessed for these?
Pain	Ask about pain symptoms in terms of: • location(s) • pattern • aggravating and easing factors • what type of pain (e.g. neurogenic, rheumatological, inflammatory, mechanical) • any relation to other symptom exacerbation (for example if it follows a pattern of PEM)
	Simple rating scales for pain are detailed in chapter 18
	Are there any pain red flags?
	Are there signs of fibromyalgia?
	Is there mention of neck and shoulder pain in a 'coat-hanger' pattern? This may be indicative of an orthostatic intolerance (see chapter 12)
	Is there pain around the temporomandibular joint and associated structures, which may indicate a temporomandibular disorder?
	Are migraines or headaches reported?
	More information about pain can be found in chapter 10, with individual co-morbidities detailed in chapter 2
Neurological impairments	Are there any reported motor impairments in terms of fasciculations, dystonia, tonal changes, unsteadiness or noticeable weakness? Have they been investigated for these symptoms?
	Are there hyper-sensitivities to light, sound, touch or smell?
	Are there any neurological red flags that may require a medical referral?

Autonomic dysfunction	Is there evidence of autonomic dysfunction? • palpitations, with or without arrhythmias • light-headedness • laboured breathing • exertional dyspnoea (breathlessness) • nausea • bladder or bowel dysfunction Look for evidence of orthostatic intolerances. Are symptoms exacerbated in an upright posture or relieved by adopting other positions such as elevated feet, crossing legs or supine postures? If a breathing pattern disorder is suspected, consider using an appropriate outcome measure (see chapter 18) More information on autonomic dysfunction can be found in chapter 12
Neuroendocrine manifestations	Do they report feeling extremes of heat or cold, or an inability to cope with changing temperatures? Do these symptoms fluctuate in response to exertion, or are they constant?
Immune dysfunction	Do they experience immune symptoms such as sore throats, flu-like symptoms or tender lymph nodes? Do these symptoms fluctuate in relation to known triggers or are they constant? Have any new symptoms been checked for presence of a new/acute infection unrelated to ME/CFS that need onward referral and investigation? Look for signs of mast cell activation syndrome (MCAS), in particular a pattern of symptoms in relation to potential triggers

Objective assessment

Typically a physiotherapy assessment involves subjective history taking followed by a physical examination, the focus of which should be influenced by what was found out in the subjective history.

In terms of potential stressors for a person with ME/CFS, consider that a physical examination would involve:

• multiple changes in posture

Mo: 'I don't remember any details from my first assessment! We had to go back over everything again on the second one. Having things in writing really helps.'

- physical exertion, often requiring maximal muscle contraction to test power and force
- sensory stimulation in the form of pressure from handling, passive movements and joint mobilizations.

Ana: 'The physiotherapists who were most helpful were those who came in with no preconceived ideas and listened to me.'

For someone with ME/CFS a typical objective assessment may negatively impact on symptoms such as pain, orthostatic intolerance and PEM. Therefore any objective assessment should be clinically reasoned for relevance to their problem, taking into account the risk of symptom exacerbation.

Necessary objective tests that specifically stress the body, such as the NASA lean test, may have to be scheduled on a different session than the initial assessment in order to minimize symptom exacerbation. Objective assessments specific to ME/CFS are shown in Table 14.2.

Table 14.2 Objective assessment of people with ME/CFS

Observation	Observe the person and any adaptations they have made in their environment, or their response to a clinic environment and your interaction
	Some signs of PEM may be observable such as pallor, declining cognitive function, speech difficulties like slurring or monosyllabic responses, declining physical abilities, increased sensitivities to sensory stimuli, and muscle twitches
	Objective measures such as heart rate, blood pressure, oxygen saturation and respiratory rate can also be measured and monitored particularly during any positional changes
	Such observations should form a continuous monitoring process throughout every interaction
Muscle, joint and skin integrity	A traditional assessment of passive range of movement will test muscle length, tone, joint range and skin integrity, with particular relevance to people who are bedbound, in order to identify the potential for tissue shortening and contractures, which will inform postural care advice. Concerns over skin integrity can be referred for pressure care support
	Assessment of joints should take into account that people with ME/CFS may be at risk of osteoporosis due to potential vitamin D deficiency from reduced exposure to sunlight and reduced weight bearing activity (1)
	Consider the potential sensitivity to touch when handling people and maintain open communication and observation throughout

Hypermobility	The Beighton Scoring system (2) is a simple and openly accessible diagnostic tool for hypermobility featuring a nine-point scale of particular movements associated with hypermobility
	Identifying hypermobile joints allows for further exploration of reported musculoskeletal pain, as well as guiding caution with handling and positioning
	Be aware of the potential for brain stem and spinal cord co-morbidities (see chapter 2)
Muscle strength	Global muscle strength testing should not be routinely used due to the potential for symptom exacerbation
	Strength testing may be indicated in the case of a specific injury for example. Consider that people with ME/CFS have muscles that are quicker to fatigue, particularly under repeated contractions (see chapter 7)
Neurological testing	Consider neurological assessments if particular neurological symptoms have been identified, taking into account potential sensitivities to touch
Neurodynamic testing	Pain symptoms could be explored using neurodynamic testing, taking into account potential sensitivities to touch and symptom exacerbation
Movement analysis	Restrict assessment only to key functional movements identified as a priority in the subjective assessment
	Generalized mobility assessments may cause symptom exacerbation and may not be a priority for the person
Orthostatic intolerance	If orthostatic intolerance is suspected, consider an objective outcome measure such as the active stand test or NASA lean test (see chapter 18)
Autonomic dysfunction	Heart rate variability is a potential objective measure of autonomic function. A number of commercially available heart rate monitors can now measure heart rate variability – see chapter 18 for more information
Dysfunctional breathing	If indicated, assess for dysfunctional breathing with observation of use of stomach verses upper chest and hands-on assessment of breathing technique. See chapter 12 for more information on breathing dysfunction
Exercise tolerance	Exercise tolerance testing is not recommended for people with ME/CFS as it is known to cause symptom exacerbation
	The subjective assessment should be enough to identify current activity limitations

Applying the assessment findings to practice

The information gained from an assessment will lead to the development of a management plan or influence treatment decisions if working with the person for a condition unrelated to ME/CFS.

When directly addressing ME/CFS symptoms

Key questions that should shape the management plan are:

- What are the person's main problems/priorities/aims?
- Are there identified triggers for symptom exacerbation and how should the management plan be adapted to avoid these?
- How will I monitor the person's response to the management plan?

Management ideas are discussed throughout this book in relation to specific symptoms or in general. There is no fixed management plan that is recommended for people with ME/CFS. All plans should be individualized and regularly monitored and evaluated. A complete assessment may take several sessions and a management plan may evolve as strategies are tried, evaluated and changed where needed.

When working with a person for an unrelated matter

Regardless of the reason for a physiotherapy intervention, any person with ME/CFS should have an assessment that determines the nature, severity and triggers of their symptoms. The key questions that should shape any management plan should be:

- Are there identified triggers for symptom exacerbation and how should the management plan be adapted to avoid these?
- How will I monitor the person's response to my management plan?

In some cases a typical intervention may not be suitable for a person with ME/CFS but there may be a number of ways to adapt it, for example if a musculoskeletal injury requires a specific exercise it could be adapted by changing the positioning of the person, altering the intensity, or finding the means to adapt a daily routine so that the exercise could be incorporated without causing excessive exertion.

More discussion on whether exercise may be appropriate for people with ME/CFS and how it could be safely approached is in chapter 17.

In other cases an intervention may not be suitable for a person with ME/CFS with no other way to adapt it, for example rehabilitation following orthopaedic surgery in a person with severe ME/CFS who does not tolerate any additional physical exertion. In these cases the focus should be on the person's priorities and minimizing symptoms as much as possible. There may not be a simple solution, so open and honest discussions with the person will allow for shared decision-making.

> **Oliver**: 'A physio assessment helped me to identify issues with my posture and address it with some gentle exercises and changing my workspace.'

SUMMARY

▶ Any physiotherapy assessment of a person with ME/CFS should determine the nature, severity and triggers of their ME/CFS symptom, regardless of the reason for physiotherapy intervention.

▶ A physiotherapy assessment itself may cause symptom exacerbation, so adaptations will be required to the whole assessment process.

▶ All management plans of people with ME/CFS should prioritize the avoidance of PEM and establish a means to monitor and evaluate for symptom exacerbation.

References

1. Berkovitz, S., Ambler, G., Jenkins, M. & Thurgood, S. (2009) 'Serum 25-hydroxy vitamin D levels in chronic fatigue syndrome: a retrospective survey.' *International Journal for Vitamin and Nutrition Research* 79 (4).
2. Remvig, L., Jensen, D.V. & Ward, R.C. (2007) 'Are diagnostic criteria for general joint hypermobility and benign joint hypermobility syndrome based on reproducible and valid tests? A review of the literature.' *Journal of Rheumatology* 34 (4).

CHAPTER 15

Energy Management

PURPOSE OF CHAPTER

Energy management is a strategy that involves managing activities to stay within available energy levels. People with ME/CFS have reported that energy management is one of the most effective forms of symptom management. However, while physiotherapists may feel familiar with the concepts of energy management, activity management and pacing, it is important to understand that there are different types of energy management, some of which may not be appropriate for people with ME/CFS.

It is also important to acknowledge that energy management is not a treatment for ME/CFS, but is a strategy that can help people with ME/CFS to manage their symptoms.

This chapter will describe energy management, activity management and pacing, and how they could be implemented appropriately in relation to ME/CFS.

Energy management/activity management

'Energy management' can be defined as a strategy that involves managing a person's activities to stay within their available energy levels (1). It is also sometimes known as 'activity management', and these two terms appear to be used interchangeably in clinical practice and research. Energy management involves strategies to minimize the amount of energy required for tasks and maximize the amount of activity that can be achieved within a person's available energy. Strategies might include using equipment or technology to adapt activities, or planning and prioritizing schedules. Further discussion of these strategies can be found later in this chapter.

Pacing

Pacing is described as an approach that balances activities and rest to help manage symptoms (2) and it is utilized by physiotherapists for many conditions that involve chronic pain and chronic fatigue (3). However, pacing is a poorly defined construct in research, without a consensus of definition or a demonstrable evidence base (4) (3). There are two identified types of pacing (3):

- 'quota-contingent pacing': undertaking activities according to an amount, distance or goal with the aim of improving function
- 'symptom-contingent pacing': activities are driven by perceived symptom levels, with the aim of avoiding symptoms and conserving energy. Terms that may describe this include 'adaptive pacing' and 'envelope theory'.

Quota-contingent pacing is associated with improving levels of function and is more commonly used than symptom-contingent pacing by health professionals working with people who have chronic pain and chronic fatigue. An online survey (3) of 92 health professionals including physiotherapists found that 50% reported they used quota-contingent pacing as part of their clinical practice, whereas just 5.4% used the envelope theory and 12% used adaptive pacing, both of which are types of symptom-contingent pacing.

A randomized controlled trial (5) compared the effectiveness of symptom-contingent pacing against quota-contingent pacing methods in ME/CFS. Over 600 people with ME/CFS diagnosed with the basic Oxford Criteria, which does not include post exertional malaise (PEM) (see chapter 1), were split into groups of:

- 'simple, non-incremental pacing' (activities are planned to balance activity and rest)
- 'simple incremental pacing' (a gradual and planned increase in physical activity or exercise)
- 'complex incremental pacing' (a combination of simple pacing, incremental pacing and targeting cognitions and behaviours to encourage extension of physical functioning)
- 'specialist medical care' (a control group).

The trial suggested that simple, non-incremental pacing was no more effective than specialist medical care, whereas incremental methods produced moderately improved outcomes. However, the pacing approaches used in this trial have been criticized as being too ambiguous (6) and there have been numerous critiques of the quality of the trial itself, leading many to disregard its findings. More discussion of these critiques can be found in chapter 17.

Quota-contingent pacing involves incremental increases in activity and therefore its principles of treatment align with those of graded exercise therapy, where gradual improvements are expected and activities should continue regardless of symptom exacerbation because the body will 'adjust' (7). While this principle may be appropriate for many conditions, if a person with ME/CFS is encouraged to increase activity levels irrespective of their symptoms the likelihood is they will repeatedly trigger PEM and experience further symptom exacerbation. More reasons why a graded approach is not suitable for people with ME/CFS are discussed in chapters 6 and 17.

Symptom-contingent pacing focuses on the reduction of symptom exacerbation. In the survey of health professionals (3), only 0.1% used pacing to conserve energy and 1.7% used it to reduce symptoms; however for people with ME/CFS the primary aim of pacing should be to reduce symptoms and allow for as much function as possible within their available energy.

Physiotherapists should therefore recognize that their typical understanding of pacing may not be the most appropriate technique for people with ME/CFS, and that for this group of people energy management is not a treatment designed to make structured improvement: it is a strategy to avoid symptom exacerbation and maximize function and quality of life.

As the concept of symptom-contingent pacing aligns with appropriate energy management strategies for people with ME/CFS, this type of pacing will be included under the term 'energy management' for the remainder of this chapter.

Energy management for people with ME/CFS

PEM is the hallmark feature of ME/CFS and involves the addition of symptoms or increase of current symptoms in response to physical, cognitive, sensory and emotional exertion (8). More information regarding PEM can be found in chapter 6. The purpose of energy management is to help people with ME/CFS use their available energy while minimizing the risk of PEM.

Energy management is a self-management strategy that involves managing a person's activities to stay within their energy envelope (1). An 'energy envelope' describes the amount of perceived energy a person has available to use without triggering an increase in their symptoms. If a person with ME/CFS only expends the energy available within their 'envelope' it is thought that they may then reduce the frequency and severity of their symptoms (9). To achieve an optimal level of activity, a person should not over-expend or under-expend their energy supplies but aim to remain within their energy boundaries (10).

The evidence base for the effectiveness of energy management in people with ME/CFS is limited. A series of case studies have suggested that staying within the energy envelope is an effective mechanism to decrease symptom exacerbation in people with ME/CFS (11) (12). Additionally, a small cohort study (13) of 30 people with ME/CFS looked at the use of a buddy to assist with basic life tasks that were too physically or cognitively demanding in order to reduce over-exertion. The results showed that those who received the buddy intervention had significantly greater reductions in fatigue severity than individuals in a control group without support, suggesting the intervention enabled people with ME/CFS to reduce over-exertion and possibly remain within their energy envelopes, although the amount of energy expenditure was not measured.

One study (10) attempted to formalize measurement of energy management by asking 110 people with ME/CFS to rate on a 100-point scale the amount of energy they perceived they had available and the amount of energy they actually expended. The researchers then created a percentage daily 'energy quotient' by dividing the expended energy by the perceived energy and multiplying this by 100. An energy quotient of less than 100 meant that individuals had expended less than their perceived energy, whereas a quotient of greater than 100 indicated that they had expended more energy than their perceived available energy. The study found that 86% of participants had a daily energy quotient greater than 100, which indicated they were expending more energy than they perceived they had available.

The study also tracked symptom severity and found statistically significant links between higher energy quotients and higher severity rankings for PEM and fatigue, which suggests that people were experiencing symptom exacerbation when they expended energy beyond their perceived energy envelope.

The 'energy quotient' was later used to track four groups totalling over 450 people with ME/CFS who demonstrated PEM, finding again that people who exceeded their energy envelope ended up with increasing symptom severity (14). This study also found that those who had a high level of functioning from a 'larger' envelope would demonstrate similar symptom severity if they exceeded the envelope compared to those with very low levels of function, suggesting that over-exertion was particularly impactful on people who had higher levels of functioning, and therefore the energy envelope theory may be of most benefit to people with milder levels of ME/CFS.

Although the evidence base for energy management is limited, the strategy is frequently reported as one of the most useful approaches by people with ME/CFS (2) (15). Online surveys have shown that of 4000 responses, 'pacing' was rated very strongly as the most effective form of management (16) and 45% of 1000 respondents reported 'pacing' improved their symptoms, although 14% reported their symptoms were made worse (17). An analysis of multiple surveys (18) gave a sample size of 18,000 and found that pacing was considered the most beneficial treatment, with 82% of people with ME/CFS reporting symptom improvement. However, surveys involve a self-selected group of respondents and therefore may contain selection bias, and it is often unclear what form of pacing or energy management was implemented or what ME/CFS diagnostic criteria was used for each respondent.

How to support energy management
Gathering information
There is no single energy management plan that will benefit every person with ME/CFS. A suitable plan will depend on many factors, so prior to a discussion on energy management the following information should be obtained:

- symptom severity
- known triggers of PEM
- current responsibilities (e.g. work, children, pets, care duties)
- level of support available to the person (e.g. family support, carers, financial stability)

- their individual priorities
- what energy management techniques have already been tried and whether they were helpful.

Establish what the person's current routine is, making sure to include activities that involve physical, cognitive, sensory and emotional exertion, as these activities may be potential causes of PEM. The person may already be able to identify which activities cause them particular problems, or there may not be an obvious cause. In this case, a longer period of activity and symptom tracking may be beneficial, and the use of a heart rate monitor may help to identify activities that cause physical exertion. More information on heart rate monitoring can be found in chapter 16.

Simply gathering this amount of information may be enough to cause cognitive exertion and trigger PEM, so consider methods of obtaining information outside of an in-person interaction, for example sending a questionnaire beforehand that can be completed within the person's own timeframe. More suggestions for pre-assessment information gathering are in chapter 14.

Energy priorities

An analogy of an 'energy savings bank' has been proposed in which a person with ME/CFS creates four energy 'accounts' (19). The 'primary account' is energy for the essential activities of daily living, such as personal care and nutrition. An 'emergency conserve' should be built in to deal with any unexpected events. A 'sharing budget' consists of energy that should be used for social interaction. And, finally, there should be an 'energy savings investment' in which good quality rest will help to minimize symptom exacerbation and 'invest in future health'. This final concept of staying within energy limits to improve future health has been demonstrated in a study that found people with ME/CFS had improved functioning over time when they adopted energy management strategies that helped them to stay within their energy envelope (10).

Rest

The concept of rest is different to that of sleep. Rest is considered to be multifaceted, with one paper describing three components (20):

- physical – a lack of movement

- mental – freedom from 'anything that wearies'
- spiritual – creating harmony and calm.

Considering that the potential triggers of PEM are physical, cognitive, sensory and emotional, it is clear that true rest can be a means to avoid symptom exacerbation. If a person with ME/CFS already schedules in rest periods, it is important to clarify what they do during this time. Some people may only recognize the physical aspects of rest and will include a cognitive or sensory activity that may involve reading, watching or listening. If cognitive or sensory exertion is a trigger of their symptoms, then they may not realize they are not actually resting and should be advised to reduce all stimulation for true restorative rest.

Rest can sometimes be resisted by people because it can be seen as too passive. A person with many responsibilities may feel incredible guilt for resting and instead push themselves. By reframing rest as a strategy for dealing with symptoms, a physiotherapist can help the person to understand the importance of rest and incorporate it into their management plan.

Energy management techniques

There are many strategies to manage activities within energy limits (8) (19) (21). The list provided in Table 15.1 should be seen as a selection of ideas rather than a rigid set of instructions, and it is important to consider that there is currently very little evidence to support the effectiveness of any of these interventions. As with any management strategy for people with ME/CFS, there should be a constant monitoring of symptoms in response to a change or addition to routine, and management should always be individualized.

Table 15.1 Energy management techniques

Adapting the schedule Changing the order of a person's routine and building in rest periods can help to lessen exertion and therefore lessen triggers for PEM	Build in rest periods between activities that have been identified as key triggers for PEM
	Alternate physical and cognitive activities (remembering that cognitive activities may be just as exertional)
	Alternate body positions, for example lying, sitting or standing

Adapting activities Activities could be adapted in several ways in order to reduce the amount of energy required to complete them	Split activities into smaller components with rests in between Reduce hours and/or location of school/work Change the position that an activity is carried out in, e.g. sitting rather than standing, avoiding overhead positions
Energy monitoring Keeping track of how much energy has been used, or how exertional a task is, can help a person to monitor their expenditure and know when they should take a break	Heart rate monitoring (see chapter 16) Step-counter 'Spoon theory' in which energy units are counted as 'spoons' with each task using up a spoon (22) Wrist bands representing available energy, moving them to the opposite wrist after each exertional task Timer/alarm Apps (several apps for smart devices now exist to help track energy expenditure) Activity and symptom diary for longer-term tracking The Borg scale of perceived exertion can provide instant subjective indication of fatigue levels (23)
Adaptive aids and equipment Specialist equipment can lessen energy expenditure. If provision of this type of equipment is outside of scope of practice, consider referral to occupational therapists for specialist input	Perching stool (bathroom/kitchen) Shower chair/stool Commode (reduce distance to toilet) Stair lift Wheelchair/mobility scooter
Assistive technology/devices These tools and gadgets can reduce the amount of energy required to complete a task, or limit how much a person would need to get up (which may also help with orthostatic intolerance symptoms)	Electric can opener Electric toothbrush Kettle tipper Smart lighting Smart doorbells Smart technology for curtains/blinds

cont.

Cognitive aids Aids and task adaptations can help to reduce cognitive exertion and account for cognitive dysfunction	Have allocated places for items such as keys, money, medication, phone Use task/'to do' lists Keep notepads in key places to jot down important information Use labels to identify where items are stored Use a journal as a memory aid Use wallcharts/calendars to track daily events and appointments Utilize smart technology to set reminders and alarms
Adaptations to meals When a person with ME/CFS does not have support for meal preparation, there are several adaptations that can be made to help lessen the energy expenditure required	Buy frozen, pre-chopped ingredients Batch-cook on quieter days so meals are ready for busy days/symptom flares Online shopping reduces physical exertion and a single shop can be split into smaller chunks to limit cognitive exertion Use a slow cooker/pressure cooker Prepare bags of ingredients in advance that can be emptied into a slow cooker/pot
Additional support Hiring people to provide support, either for personal care or general household tasks, may be a necessity for some people with ME/CFS but also involves significant cost. Supporting access to financial aid may be beneficial	Carers or personal assistants for personal care or administration tasks Cleaners/gardeners

Kim: 'My physiotherapist has given me pacing advice, reminders and practical tips. If events or commitments are coming up, I ensure I rest in advance and have recovery time afterwards.'

It is important to note that energy management requires a great deal of patience and dedication. A person with ME/CFS may have to sacrifice or compromise on activities that are very meaningful to them, so any discussion about energy management techniques should be carried out with professionalism, compassion and an understanding that while the advice being provided may help the person to manage their symptoms, it may also result in a complete change to their life.

Energy management during relapse/remission

As discussed in chapter 1 it is common for symptoms of ME/CFS to fluctuate over time. The energy envelope may be changeable and a person with ME/CFS may experience periods of time in which they are able to achieve more, and periods when they are unable to manage as much. Strategies for energy management are therefore not fixed, and a physiotherapist can have a beneficial role by providing guidance and support over time, depending on how symptom severity fluctuates.

Oliver: 'Pacing is hard to describe because it is not something that just happens instantly – it is a constant thing that you have to work on, and lots of trial and error.'

A person with ME/CFS may need support to further adapt activities during a period of increased symptom severity, or they may seek guidance on ways to increase their activity safely if their energy envelope has increased. Symptoms should always be closely monitored and evaluated with any changes to a person's activity levels to check that PEM is not being triggered.

Limitations of energy management

While energy management has been identified as one of the most beneficial strategies for people with ME/CFS, there are limitations. Estimating the energy available can be very difficult (19), demonstrated by the study detailed earlier in this chapter in which 86% of 110 people with ME/CFS were found to have exceeded their perceived energy limits (10). Relying on symptom behaviour to know when a person is exerting too much is not possible considering PEM is usually a delayed response, often by days, and a perception of effort can be altered in some people with ME/CFS, which is discussed further in chapter 7. Heart rate monitoring can be a useful real-time measure of exertion, although this is also not without its limitations. Further information on heart rate monitoring is in chapter 16.

While planning and prioritizing is recommended, the approach is not so simple considering the fluctuating nature of ME/CFS combined with potential unexpected events such as new infections or situations requiring urgent action. A person may have responsibilities, child or elder care for example, that make many energy management practices completely infeasible.

Energy management techniques may also be irrelevant for people with severe or very severe ME/CFS, where symptom severity is so extreme that they are unable to carry out any activities of daily living without causing symptom exacerbation. People with severe and very severe ME/CFS do not appear to have been included in any of the research around energy management and pacing, so all conclusions from current evidence cannot be applied to this group. Severe and very severe ME/CFS are discussed further in chapter 3.

Mo: 'My energy management involves batch cooking and online shopping, using alarms as reminders to take a break from the computer, and equipment like a shower chair and perching stool to make tasks easier.'

A physiotherapist should understand that energy management is one tool for helping people with ME/CFS maximize their quality of life while minimizing symptom exacerbation, but it is not always easy, practical or beneficial.

SUMMARY

- ▸ 'Energy management', 'activity management' and 'symptom-contingent pacing' are all terms that describe the same strategy: to minimize energy expenditure in order to reduce symptom exacerbation while maximizing their functional abilities.
- ▸ Other types of pacing are commonly used by physiotherapists that focus on increasing activity, often in set increments. This type of pacing is not appropriate for people with ME/CFS due to the nature of PEM.
- ▸ Energy management involves strategies to adapt activities to lessen energy expenditure, which may include use of aids, equipment and technology.

APPLICATION TO PRACTICE

- ▸ Energy management is one potential tool to consider for symptom management when working with people who have ME/CFS.
- ▸ The aim of energy management is to reduce symptom exacerbation by working within the energy envelope.

▶ Planning energy management strategies should be a collaborative project between the physiotherapist and the person with ME/CFS.

References

1. National Institute for Health and Care Excellence (2021) 'Myalgic encephalomyelitis (or encephalopathy)/chronic fatigue syndrome: diagnosis and management.' Accessed on 2/12/2022 at www.nice.org.uk/guidance/ng206.
2. Goudsmit, E.M., Nijs, J., Jason, L.A. & Wallman, K.E. (2012) 'Pacing as a strategy to improve energy management in myalgic encephalomyelitis/chronic fatigue syndrome: a consensus document.' *Disability and Rehabilitation 34* (13).
3. Antcliff, D., Keenan, A.M., Keeley, P., Woby, S. & McGowan, L. (2019) 'Survey of activity pacing across healthcare professionals informs a new activity pacing framework for chronic pain/fatigue.' *Musculoskeletal Care 17* (4).
4. Gill, J.R. & Brown, C.A. (2009) 'A structured review of the evidence for pacing as a chronic pain intervention.' *European Journal of Pain 13* (2).
5. White, P.D., Goldsmith, K.A., Johnson, A.L., Potts, L., Walwyn, R. & DeCesare, J.C. (2011) 'Comparison of adaptive pacing therapy, cognitive behaviour therapy, graded exercise therapy, and specialist medical care for chronic fatigue syndrome (PACE): a randomised trial.' *The Lancet 377* (9768).
6. Jason, L.A. (2017) 'The PACE trial missteps on pacing and patient selection.' *Journal of Health Psychology 22* (9).
7. Bavinton, J., Darbishire, L. & White, P.D. (2004) *Graded Exercise Therapy for CFS/ME: Manual for Therapists.* Final Trial Version: Version 7 (MREC Version 2). Accessed on 12/01/2023 at https://me-pedia.org/wiki/PACE_trial_documents.
8. Bateman, L., Bested, A.C., Bonilla, H.F., Chheda, B.V., *et al.* (2021) 'Myalgic encephalomyelitis/chronic fatigue syndrome: essentials of diagnosis and management.' *Mayo Clinic Proceedings 96* (11).
9. Jason, L., Muldowney, K. & Torres-Harding, S. (2008) 'The energy envelope theory and myalgic encephalomyelitis/chronic fatigue syndrome.' *American Association of Occupational Health Nurses Journal 56* (5).
10. Jason, L. & Benton, M. (2009) 'The impact of energy modulation on physical functioning and fatigue severity among patients with ME/CFS.' *Patient Education and Counseling 77* (2).
11. Pesek, J.R., Jason, L.A. & Taylor, R.R. (2000) 'An empirical investigation of the envelope theory.' *Journal of Human Behavior in the Social Environment 3* (1).
12. Jason, L.A., Melrose, H., Lerman, A., Burroughs, V., *et al.* (1999) 'Managing chronic fatigue syndrome: overview and case study.' *American Association of Occupational Health Nurses Journal 47* (1).
13. Jason, L.A., Roesner, N., Porter, N., Parenti, B., Mortensen, J. & Till, L. (2010) 'Provision of social support to individuals with chronic fatigue syndrome.' *Journal of Clinical Psychology 66* (3).
14. O'Connor, K., Sunnquist, M., Nicholson, L., Jason, L.A., Newton, J.L. & Strand, E.B. (2019) 'Energy envelope maintenance among patients with myalgic encephalomyelitis and chronic fatigue syndrome: implications of limited energy reserves.' *Chronic Illness.*
15. Jason, L.A., Brown, M., Brown, A., Evans, M., *et al.* (2013) 'Energy conservation/envelope theory interventions to help patients with chronic fatigue syndrome.' *Fatigue 1* (1–2).
16. ME Association (2008) *Managing My ME. What People with ME and Their Carers Want from the UK's Health and Social Services.* London: ME Association.
17. ME Association (2015) *ME/CFS Illness Management Survey Results: No Decision about Me without Me.* London: ME Association.

18. Geraghty, K., Hann, M. & Kurtev, S. (2019) 'Myalgic encephalomyelitis/chronic fatigue syndrome patients' reports of symptom changes following cognitive behavioural therapy, graded exercise therapy and pacing treatments: analysis of a primary survey compared with secondary surveys.' *Journal of Health Psychology 24* (10).

19. Carruthers, B.M., van de Sande, M.I., De Meirleir, K.L., Klimas, N.G., *et al.* (2012) *Myalgic Encephalomyelitis – Adult & Paediatric: International Consensus Primer for Medical Practitioners.* Accessed on 12/01/2023 at www.investinme.org/Documents/Guidelines/Myalgic Encephalomyelitis International Consensus Primer -2012-11-26.pdf.

20. Nurit, W. & Michal, A.B. (2003) 'Rest: a qualitative exploration of the phenomenon.' *Occupational Therapy International 10* (4).

21. Friedberg, F., Sunnquist, M. & Nacul, L. (2019) 'Rethinking the standard of care for myalgic encephalomyelitis/chronic fatigue syndrome.' *Journal of General Internal Medicine 35* (3).

22. Miserandino, C. (2003) *The Spoon Theory: But You Don't Look Sick.* Accessed on 2/12/2022 at https://cdn.totalcomputersusa.com/butyoudontlooksick.com/uploads/2010/02/BYDLS-TheSpoonTheory.pdf.

23. Balady, G.J., Arena, R., Sietsema, K., Myers, J., *et al.* (2010) 'Clinician's guide to cardiopulmonary exercise testing in adults: a scientific statement from the American Heart Association.' *Circulation 122* (2).

CHAPTER 16

Pacing with a Heart Rate Monitor

PURPOSE OF THIS CHAPTER

Energy management is a key strategy for people with ME/CFS to manage their daily activities within their energy envelope (see chapter 15) to avoid triggering post exertional malaise (PEM). However, staying within energy limits can be difficult as PEM is often a delayed response to exertion. Pacing with a heart rate monitor offers people with ME/CFS an objective way of managing activity in 'real time' to reduce PEM, and the approach can be utilized either as a long-term management strategy or as part of a physiotherapy assessment process.

This chapter describes the physiological basis of pacing with heart rate monitors, how to use this approach and the potential benefits and difficulties. A physiotherapist needs to understand the principles of pacing with a heart rate monitor in order to support people with ME/CFS to successfully use this management strategy.

Physiological basis for heart rate monitoring

Pacing with a heart rate monitor is an approach that involves the use of a wearable device to monitor the heart rate during activity with the aim to either remain below or minimize the time spent in anaerobic metabolism. As repeated exertion at this level appears to cause further deterioration in performance that is reflective of PEM, then theoretically if a person with ME/CFS avoids or minimizes activity levels that cause them to work anaerobically, they may help to avoid or minimize PEM.

The transition from aerobic to anaerobic metabolism is referred to by terms such as 'lactate threshold', 'heart rate deflection point' and 'ventilatory anaerobic threshold' (VAT) (1). This threshold can be observed using cardiopulmonary exercise testing (CPET) (2), which is discussed further in chapter 6.

Faith: 'I set off my heart rate monitor doing basic things like brushing my teeth! It is almost impossible to live my life within a set limit, but the monitor has helped me to identify when I need to take a moment to rest, and I use it as an objective marker to show my family how I'm feeling, which helps them to understand why I might have to stop an activity.'

During exercise testing, people with ME/CFS transition into anaerobic metabolism more quickly compared to controls who are age and sex matched, and they show further deterioration in performance on a repeated test 24 hours later (3). This deterioration in performance is the hallmark feature of people with ME/CFS and may be indicative of PEM (4).

It is not possible to identify the levels of gaseous exchange to determine when a person is using anaerobic metabolism without appropriate equipment and analysis from a CPET. However, the rate at which the heart beats, measured in number of beats per minute, tends to increase linearly with all other measures of cardiovascular function (4) (5) and the heart rate can be measured using accessible wearable devices. Therefore, monitoring the heart rate can be a practical 'real-time' measure to estimate when a person is working towards anaerobic metabolism.

It is important to recognize that using a heart rate monitor for people with ME/CFS is very different to using a heart rate monitor for exercise prescription in other populations. For example, in most populations exercise intensity can be set using 'target heart rate zones' with the aim to train at or around the anaerobic threshold to improve cardiovascular fitness (6) (1). Exercise prescription for the general population suggests working at 40–60% of maximal heart rate for 'moderate intensity' and exceeding 60% for 'vigorous intensity' (5).

However, for people with ME/CFS, heart rate monitors are used for the opposite reason: to inform when a person may be exerting too much so that they can reduce their workload to avoid or minimize the time spent in anaerobic metabolism. This enables them to identify when to reduce activity levels to avoid or minimize PEM.

Evidence for pacing with a heart rate monitor

There is currently limited evidence for pacing with a heart rate monitor. A published case study (7) determined the VAT of a person with ME/CFS using a two-day CPET, then implemented pacing with a heart rate monitor alongside a flexibility and strengthening programme. After one year the participant was able to complete daily activities without symptoms, with improvements in maximum oxygen consumption (VO_2) and maximum minute ventilation (VE). As this is a single case study the results cannot be generalized to the wider population of people with ME/CFS.

Despite the current lack of research, pacing with a heart rate monitor is an approach used by many people with ME/CFS. An international survey sought experiences of using a heart rate monitor to pace from people with ME/CFS (8) and received 488 responses with over 30 benefits reported, including:

- the approach allowed them to understand their PEM triggers (72%)
- the approach helped them to minimize PEM (57%)
- the use of heart rate monitors helped to raise the awareness of those around them of the effects of activity on their heart rate (52%).

One of the main negatives reported in the survey was the cost of buying a wearable device (43%) and the lack of support from healthcare providers in setting up and managing a heart rate monitor as part of an energy management plan (57%).

Using a heart rate monitor to pace is an area that requires more research in order to understand the approach further so that health professionals such as physiotherapists can provide evidence-based support to people with ME/CFS.

Determining a heart rate limit for use in pacing

There is limited evidence supporting a definitive approach to the use of heart rate monitors to pace. The first parameter is determining the level of heart rate at which a limit will be set, and whether the person will try to always keep below the limit or aim to minimize the time spent above the limit. People with ME/CFS have reported using a variety of methods to determine the heart rate at which they set a limit (8).

Cardiopulmonary exercise test (CPET)

A CPET can be used to estimate the heart rate at which a person enters anaerobic metabolism (2). To more closely reflect PEM a repeated two-day CPET is required with measurements taken on the second test to determine heart rate limits. However, the nature of a CPET would push a person with ME/CFS into a level of physical exertion that would cause PEM and could therefore be detrimental.

A CPET can only give information about the person's response to that particular task, often a treadmill or exercise bike with increasing speed or resistance, and only provide information about the person on the day of testing. The results may therefore not necessarily be generalizable to typical activities of daily life or reflect the fluctuating nature of ME/CFS. The resources for a CPET are also not generally available in clinical practice. In the international survey just 3.8% of respondents had used a CPET to determine their heart rate limit (8).

Resting heart rate plus 15 beats per minute

The Workwell Foundation, a team of exercise physiologists based in the USA who are specialists in ME/CFS, report based on their experience that people with ME/CFS enter anaerobic metabolism at just 15 beats above their resting heart rate (9). They recommend determining the resting heart rate from an average of measurements taken over seven days, with the person measuring their heart rate after waking when they are still flat in bed. In the international survey 13.7% of respondents used this method (8). However, limiting activities to just 15 beats per minute above resting heart rate may be very restrictive and potentially impractical, which is discussed in the 'Limitations' section of this chapter.

Percentage of maximal heart rate

A limit can be set by working out a percentage of the maximum heart rate. The maximal heart rate is the highest number of beats per minute that a heart can contract in an individual, which will vary across age, sex and fitness levels. A common method of calculating maximal heart rate (10) is using the equation: 220 − age. For example, a 50-year-old's maximal heart rate would be: 220 − 50 = 170.

However, this calculation was based on data from stress tests on healthy young males and cannot therefore be generalized to women or older adults (10)(11). A revised calculation based on a wider spread of data was developed (10) that included both sexes and is presented as: 208 − (0.7 × age). For example, the maximal heart rate of a 50-year-old would be: 208 − (0.7 × 50) = 173.

A later calculation was developed specifically for women and presented as (11): 206 − (0.88 × age). For example, the maximal heart rate of a 50-year-old woman would be: 206 − (0.88 × 50) = 162.

Some people may take medications that act to lower the rate heart such as beta-adrenergic blockade therapy (beta blockers). A subsequent calculation (12) was devised for people on this type of medication as: 164 − (0.7 × age). For example, the maximal heart rate of a 50-year-old on beta blockers would be: 164 − (0.7 × 50) = 129.

In the international survey, people with ME/CFS reported setting a limit using a percentage of their maximum heart rates (using the standard calculation of 220 − age), with a variety of percentages reported including 60% of the maximum heart rate (used by 19% of respondents), 55% (used by 10.3%) and 50% (used by 11.7%) (8).

Given the lack of specificity of calculating an accurate maximum heart rate, as well as no defined guidance on what percentage of the maximum heart rate should be used, these calculations should be seen as suggestions rather than prescriptions.

Heart rate variability

Heart rate variability (HRV) describes the variability of the interval between consecutive heart beats (13). HRV has been shown to have good reliability in measuring autonomic function, with a high variability indicating a healthy system and a low variability suggesting some autonomic dysfunction (14). HRV is discussed in more detail in chapter 12.

Some wearable devices can measure HRV and some people with ME/CFS have used this measurement as part of their energy management strategies. In the international survey (8) 53.7% of respondents used HRV to help guide their pacing by taking a reading on waking and comparing it to their normal values, with a lower than normal reading suggesting they may need to prioritize rest more that day. However, there is currently no published research on the use of HRV in pacing for people with ME/CFS, and some respondents in the survey report that the method can be inconsistent with their symptoms or simply too complicated to analyse (8).

Physiotherapy support for pacing with a heart rate monitor

While pacing with a heart rate monitor is currently not an evidence-based strategy, it is still beneficial for a physiotherapist to consider because it provides a non-invasive method of obtaining objective data and it is already being used successfully by some people with ME/CFS. In the international survey (8) the biggest limitation of using a heart rate monitor to pace was the lack of support from medical professionals for the approach, which was identified by 57% of respondents. If physiotherapists incorporated the approach into their management plans then they could offer further support to people with ME/CFS.

Given there are no set protocols for pacing with a heart rate monitor, a physiotherapist should use a collaborative approach with the person with ME/CFS to determine how heart rate monitors may add the most value to their lives.

How will the heart rate monitor be used?

A heart rate monitor could be utilized in two ways:

1. as part of an assessment process, worn in the short-term to allow the person to learn about their physical limitations and abilities with objective real-time information (this process may allow the person to identify key activities that may be causing exertion, which could then be modified as part of the energy management plan).
2. as a component of an energy management plan, used long term to manage daily activities.

A trial period may be required before the person with ME/CFS decides whether the approach will suit them in the long term. Even used short term, a heart rate monitor can be helpful to validate the person's experiences with objective data, providing real-time feedback on the effects of daily activities (8).

A heart rate monitor could also provide real-time information on whether a person with ME/CFS is tolerating a physiotherapy intervention, which could be helpful if introducing anything new to the person's routine or trying a new strategy for symptom management.

Selecting a wearable device

Heart rate monitors are widely available and can vary significantly in price and function. There is currently no wearable device designed specifically for people with ME/CFS. In the international survey over 100 different types of wearable device were reported (8).

Heart rate monitors can be worn on the wrist or paired with a strap across the chest or arm. In terms of accuracy, wrist-worn devices can measure accurate heart rate at rest but lose accuracy as the intensity of exertion increases (15). Chest straps have been shown to have more accuracy, particularly during vigorous exercise (15) (16). However, these studies involved healthy adults tested during strenuous exercise and will not be reflective of the daily activities of a person with ME/CFS.

Kim: 'I take heart rate variability measurements each morning as an objective measure of my level of energy. I use this to adjust my usual pacing regime and have found it very helpful as a way to get some objective feedback.'

In the international survey (8) 83% of respondents used a wrist-worn device, whereas only 12.3% paired a wrist device with a chest strap. Some respondents found chest straps uncomfortable to wear or struggled with more complex technology due to their cognitive dysfunction (8).

It is important for a physiotherapist to understand the variety of wearable devices so that they can support a person with ME/CFS in selecting a wearable device that would be more appropriate for them.

Setting a limit/measurement

As described earlier in this chapter there is no standardized method for determining the level of heart rate that will be used as a limit. A physiotherapist should collaborate with the person with ME/CFS to decide which method to use. This may depend on the severity of the person's symptoms, their priorities and responsibilities, whether they have any co-morbidities or are on any medications that affect their heart rate, and their personal approach to risk.

It is helpful to establish a way to collect data on symptoms and activities, for example a diary or brief notes, so that they can be analysed after a few weeks of trying pacing with a heart rate monitor. At this point the current settings can be evaluated and adapted based on information such as:

- Were symptoms reduced or exacerbated, or was there no change?
- Were activities limited too much?
- Did they feel they could increase their workload without triggering symptoms, or was the limit at a point that caused PEM and needs to be lowered further?
- Did the person find the use of a heart rate monitor helpful?

This information may indicate whether the heart rate limit should be altered, identify any key activities that could be modified as part of an energy management plan, and facilitate a discussion about whether heart rate monitoring would be a beneficial approach for that individual going forwards.

Limitations of pacing with a heart rate monitor

As well as the lack of evidence base for this approach, there are several limitations of pacing with a heart rate monitor.

- Wearable devices incur a sizeable cost, and in the international survey of people with ME/CFS, 43% reported this as a negative of using a heart rate monitor to pace (8).
- Using heart rate as a limit can place significant restrictions on a person's daily life, and 43% of respondents in the international survey found this a negative aspect of the approach, while 31% reported they found the device was continually alerting them (8).
- Cognitive exertion is rarely identified with heart rate monitors (8), so while this approach can be useful for managing physical exertion, a wider energy management approach should also consider cognitive, sensory and emotional triggers. See chapter 15 for more information regarding energy management.
- Orthostatic intolerances such as postural orthostatic tachycardia syndrome (POTS) are a common co-morbidity of people with ME/CFS and can involve altered or exaggerated heart rates

in standing – see chapter 2 for more information. Common medications for POTS, such as beta blockers, work to lower the heart rate. In these situations, determining a suitable heart rate limit can be challenging and limits may need to be over - or under-exaggerated depending on symptoms and medications.

· Some people with ME/CFS have sensory intolerances and can find wearing something around their chest, arm or wrist too uncomfortable to tolerate.

· The constant monitoring of heart rate can cause heightened anxiety or become an obsession for some people, with 27% reporting that they found the alerts they received when exceeding their limits too stressful (8).

SUMMARY

▸ People with ME/CFS may experience PEM after physical exertion, often when they have worked in anaerobic metabolism.

▸ People with ME/CFS may work in anaerobic metabolism at a lower level of exertion than the healthy population, and with repeated exertion they may experience further deterioration in their symptoms.

▸ Pacing with a heart rate monitor is an approach that involves the use of a wearable device to monitor the heart rate in order to minimize or avoid time spent in anaerobic metabolism, and potentially minimize or avoid PEM.

▸ Heart rate variability can also be used as a daily comparison to anticipate PEM and monitor dysfunction in the autonomic nervous system.

▸ There are many benefits to using heart rate monitors for pacing, including understanding exertional triggers and reducing PEM, but there are also a number of limitations.

APPLICATION TO PRACTICE

▸ A heart rate monitor could be an objective measure of the suitability of any physiotherapy intervention.

▶ Using a heart rate monitor to pace could be an assessment tool, or a longer-term approach as part of an energy management plan.

▶ There is no standard protocol for pacing with a heart rate monitor, therefore the approach should be devised in collaboration with the person with ME/CFS and regularly monitored and evaluated so that the most beneficial set-up is established.

References

1. Ghosh, A.K. (2004) 'Anaerobic threshold: its concept and role in endurance sport.' *Malaysian Journal of Medical Sciences 11* (1).
2. Albouaini, K., Egred, M., Alahmar, A. & Wright, D.J. (2007) ' Cardiopulmonary exercise testing and its application.' *Postgraduate Medical Journal 83* (985).
3. Davenport, T.E., Stevens, S.R., Stevens, J., Snell, C.R. & Van Ness, J.M. (2020) 'Properties of measurements obtained during cardiopulmonary exercise testing in individuals with myalgic encephalomyelitis/chronic fatigue syndrome.' *Work 66* (2).
4. Davenport, T.E., Lehnen, M., Stevens, S.R., VanNess, J.M., Stevens, J. & Snell, C.R. (2019) 'Chronotropic intolerance: an overlooked determinant of symptoms and activity limitation in myalgic encephalomyelitis/chronic fatigue syndrome?' *Frontiers in Pediatrics 7* (82).
5. Balady, G.J., Arena, R., Sietsema, K., Myers, J., *et al.* (2010) 'Clinician's guide to cardiopulmonary exercise testing in adults: a scientific statement from the American Heart Association.' *Circulation 122* (2).
6. Davis, J.A., Frank, M.H., Whipp, B.J. & Wasserman, K. (1979) 'Anaerobic threshold alterations caused by endurance training in middle-aged men.' *Journal of Applied Physiology 46* (6).
7. Stevens, S.R. & Davenport, T.E. (2010) 'Functional outcomes of anaerobic rehabilitation in an individual with chronic fatigue syndrome: case report with 1-year follow-up.' *Bulletin of the International Association for Chronic Fatigue Syndrome/ Myalgic Encephalomyelitis 18* (3).
8. Clague-Baker, N., Davenport, T., Mohammad, M., Dickinson, K., Leslie, K., Bull, M. & Hilliard, N. (2023) 'An international survey of experiences and attitudes towards pacing using a heart rate monitor for people with myalgic encephalomyelitis/ chronic fatigue syndrome.' Pre-press: 1–10. Accessed on 19/04/2022 at https:// content.iospress.com/articles/work/wor220512.
9. Workwell Foundation (2022) 'ME/CFS activity management with a heart rate monitor.' Workwell Foundation. Accessed on 3/12/2022 at https://workwellfoundation. org/wp-content/uploads/2021/03/HRM-Factsheet.pdf.
10. Tanaka, H., Monahan, K.D. & Seals, D.R. (2001) 'Age-predicted maximal heart rate revisited.' *Journal of the American College of Cardiology 37* (1).
11. Gulati, M., Shaw, L.J., Thisted, R.A., Black, H.R., Bairey Merz, C.N. & Arnsdorf, M.F. (2010) 'Heart rate response to exercise stress testing in asymptomatic women: the St. James Women Take Heart Project.' *Circulation 122* (2).
12. Brawner, C.A., Ehrman, J.K., Schairer, J.R., Cao, J.J. & Keteyian, S.J. (2004) 'Predicting maximum heart rate among patients with coronary heart disease receiving beta-adrenergic blockade therapy.' *American Heart Journal 148* (5).
13. Tracy, L.M., Ioannou, L., Baker, K.S., Gibson, S.J., Georgiou-Karistianis, N. & Giummarra, M. (2016) 'Meta-analytic evidence for decreased heart rate variability in chronic pain implicating parasympathetic nervous system dysregulation.' *Pain 157* (1).

14. Bertsch, K., Hagemann, D., Naumann, E., Schächinger, H. & Schulz, A. (2012) 'Stability of heart rate variability indices reflecting parasympathetic activity.' *Psychophysiology 49* (5).
15. Pasadyn, S.R., Soudan, M., Gillinov, M., Houghtaling, P., *et al.* (2019) 'Accuracy of commercially available heart rate monitors in athletes: a prospective study.' *Cardiovascular Diagnosis and Therapy 9* (4).
16. Wang, R., Blackburn, G., Desai, M., Phelan, D., *et al.* (2017) 'Accuracy of wrist-worn heart rate monitors.' *JAMA Cardiology 2* (1).

CHAPTER 17

Exercise

PURPOSE OF THIS CHAPTER

All physiotherapists should be aware that a person with ME/CFS may be adversely affected by exercise.

Exercise can be defined as a purposeful and structured activity focused on the improvement or maintenance of physical fitness (1). Exercise is an example of physical activity, which is any use of the skeletal muscles that expends energy (2).

Exercise is one of the key interventions that physiotherapists use for almost any disease or presentation. Countless studies demonstrate its benefits for health, including lowering the risk of cardiovascular disease (3), preventing the deterioration of muscle mass with age (4), improving the strength and stamina of people with chronic obstructive pulmonary disease (5) and chronic heart disease (6), and even alleviating the symptoms of clinical depression (7). But for all its benefits, exercise also has the potential to cause a stress response that, when dysregulated, can be detrimental to health, for example in the form of anaphylaxis, exercise-induced asthma, overuse syndrome and an exacerbation of co-morbid conditions (8).

Given the hallmark feature of ME/CFS is post exertional malaise (PEM), which is additional symptoms or an exacerbation of current symptoms following exertion, a typical exercise-based approach has a high chance of worsening symptoms and causing harm (9). Therefore, all physiotherapists must understand the risks of exercise for people with ME/CFS regardless of whether they are working with the person directly for their ME/CFS symptoms or for an unrelated problem, for example a musculoskeletal injury or to recover from orthopaedic surgery. A physiotherapist should also make sure the person with ME/

CFS is aware of these risks to enable them to give informed consent for any intervention.

This chapter summarizes the physiological processes that occur in people with ME/CFS in response to physical exertion, explores the evidence base for different types of exercise, and discusses the key questions any physiotherapist should consider before implementing any form of exercise for a person with ME/CFS.

Effects of physical exertion on people with ME/CFS

The physiological effects of physical exertion in people with ME/CFS have been studied in laboratory conditions, usually in tests that involve working towards or at maximum effort on stationary bicycles or treadmills. Such physical exertion has been shown to elicit the following in people with ME/CFS:

- deterioration in cardiopulmonary function (10)
- early intracellular acidosis (11)
- increased intramuscular acidosis and prolonged recovery (12)
- abnormal increases in lactic acid (13)
- abnormally increased levels of oxidative stress with prolonged recovery (14)
- early fatigue with prolonged recovery (15) (16)
- decrease in general function (17)
- altered ion transport and ion channel activity (18)
- rapid increase in gene expression for detection of muscle metabolites, sympathetic nervous system processing and immune function (19)
- significant increases in activators of inflammatory immune cells (20)
- altered gut microbiome and increased bacterial translocation (21)
- reduced oxygenation of the prefrontal cortex (22)
- impaired cognitive processing (23) (17)
- decreased pain threshold (24).

More information on these responses and their role in PEM can be found in chapter 6.

Exercise as a 'treatment' for ME/CFS: graded exercise therapy

Graded exercise therapy (GET) is based on the theory that ME/CFS symptoms are maintained by physical inactivity, which causes deconditioning, further symptoms and an altered perception of effort leading to active avoidance of activity (25). Deconditioning describes a progressively reduced exercise capacity often caused by reduced physical activity (26). Exercise is used by physiotherapists as an effective method to prevent or reverse deconditioning in presentations such as post-operative deconditioning in the elderly (27), people with spinal cord injury (28) and stroke (29). Therefore the principle of GET is to reverse the deconditioning of a person with ME/CFS and subsequently increase their tolerance of physical activity (26).

Ana: 'An in-patient programme made me do 40 minutes of exercise on my first day. I relapsed so severely that I became completely bedbound and was discharged. The relapse lasted for nine months.'

GET involves establishing a baseline of physical activity then incrementally increasing the frequency, duration and intensity of physical activity and aerobic exercise (30) (25). GET uses an incremental approach, with the manual for therapists advising that people with ME/CFS should maintain exercise as much as possible during any increase of symptoms under the assurance that the body would 'habituate to the increase in activity' (25).

Compared against standard medical care, GET was reported to improve the subjective fatigue and physical function of people with ME/CFS when carried out under guidance of a trained physiotherapist (30) and shown to improve fatigue when delivered as a self-directed programme (31). On a 12-month follow-up of a randomized trial (the 'PACE' trial) a reported 22% of participants who underwent GET had made a full recovery, compared to 7% in standard care (32).

However, the quality of the evidence for the effectiveness of graded exercise therapy and its safety for people with ME/CFS has been repeatedly called into question (33) and while GET was historically included in clinical guidelines it has been subsequently removed as a treatment recommendation from guidelines in the USA (34) and the UK (1).

The effectiveness of GET is questionable on the understanding that deconditioning is not considered to be a primary cause of ME/CFS, which is discussed in chapter 7. There are also several key points of criticism for the evidence base as follows.

Participant diagnosis

Diagnosis of ME/CFS is problematic and many criteria do not include the hallmark symptom of PEM. How this affects the generalizability of results from research is discussed in detail in chapter 1.

A systematic review in 2021 grouped studies of physiotherapeutic interventions on people with ME/CFS according to the diagnostic criteria used and found no studies on GET have been carried out using a diagnostic criteria that includes PEM (35). Of note is that the large randomized controlled trial (PACE) used the Oxford Criteria (32), which do not mention PEM and are so basic they have since been recommended to be 'retired' (36).

Mirroring these findings, a Cochrane review (37) of evidence for exercise therapy in ME/CFS included eight randomized controlled trials with data from 1518 participants and concluded that while exercise therapy 'probably has a positive effect on fatigue' compared to usual care, all studies were conducted with participants diagnosed with either the Fukuda Criteria or the Oxford Criteria, and therefore people diagnosed with other criteria may experience different effects.

Outcome measures

While self-reported fatigue and physical function were reported as improved following GET in the PACE trial, the data was reanalysed by an independent group and any reported treatment effects were erased when objective measures were taken into account (33). This discrepancy between subjective and objective measures has been seen in several other studies, suggesting subjective gains do not necessarily translate into objective improvements (38). A systematic review of the evidence also noted that there was often a lack of discussion as to the clinical significance of any reported subjective gains (35).

Another outcome measure used in the PACE trial was 'return to work'. The groups involved were followed up 12 months later and there was no clear difference in lost employment levels and welfare payments between any of the interventions (39). A literature review of the effectiveness of GET was carried out in 2022 and concluded that more people were unable to work after treatment with GET (and cognitive behavioural therapy) than before (40).

Carry-over

The reported benefits of graded exercise therapy for ME/CFS fail to demonstrate significant long-term carry-over. The claims of recovery in the PACE trial have been questioned due to alterations in selection criteria midway through the study, which meant that technically a participant could deteriorate from baseline but still be counted as 'recovered' according to the study's revised parameters (9).

The improvements found with self-directed exercise have been shown to maintain on long-term follow-up, but similar improvements were also seen in a standard medical care group, meaning there was no longer a significant difference between intervention and control (41) (42).

Interpreting how improvements may happen over time is key. One study found that people with ME/CFS were able to increase their daily physical activity for four weeks (43) but when the research team reanalysed their data they realized that it was only in the first four to ten days that participants were able to meet activity targets, with a reduction in activity in the following weeks. This was compared to healthy controls who were able to increase and then maintain their activity (44).

So graded exercise therapy, or any exercise programme involving incremental increases, does not appear to have long-term benefits or carry-over for people with ME/CFS.

Adverse events

Some studies conclude that improvements can be made with exercise interventions for people with ME/CFS, but also note that many people were not able to complete the intervention. For example, one study found an individualized exercise plan reduced fatigue and improved function in people with ME/CFS but also mentioned that over 50% of participants did not tolerate the treatment (45). Another showed improved visual attention following 16 weeks of structured exercise but reported that 36% of participants were not able to complete the programme (46). This issue with adherence, alongside the discrepancies in diagnostic criteria described previously, could suggest that those who present with PEM may not be tolerating the exercise programme, whereas those who may perhaps have fatigue symptoms due to any number of other causes could be responding more favourably.

People with ME/CFS have reported deterioration resulting from GET and it has been called 'unethical' and 'potentially harmful' (47).

A review of ten surveys of people with ME/CFS from across the world found 51% of respondents reported that GET made their health worse (9), although some researchers have attributed these qualitative findings to exercise therapy delivered inappropriately under the guidance of inadequately trained physiotherapists (48).

There is currently not enough evidence to suggest that GET is a beneficial treatment for people with ME/CFS, and the underlying principles of the treatment do not align with the known pathophysiology of the condition. Therefore GET should not be implemented for people with ME/CFS.

Can people with ME/CFS exercise?

While exercise for ME/CFS does not provide a cure or treatment (49), there may still be benefits of exercise in relation to specific symptom management, as a treatment for an unrelated condition, or because exercise is important to the person. In this regard, a physiotherapist must work with the person to explore whether exercise is an appropriate intervention and in what form this will take to be safe.

Considering that the adverse physiological effects detailed in this chapter all involve exercise to the point of maximum exertion in anaerobic metabolism, it is feasible that an exercise regime working below anaerobic threshold could be tolerated by a person with ME/CFS (50). As discussed in chapter 6, it is important to note that people with ME/CFS have been found to enter anaerobic metabolism at much lower levels of exertion than the general population, with further deterioration in performance on repeated exertion. Any additional exertion to a person's daily routine should be very carefully considered within the overall approach of energy management discussed in chapter 15.

The structure of any exercise programme should also consider the fluctuating nature of ME/CFS symptoms (51). Flexibility is key. For example, one study (52) took 32 people diagnosed with ME/CFS using the Fukuda Criteria (which do not include PEM as essential) and enrolled them on a 12-week exercise programme in which the exercise session was an aerobic activity such as walking, cycling or swimming and was undertaken for between 5 and 15 minutes at a time, every other day. The programme was designed so that if a participant experienced an exacerbation of symptoms they would postpone the subsequent exercise session and reduce the intensity of follow-up sessions according to what they could manage. The study reported participants were able to adhere to the protocol. They also compared the exercise group to a stretching and relaxation programme and reported improvements in a reduction of perceived effort scores during exercise testing in the exercise group, although no significant difference in a self-rated scale of improvement between groups, final oxygen uptake values or activity levels were recorded. Of note with this study is that it used the term 'graded exercise therapy' to describe the intervention, when the intervention did not follow a structured grading programme and was instead flexible according to symptoms. Care should be taken to interpret abstracts and titles of studies in relation to 'graded exercise therapy' as the term may be applied broadly and incorrectly.

It is important to acknowledge that there is still very little evidence showing the safety and effectiveness of exercise for people with ME/CFS, even if exercise is prescribed at a level below the anaerobic threshold. As such, if a physiotherapist is considering an exercise prescription for a person with ME/CFS, whether to treat a symptom of ME/CFS directly or for an unrelated issue, they must consider several key questions.

1   What is the purpose of the exercise?

Exercise will not directly treat or cure ME/CFS, but an exercise may be prescribed to address a specific problem, for example weakness, pain or stiffness. Alternatively, exercise may be important for maintenance of joint and muscle health, and quality of life.

For people with ME/CFS, exercise could be considered as part of a management plan:

- to strengthen a muscle group that can be used for a relevant functional activity, e.g. quadriceps to improve sit to stand (53)
- to improve the lower limb muscle pump and increase venous return in upright positions (54), helping to manage symptoms of orthostatic intolerance (see chapter 12)
- to address an unrelated problem to ME/CFS, for example a musculoskeletal injury or following surgery
- to address pain, for example to strengthen muscles to improve joint stability in the case of hypermobility; care must be taken with regards to pain given physical exertion can also further

decrease pressure pain thresholds and potentially increase pain (see chapter 10)

· to provide psychological benefits such as a sense of accomplishment and wellbeing (50)

· because exercise is important to that person and they want to find a safe way to include it in their life.

When prescribing an exercise, the physiotherapist should first clinically reason the purpose of the exercise and its intended outcome.

2 What type of exercise is best for this person?

Exercise comes in many forms, with the aim to stretch or strengthen parts of the body or stress the cardiovascular system. Deciding on what type of exercise might be suitable for a person with ME/CFS should be a joint discussion, taking into account what the person enjoys, what they may have tried previously, and what their specific goals are.

An exercise may be specific to a problem unrelated to ME/CFS, for example a musculoskeletal injury. In this case the physiotherapist must still consider whether the exercise is suitable in respect of ME/CFS, or if adaptations need to be made. The positioning of a person (lie, sit, stand) or an involvement of overhead activity will influence the level

Oliver: 'I couldn't exercise for a really long time; it was only when I'd got my energy management sorted that I could start to do a little. I exercise to keep my current level constant: a light walk and a little strengthening so I can maintain my muscle mass. But I can't do as much as a normal person.'

of physical exertion required. Upright positions may also increase symptoms in relation to orthostatic intolerance (see chapter 12).

There are few studies (55) (56) (57) (49) that have investigated the safety and effectiveness of various types of exercise for people with ME/CFS. People with severe or very severe ME/CFS tend to be excluded from this research so application of any findings to this particular group is not possible. More information on working with people who have severe or very severe ME/CFS can be found in chapter 3. Additionally no research defines the severity of the participants and it appears that most participants would be defined as 'mild' considering the nature of the interventions being investigated. More information on levels of severity can be found in chapter 1.

Strengthening and endurance programmes

The World Health Organization recommends healthy adults and adults with chronic conditions (not listing ME/CFS) should involve either 150 to 300 minutes of moderate-intensity aerobic physical activity, or 75 to 100 minutes of vigorous-intensity aerobic physical activity, each week, alongside muscle strengthening activities twice a week (2). However, some studies have found that there are still benefits for cardiorespiratory fitness from performing very short bursts of high-intensity activity in the healthy population, such as three sessions per week of a 60-second intensive cycle (58) (59), even finding that 10-minute bursts of high-intensity cycling were more effective at improving cardiovascular fitness than moderate-intensity cycling for 30 minutes (60). Therefore, even small amounts of activity may have beneficial effects without having to increase the intensity beyond the capabilities of a person with ME/CFS.

The Workwell Foundation, a team of exercise physiologists in the USA who specialize in working with people with ME/CFS, recommend parameters that allow a person to exercise within their metabolic limits:

- very brief periods of activity, no more than two minutes at a time
- at least one minute of rest between each activity
- a single session should last no longer than 20 minutes.

However, these parameters are not evidence based and therefore any intervention should be individualized and monitored for adverse responses, keeping in mind that PEM can be delayed by several days, and considering the remaining prompts in this chapter regarding both measurement of outcome and whether the activity is an appropriate use of energy.

The Workwell Foundation recommend that a regime starts with static stretching and an active range of movement activities with time to assess whether these are tolerated before considering the addition of strengthening and endurance exercises (53).

A case study (55) presents a person with ME/CFS who used heart rate monitoring to pace their daily activities and an individualized exercise programme three times a week, which addressed flexibility, resistance training and short-term endurance. The outcome after one year was that the person had maintained participation in the exercise programme, was able to manage more activities of daily living without triggering PEM, and on cardiopulmonary exercise testing demonstrated a reduced recovery time by 75%. This is, however, a single case study and so it is not possible to generalize the results to the wider population.

If considering strength or endurance training it is important to recognize that people with ME/CFS have been shown to have poorer performance on repeated strength testing (15) (16) so high numbers of repetitions may be counter-productive. More detail on peripheral fatigue is in chapter 8.

Yoga and qigong exercises

Yoga and qigong are styles of exercise that involves static poses, slow movements and breathing control, and their impact on people with ME/CFS has been explored in a series of small trials (56). Subjective mental and physical fatigue scores have improved with these interventions; however trials have also noted adverse events such as a deterioration in symptoms and increased pain and fatigue (56). It is therefore not possible to conclude whether this type of exercise is suitable and an individual approach with constant monitoring should always be applied.

Aquatic exercise

A pilot study (57) of 11 people with ME/CFS looked at a five-week aquatic exercise programme with two self-paced sessions a week to explore whether they would benefit from the typical effects of aquatic exercise such as pain relief, improved blood flow and physical function. Participants were selected with a diagnosis based either on the Canadian Criteria (which do include PEM) or the Fukuda Criteria (which do not include PEM), and their symptoms were very closely monitored each day for signs of PEM. While some symptom increase was noted one to two days after each session, an overall trend of decreased severity of symptoms emerged after three weeks. However, this was a very small study without a control group so further research would be required on a larger scale.

Walking

Walking programmes for people with ME/CFS have been explored in several small studies. An increase in 'perception of wellness' was reported in a study of 20 people with ME/CFS who undertook a 20-week walking programme with the intensity set at 50% of the maximum heart rate (49). No other outcomes or benefits were noted and the set of criteria used for participants was Fukuda, which does not include PEM.

Another study (61) looked at whether intermittent walking would be tolerated by ten people with ME/CFS. A 30-minute treadmill walk was split into ten periods of 3-minute walks with 3 minutes of rest and recovery between each set. Participants were able to complete the activity without any change to their level of disability over a week of monitoring after the session. However, this study used ten participants who met the Fukuda Criteria (which do not include PEM), and they did not report any beneficial effects of the intervention. While the paper concludes that intermittent walking was not responsible for any significant symptom exacerbation, it also states that participants reported symptoms of headache, leg pain, fatigue and sore throats after the exercise, which does suggest a level of symptom exacerbation and signs of PEM.

Both of these studies used an approach that worked within energy limits and avoided anaerobic metabolism. In contrast, one study (43) attempted to increase activity levels by 30% with a prescribed walking programme over four weeks. The study involved six participants, four of which did not achieve the prescribed increase in activity, and all participants reported a worsening of mood and increased pain and fatigue over the course of the programme.

Walking may be seen as a gentle exercise, but a small study (62) looked at the 'physiological cost' of walking in 17 people with ME/CFS compared to matched-controls, observing the oxygen uptake when participants walked for 5 minutes at the same speed. People with ME/CFS had significantly less oxygen uptake than healthy controls leading the researchers to conclude that they had higher energy demands and the 'physiological cost' of walking was much higher.

While walking within energy limits may have positive effects on mood in people with ME/CFS, the evidence base consists of small pilot studies so their outcomes cannot be applied to clinical practice. It is also important to consider that general activities of daily living may already involve regular walking, and any additional walking needs to be balanced against the person's priorities and the potential for symptom exacerbation.

3   How will I monitor whether this person can tolerate this exercise?

A mandatory measure for any physiotherapy intervention in people with ME/CFS is to monitor for signs of PEM, which is additional symptoms or the exacerbation of current symptoms following exertion (see chapter 6). Measuring PEM is difficult because it is an individual experience covering a range of symptoms with a variety of timescales. Subjective methods of measuring PEM are discussed in detail in chapter 18.

Kim: 'Gentle movement in lying within my limits has been beneficial. I have been able to slowly build core strength and flexibility.'

PEM can be a delayed response, most commonly by one to two days after an activity (63), so it may not be obvious that the intervention is not being tolerated until it is too late. Using an objective measure such as a heart rate monitor may allow for real-time monitoring of a person's response to exercise and allow the intensity of an activity to be moderated. Heart rate variability can also be a tool to measure how exercise is being tolerated. See chapter 16 for more details on using heart rate monitors for people with ME/CFS. Additionally, it may also be helpful to monitor blood pressure and oxygen saturation and keep a daily activity and symptom record.

The potential for symptom fluctuation should be taken into account. An exercise may be tolerated on a 'good' week, but then be intolerable during a symptom flare. Any intervention should be carefully monitored and evaluated for signs of symptom exacerbation over a number of weeks before an additional activity is added, or any modification to the current level of exercise is considered.

4   How will I measure whether the exercise is benefiting this person?

An appropriate outcome measure should be put in place to provide information as to the effectiveness of an exercise. There are a wide range of outcome measures that can be used in relation to the symptoms of ME/CFS (see chapter 18), as well as linked to a condition-specific intervention such as a musculoskeletal injury, so it is important to select one that measures the desired outcome of the exercise, as well as one that measures the symptoms of ME/CFS that may be exacerbated by the increase in activity.

'Maintenance' exercises that are used for general health and quality of life can be measured by adherence and tolerance as well as symptom stability, so an outcome measure that captures the spectrum of symptoms experienced in ME/CFS, such as the DePaul Symptom Questionnaire (64), may be suitable.

As well as capturing the effectiveness of an intervention, an outcome measure could also highlight deterioration, which may indicate that the exercise is not appropriate.

5   Is exercise an appropriate use of energy for this person?

It is important to consider whether the use of exercise is appropriate for each individual. An unrelated injury may become a priority for that person due to the consequences of pain or reduced function. Some people value exercise as an enjoyable daily activity and would prioritize it in their energy expenditure if able. Others may have hobbies and activities that require physical activity (not structured exercise) which are of greater importance to that person's quality of life, for example gardening, playing a musical instrument or arts and crafts.

Some people with ME/CFS must unfortunately rely on their limited energy to carry out essential activities of daily living, and any additional energy expenditure causes symptom exacerbation. As discussed in chapter 6, physical exertion is not the only trigger of PEM, so a physiotherapist should be aware of other demands on a person that may be cognitive, sensory and emotional. In these cases there must be sound clinical reasoning behind the choice to add any formal exercise programme.

Given that a single exercise will not address any of the complex physiological processes that are involved with ME/CFS, a physiotherapist must determine what the value of each exercise is to that individual person and whether it is an appropriate use of their energy. Open and honest discussion with the person about the benefits and potential adverse effects of exercise is essential so that a plan is developed with shared decision-making.

SUMMARY

▸ Exercise is not a treatment or cure for ME/CFS and may make symptoms worse.

▸ Maximal physical exertion has been shown to cause adverse physiological effects.

▸ The evidence base for all exercise studies in ME/CFS is limited.

▸ Individually tailored exercise programmes may have beneficial effects on function, pain, mood and quality of life, but the evidence base is limited.

▸ Research on exercise for people with ME/CFS appears to recruit people with milder presentations of ME/CFS, therefore any conclusions cannot be applied to those with moderate and severe ME/CFS.

APPLICATION TO PRACTICE

The introduction of any exercise for a person with ME/CFS must be clinically reasoned, taking into account the key questions:

1. What is the purpose of the exercise?
2. What type of exercise is best for this person?
3. How will I monitor whether this person can tolerate this exercise?
4. How will I measure whether the exercise is benefiting this person?
5. Is exercise an appropriate use of energy for this person?

Given the laboratory data showing adverse physiological responses to exertion, and the sparsity of evidence showing any significant benefits of exercise for people with ME/CFS, physiotherapists should have an open discussion with the person to decide together whether the rewards of introducing exercise outweigh the risks.

References

1. National Institute for Health and Care Excellence (2021) 'Myalgic encephalomyelitis (or encephalopathy)/chronic fatigue syndrome: diagnosis and management.' Accessed on 2/12/2022 at www.nice.org.uk/guidance/ng206.
2. World Health Organization (2020) 'Physical activity.' Accessed on 3/12/2022 at www.who.int/news-room/fact-sheets/detail/physical-activity.
3. Nystoriak, M.A. & Bhatnagar A. (2018) 'Cardiovascular effects and benefits of exercise.' *Frontiers in Cardiovascular Medicine 5.*
4. Fragala, M.S., Cadore, E.L., Dorgo, S., Izquierdo, M., *et al.* (2019) 'Resistance training for older adults: position statement from the national strength and conditioning association.' *Journal of Strength and Conditioning Research 33* (8).
5. Vogiatzis, I. (2011) 'Strategies of muscle training in very severe COPD patients.' *European Respiratory Journal 38.*
6. Cornish, A.K., Broadbent, S. & Cheema, B.S. (2011) 'Interval training for patients with coronary artery disease: a systematic review.' *European Journal of Applied Physiology 111.*
7. Craft, L.L. & Perna, F.M. (2004) 'The benefits of exercise for the clinically depressed.' *Primary Care Companion Journal of Clinical Psychiatry 6* (3).
8. Cooper, D.M., Radom-Aizik, S., Schwindt, C. & Zaldivar, F., Jr. (2007) 'Dangerous exercise: lessons learned from dysregulated inflammatory responses to physical activity.' *Journal of Applied Physiology [1985] 103* (2).
9. Kindlon, T. (2011) 'Reporting of harms associated with graded exercise therapy and cognitive behavioural therapy in myalgic encephalomyelitis/chronic fatigue syndrome.' *Bulletin of the IACFS/M 19* (2).
10. Davenport, T.E., Lehnen, M., Stevens, S.R., VanNess, J.M., Stevens, J. & Snell, C.R. (2019) 'Chronotropic intolerance: an overlooked determinant of symptoms and activity limitation in myalgic encephalomyelitis/chronic fatigue syndrome?' *Frontiers in Pediatrics 22* (7).
11. Chaudhuri, A. & Behan, P.O. (2004) 'In vivo magnetic resonance spectroscopy in chronic fatigue syndrome.' *Prostaglandins, Leukotrienes & Essential Fatty Acids (PLEFA) 71* (3).
12. Jones, D.E., Hollingsworth, K.G., Jakovljevic, D.G., Fattakhova, G., *et al.* (2012) 'Loss of capacity to recover from acidosis on repeat exercise in chronic fatigue syndrome: a case-control study.' *European Journal of Clinical Investigation 42* (2).
13. Lien, K., Johansen, B., Veierød, M.B., Haslestad, A.S., *et al.* (2019) 'Abnormal blood lactate accumulation during repeated exercise testing in myalgic encephalomyelitis/chronic fatigue syndrome.' *Physiology Reports 7* (11).
14. Jammes, Y., Steinberg, J.G., Mambrini, O., Brégeon, F. & Delliaux, S. (2005) 'Chronic fatigue syndrome: assessment of increased oxidative stress and altered muscle excitability in response to incremental exercise.' *Journal of Internal Medicine 257* (3).
15. Jäkel, B., Kedor, C. & Grabowski, P. (2021) 'Hand grip strength and fatigability: correlation with clinical parameters and diagnostic suitability in ME/CFS.' *Journal of Translational Medicine 19* (159).
16. Paul, L., Wood, L., Behan, W.M. & Maclaren, W.M. (1999) 'Demonstration of delayed recovery from fatiguing exercise in chronic fatigue syndrome.' *European Journal of Neurology 6* (1).
17. Mateo, L.J., Chu, L., Stevens, S., Stevens, J., *et al.* (2020) 'Post-exertional symptoms distinguish myalgic encephalomyelitis/chronic fatigue syndrome subjects from healthy controls.' *Work 66* (2).
18. Whistler, T., Jones, J.F., Unger, E.R. & Vernon, S.D. (2005) 'Exercise responsive genes measured in peripheral blood of women with chronic fatigue syndrome and matched control subjects.' *BMC Physiology 5* (1).
19. Light, A.R., White, A.T., Hughen, R.W. & Light, K.C. (2009) 'Moderate exercise increases expression for sensory, adrenergic, and immune genes in chronic fatigue syndrome patients but not in normal subjects.' *Journal of Pain 10* (10).

20. Sorensen, B., Streib, J.E., Strand, M., Make, B., *et al.* (2003) 'Complement activation in a model of chronic fatigue syndrome.' *Journal of Allergy and Clinical Immunology 112* (2).

21. Shukla, S.K., Cook, D., Meyer, J., Vernon, S.D., *et al.* (2015) 'Changes in gut and plasma microbiome following exercise challenge in myalgic encephalomyelitis/ chronic fatigue syndrome (ME/CFS).' *PLOS ONE 10* (12).

22. Neary, P.J., Roberts, A.D., Leavins, N., Harrison, M.F., Croll, J.C. & Sexsmith, J.R. (2008) 'Prefrontal cortex oxygenation during incremental exercise in chronic fatigue syndrome.' *Clinical Physiology and Functional Imaging 28* (6).

23. LaManca, J.J., Sisto, S.A., DeLuca, J., Johnson, S.K., *et al.* (1998) 'Influence of exhaustive treadmill exercise on cognitive functioning in chronic fatigue syndrome.' *American Journal of Medicine 28* (105).

24. Van Oosterwijck, J., Nijs, J., Meeus, M., Lefever, I., *et al.* (2010) 'Pain inhibition and postexertional malaise in myalgic encephalomyelitis/chronic fatigue syndrome: an experimental study.' *Journal of Internal Medicine 268* (3).

25. Bavinton, J., Darbishire, L. & White, P.D. (2002) *Graded Exercise Therapy for CFS/ME: Manual for Therapists.* Final Trial Version: Version 7 (MREC Version 2). Accessed on 12/01/2023 at www.qmul.ac.uk/wiph/centres/centre-for-psychiatry-and-mental-health/research/pace-trial.

26. Fulcher, K.Y. & White, P.D. (1998) 'Chronic fatigue syndrome: a description of graded exercise treatment.' *Physiotherapy 84* (5).

27. Wu, Y., Hu, X. & Chen, L. (2020) 'Chronic resistance exercise improves functioning and reduces toll-like receptor signaling in elderly patients with postoperative deconditioning.' *Journal of Manipulative and Physiological Therapeutics 43* (4).

28. Maher, J.L., McMillan, D.W. & Nash, M.S. (2017) 'Exercise and health-related risks of physical deconditioning after spinal cord injury.' *Topics in Spinal Cord Injury Rehabilitation 23* (3).

29. Ivey, F.M., Hafer-Macko, C.E. & Macko, R.F. (2008) 'Exercise training for cardiometabolic adaptation after stroke.' *Journal of Cardiopulmonary Rehabilitation and Prevention 28* (1).

30. White, P.D., Goldsmith, K.A., Johnson, A.L., Potts, L., Walwyn, R. & DeCesare, J.C. (2011) 'Comparison of adaptive pacing therapy, cognitive behaviour therapy, graded exercise therapy, and specialist medical care for chronic fatigue syndrome (PACE): a randomised trial.' *The Lancet 377* (9768).

31. Clark, L., Pesola, F., Thomas, J.M., Vergara-Williamson, M., Beynon, M. & White, P.D. (2017) 'Guided graded exercise self-help plus specialist medical care versus specialist medical care alone for chronic fatigue syndrome (GETSET): a pragmatic randomised controlled trial.' *The Lancet 390* (10092).

32. White, P.D., Goldsmith, K., Johnson, A.L., Chalder, T. & Sharpe, M. (2013) 'Recovery from chronic fatigue syndrome after treatments given in the PACE trial.' *Psychological Medicine 43* (10).

33. Stouten, B. (2017) 'PACE-GATE: An alternative view on a study with a poor trial protocol.' *Journal of Health Psychology 22* (9).

34. Centers for Disease Control and Prevention (2022) 'Myalgic encephalomyelitis/ chronic fatigue syndrome.' Accessed on 4/12/2022 at www.cdc.gov/me-cfs/index. html.

35. Wormgoor, M.E.A. & Rodenburg, S.C. (2021) 'The evidence base for physiotherapy in myalgic encephalomyelitis/chronic fatigue syndrome when considering post-exertional malaise: a systematic review and narrative synthesis.' *Journal of Translational Medicine 19* (1).

36. Smith, M.E.B., Nelson, H.D., Haney, E., Pappas, M., *et al.* (2014) 'Diagnosis and treatment of myalgic encephalomyelitis/chronic fatigue syndrome.' *Evidence Report/Technology Assessment (Full Rep.) 219.*

37. Larun, L., Brurberg, K.G., Odgaard-Jensen, J. & Price, J.R. (2019) 'Exercise therapy for chronic fatigue syndrome.' *Cochrane Database of Systematic Reviews 10.*

38. Geraghty, K.J. & Blease, C. (2019) 'Myalgic encephalomyelitis/chronic fatigue syndrome and the biopsychosocial model: a review of patient harm and distress in the medical encounter.' *Disability and Rehabilitation 41* (25).
39. McCrone, P., Sharpe, M., Chalder, T., Knapp, M., *et al.* (2012) 'Adaptive pacing, cognitive behaviour therapy, graded exercise, and specialist medical care for chronic fatigue syndrome: a cost-effectiveness analysis.' *PLOS ONE 7* (8).
40. Vink, M. & Vink-Niese, F. (2022) 'Is it useful to question the recovery behaviour of patients with ME/CFS or Long Covid?' *Healthcare 10.*
41. Clark, L.V., McCrone, P., Pesola, F., Vergara-Williamson, M. & White, P.D. (2021) 'Guided graded exercise self-help for chronic fatigue syndrome: long term follow up and cost-effectiveness following the GETSET trial.' *Journal of Psychosomatic Research 146.*
42. Wearden, A.J., Dowrick, C., Chew-Graham, C., Bentall, R.P., Morriss, R.K. & Peters, S. (2010) 'Nurse led, home based self help treatment for patients in primary care with chronic fatigue syndrome: randomised controlled trial.' *British Medical Journal 340.*
43. Black, C.D., O'Connor, P.J. & McCully, K.K. (2005) 'Increased daily physical activity and fatigue symptoms in chronic fatigue syndrome.' *Dynamic Medicine 4* (1).
44. Black, C.D. & McCully, K.K. (2005) 'Time course of exercise induced alterations in daily activity in chronic fatigue syndrome.' *Dynamic Medicine 4* (10).
45. Kujawski, S., Cossington, J., Słomko, J., Zawadka-Kunikowska, M., *et al.* (2021) 'Relationship between cardiopulmonary, mitochondrial and autonomic nervous system function improvement after an individualised activity programme upon chronic fatigue syndrome patients.' *Journal of Clinical Medicine 10* (7).
46. Zalewski, P., Kujawski, S., Tudorowska, M., Morten, K., *et al.* (2020) 'The impact of a structured exercise programme upon cognitive function in chronic fatigue syndrome patients.' *Brain Science 10* (4).
47. Twisk, F.N. & Maes, M. (2009) 'A review on cognitive behavioral therapy (CBT) and graded exercise therapy (GET) in myalgic encephalomyelitis (ME) / chronic fatigue syndrome (CFS): CBT/GET is not only ineffective and not evidence-based, but also potentially harmful.' *Neuroendocrinology Letters 30* (3).
48. HANDI Working Group (2020) 'Graded exercise therapy: chronic fatigue syndrome.' *InnovAiT 13* (12).
49. Coutts, R., Weatherby, R. & Davie, A. (2001) 'The use of a symptom "self-report" inventory to evaluate the acceptability and efficacy of a walking program for patients suffering with chronic fatigue syndrome.' *Journal of Psychosomatic Research 51* (2).
50. VanNess, J.M., Snell, C.R. & Stevens, S.R. (2000) 'A realistic approach to exercise for CFS patients.' *CFS Research Review 1* (4).
51. Nijs, J., Paul, L. & Wallman, K. (2008) 'Chronic fatigue syndrome: an approach combining self-management with graded exercise to avoid exacerbations.' *Journal of Rehabilitation Medicine 40* (4).
52. Wallman, K.E., Morton, A.R., Goodman, C., Grove, R. & Guilfoyle, A.M. (2004) 'Randomised controlled trial of graded exercise in chronic fatigue syndrome.' *Medical Journal of Australia 180* (9).
53. Davenport, T.E., Stevens, S., VanNess, M.J., Snell, C.R. & Little, T. (2010) 'Conceptual model for physical therapist management of chronic fatigue syndrome/myalgic encephalomyelitis.' *Physical Therapy 90* (4).
54. Fu, Q. & Levine, B.D. (2018) 'Exercise and non-pharmacological treatment of POTS.' *Autonomic Neuroscience 215.*
55. Stevens, S.R. & Davenport, T.E. (2010) 'Functional outcomes of anaerobic rehabilitation in an individual with chronic fatigue syndrome: case report with 1-year follow-up.' *Bulletin of the International Association for Chronic Fatigue Syndrome/Myalgic Encephalomyelitis (IACFSME) 18* (3).

56. Khanpour Ardestani, S., Karkhaneh, M., Stein, E., Punja, S., *et al.* (2021) 'Systematic review of mind-body interventions to treat myalgic encephalomyelitis/chronic fatigue syndrome.' *Medicina 57* (7).

57. Broadbent, S., Coetzee, S., Beavers, R. & Horstmanshof, L. (2020) 'Patient experiences and the psychosocial benefits of group aquatic exercise to reduce symptoms of myalgic encephalomyelitis/chronic fatigue syndrome: a pilot study.' *Fatigue: Biomedicine, Health & Behavior 8.*

58. Gillen, J.B., Percival, M.E., Skelly, L.E., Martin, B.J., *et al.* (2014) 'Three minutes of all-out intermittent exercise per week increases skeletal muscle oxidative capacity and improves cardiometabolic health.' *PLOS ONE 9* (11).

59. Little, J.P., Langley, J., Lee, M., Myette-Côté, E., *et al.* (2019) 'Sprint exercise snacks: a novel approach to increase aerobic fitness.' *European Journal of Applied Physiology 119* (5).

60. Cuddy, T.F., Ramos, J.S. & Dalleck, L.C. (2019) 'Reduced exertion high-intensity interval training is more effective at improving cardiorespiratory fitness and cardiometabolic health than traditional moderate-intensity continuous training.' *International Journal of Environmental Research and Public Health 16* (3).

61. Clapp, L.L., Richardson, M.T., Smith, J.F., Wang, M., Clapp, A.J. & Pieroni, R.E. (1999) 'Acute effects of thirty minutes of light-intensity, intermittent exercise on patients with chronic fatigue syndrome.' *Physical Therapy 79* (8).

62. Paul, L., Rafferty, D. & Marshal, R. (2009) 'Physiological cost of walking in those with chronic fatigue syndrome (CFS): a case-control study.' *Disability Rehabilitation 31* (19).

63. Holtzman, C.S., Bhatia, S., Cotler, J. & Jason, L.A. (2019) 'Assessment of post-exertional malaise (PEM) in patients with myalgic encephalomyelitis (ME) and chronic fatigue syndrome (CFS): a patient-driven survey.' *Diagnostics (Basel) 9* (1).

64. Jason, L.A. & Sunnquist, M. (2018) 'The development of the DePaul Symptom Questionnaire: original, expanded, brief, and pediatric versions.' *Frontiers in Pediatrics 6* (6).

CHAPTER 18

Outcome Measures

PURPOSE OF THIS CHAPTER

This chapter gives an overview of the main outcome measures and screening tools used clinically and in research in relation to ME/CFS and provides a brief summary as to the appropriateness of each measure. Not every outcome measure used routinely in ME/CFS is necessarily appropriate.

It is important to note that none of these measures are used as a tool for diagnosis of ME/CFS. Diagnosis is made on detailed history in relation to selected criteria and more information on this can be found in chapter 1.

Many different outcome measures have been used in research on ME/CFS. A systematic review (1) looked at randomized controlled trials for physiotherapy-based interventions for ME/CFS and found that within 18 studies there were 37 different outcome measures. The plethora of outcome measures used in relation to ME/CFS reflects the many varied symptoms and systems impacted by the disease.

This chapter provides a reference list of potential outcome measures and screening tools that can be used clinically by a physiotherapist in two ways:

1. a standardized method to assess and measure the effectiveness of a treatment when directly addressing ME/CFS symptoms
2. a standardized method to monitor ME/CFS symptoms when treating someone for an unrelated issue, to ensure treatment does not cause additional symptoms or the exacerbation of current symptoms.

The vast array of outcome measures available also highlights a key issue when appraising any research in relation to ME/CFS. First, it becomes difficult to compare the results of a series of studies when there is no consistency in the measures being used. And, second, if a study claims that an intervention has benefited someone with ME/CFS, it is important to determine which outcome measures were used to demonstrate these benefits and whether they are clinically relevant. In some research on ME/CFS, outcome measures are routinely used that have major flaws in validity or reliability, and these measures are highlighted where applicable throughout this chapter.

Outcome measures and screening tools

Outcome measures can be used to grade the severity of a person's symptoms or disability (2) and to describe the effect of an intervention (3) in either clinical practice or research.

An outcome measure should be valid (it measures what it is supposed to measure) and reliable (it can reproduce results in different situations and when delivered by different people) (3). A measure of reliability ('coefficient') is provided in research as a number up to 1.00, with closest to 1.00 being the most reliable. Wherever possible these numbers are provided throughout this chapter. The coefficient of reliability estimates the proportion of variation that is not due to an error in measurement and can be reproduced from repeated measurements (4).

Screening tools are a brief measure to capture symptoms that may require further investigation. They cannot provide diagnosis. There are no screening tools for ME/CFS as a disease, but there are some screening methods for specific symptoms, such as orthostatic intolerances, which may be performed by a physiotherapist.

Types of outcome measure

Outcome measures can either be objective or patient-reported (PRO). A typical objective outcome measure may include a standardized observation or measure of performance (5). A PRO provides information relating to the person's health, quality of life or current function as reported by the person and without interpretation by the clinician (6). A PRO may be specific to a disease experience or capture a more generic picture of that person's health and quality of life. Using PROs in clinical practice can help with the discussion and detection of health-related quality of life problems as well as monitoring the quality of care (7). However, a systematic review of patient reported outcome measures used in the assessment of adults with ME/CFS found limited quality and clear discrepancies between what the outcome measures reported and how people with ME/CFS defined their own experiences (8). While outcome measures can be beneficial, it is also important to draw on subjective and objective assessment skills as described in chapter 14 in order to gain the full picture.

Objective and patient-reported outcomes provide different aspects of information relating to the person and their health (5) and using a combination of these measures allows a clinician to understand the clinical effectiveness of an intervention alongside how the person feels they have benefited (6). However, these measures will be limited by capturing information about the person in the moment the measures are taken and may not always be reflective of the fluctuating nature of ME/CFS symptoms.

Selecting an outcome measure or screening tool for people with ME/CFS

Selecting which outcome measure or screening tool to use in practice is an important decision and depends largely on the nature of the physiotherapy intervention.

A mandatory measure for any interaction is to monitor for signs of post exertional malaise (PEM, see chapter 6), which is additional symptoms or an exacerbation of current symptoms due to exertion. If a physiotherapy intervention causes PEM then it will not be appropriate for that person and the physiotherapist must adopt their practice immediately. The experience of PEM is individual and covers a wide range of potential symptoms, so creating a standardized objective measure is almost impossible. The DePaul Symptom Questionnaire (discussed later in this chapter) is a patient-reported outcome that contains a section relating to PEM. Alternatively, a basic numerical rating scale, for example 'Rate the severity of your PEM symptoms from 0 to 10', could be a quick way to monitor symptom experience in clinical practice, although it is not established if this method would give reliable and valid data over time.

Other outcome measures or screening tools may be selected to monitor a specific symptom or take a more holistic view of the person's quality of life as a whole. Considering the number of potential symptoms presented by a person with ME/CFS, it is not feasible to include an outcome measure to capture every single one. The physiotherapist must determine which outcomes are the priority and would give the most accurate impression of how their intervention is affecting that person.

Goal attainment may be another way of monitoring the effectiveness of an intervention, for example whether the person achieves their desired outcome. This can become difficult if the intervention is part of a maintenance programme, aiming to prevent deterioration and preserve function.

Finally, careful consideration should be given to the nature of any outcome measure used, whether to directly monitor ME/CFS symptoms or as part of an unrelated intervention. Some objective outcome measures will involve physical exertion and many exercise tolerance tests will not be appropriate at all for people with ME/CFS. Subjective measures in the form of questionnaires should also be used with caution, taking into account the length and complexity of a questionnaire and the resulting cognitive exertion. Simply carrying out an outcome measure or screening tool may inadvertently cause PEM and symptom exacerbation in a person with ME/CFS.

ME/CFS specific outcome measures

The symptoms and severity of ME/CFS are very varied and individual. It is therefore difficult to create a standardized outcome measure to capture the entire experience of ME/CFS. This causes issues in both appraising and comparing the evidence base, as well as in managing clinical practice.

There is currently no objective measure of ME/CFS, but two specific patient reported outcomes have been created:

The DePaul Symptom Questionnaire

A measure created specifically to capture ME/CFS symptoms is the DePaul Symptom Questionnaire (DSQ) (9), a self-reported measure that asks people to rate the frequency and severity of their symptoms. These scores are standardized and averaged to create composite scores that cover eight domains:

1. sleep dysfunction
2. post exertional malaise
3. neurocognitive dysfunction
4. immune dysfunction
5. neuroendocrine dysfunction
6. pain
7. gastrointestinal distress
8. orthostatic intolerance.

The DSQ has reported test-retest reliability with Pearson's or kappa correlation coefficients of 0.70 or higher and is considered to have good face and content validity (10). However, one study looked at people with severe ME/CFS using the DSQ to differentiate between those who were bedridden (very severe) and those who were housebound (severe). They found there were limitations in the measurement of PEM because people who were bedridden were less likely to be able to carry out activities that triggered PEM according to the scale and would therefore score lower despite having more severe symptoms (11).

The first version of the DSQ was revised in response to patient feedback and a new version, the DSQ-2, was created to give a more thorough understanding of symptom experience, with good internal consistency reliability (Cronbach's alpha 0.73 to 0.91) for each symptom measured (12).

A shorter screening version was developed called the DSQ-SF (Short Form), which reduced symptoms to a quick list of 14 and may therefore be an effective tool for time-limited research and clinical practice (9). The Short Form was able to identify a similar number of people in a multisite sample compared to the longer form (9).

Finally, a paediatric instrument was created, called the DSQ-Ped (paediatric), featuring forms for both the child and the parent, with good internal reliability reported (Cronbach's alpha 0.83) (9).

The Chronic Fatigue and Immune Dysfunction Syndrome Disability Scale

The Chronic Fatigue and Immune Dysfunction Syndrome (CFIDS) Disability Scale, also known as the Bell Disability Scale, was designed to measure symptom severity and the degree of functional impairment from ME/CFS, with the focus on symptom severity being related to exertion (13).

People are asked to rate themselves on a 10-point scale (marked 0–100) with 0 being 'severe symptoms on a continuous basis; bedridden constantly; unable to care for self' and 100 being 'no symptoms at rest; no symptoms with exercise; normal overall activity level; able to work full-time without difficulty'.

While the scale is simple to use and was created specifically for people with ME/CFS, it has not been validated in large trials.

Symptom-specific outcome measures

If an intervention is being used to address a specific symptom of ME/CFS, then a symptom-specific outcome measure may be appropriate.

Fatigue

As discussed in chapter 7, 'fatigue' is a vague term that can be used to describe the symptoms of a wide variety of disease states as well as something experienced by the general population. Unfortunately, many outcome measures that measure fatigue do not accurately represent the type of fatigue uniquely experienced by people with ME/CFS (14) and therefore lack face validity. Consequently, if considering a fatigue scale when working with a person with ME/CFS it is important to use a scale that can differentiate between general fatigue and the symptoms specifically experienced by people with ME/CFS (15). There are over 50 measures of fatigue. Table 18.1 is a summary of the main fatigue scales used in research specifically for people with ME/CFS.

Table 18.1 Subjective measurements of fatigue

Measure	Description	Comment
Fatigue Severity Scale (FSS)	A nine-item questionnaire (16)	Internal consistency, test-retest reliability, (ICC = 0.81–0.89) for multiple sclerosis and lupus (17)
		Found to differentiate ME/CFS fatigue from healthy controls (15)
		Able to distinguish between fatigue experienced with lupus, multiple sclerosis and healthy population (16)
		Criticism that it does not represent the more severe forms of ME/CFS with a 'ceiling effect' occurring as maximum scores too easily reached (14)

cont.

Measure	Description	Comment
The Patient Reported Outcome Measurement Information System (PROMIS) Fatigue-Short Form (PROMIS F-SF)	'PROMIS' is a series of outcome measures created by the National Institute for Health in the USA. The Fatigue Short Form features eight prompts for self-reported measures of fatigue (18)	For people with ME/CFS the PROMIS-F-SF was found to have good internal reliability (Cronbach's alpha 0.84) and validity in measuring fatigue (18) Good reliability (Cronbach's alpha 0.72–0.88) in people with fibromyalgia, sickle cell disease, cardiometabolic risk, pregnancy and healthy controls (19)
Fatigue Impact Scale (FIS)	A 40-item scale exploring ways in which fatigue symptoms affect cognitive, physical and psychosocial functioning (20)	Good internal consistency (0.87). Scored 80% accuracy in discriminant function analysis of 'chronic fatigue' (20) For multiple sclerosis, good test-retest reliability (0.68 to 0.85) but a low correlation found with the Fatigue Severity Scale (21)
Chalder Fatigue Scale	A 14-item questionnaire to measure the extent and severity of fatigue (22)	Not possible to distinguish ME/CFS from lupus or multiple sclerosis (23) Not possible to distinguish ME/CFS from severe depression (24) Found to have a 'ceiling effect' in people with ME/CFS (14) and not a good indicator of change (25) Overlap in scores between people who rated themselves as moderately or severely ill with ME/CFS (26) The scale was found to be reliable (Cronbach's alpha 0.88–0.90) and valid in the general population (27) Able to distinguish ME/CFS from healthy control sample (23) In spite of identified limitations, 56% of randomized controlled tests (RCTs) into physiotherapy treatment of ME/CFS used this scale (1). These limitations should be taken into account when appraising research outcomes

Checklist Individual Strength (CIS)	Measures four dimensions of fatigue: severity, concentration problems, reduced motivation and activity (28)	A reliable and valid measure of fatigue in the general population, with good internal consistency (alpha 0.84–0.95) and test-retest reliability (r = 0.74–0.86) (28) 'Ceiling effect' found in more severe levels of fatigue with ME/CFS (14) 25% of RCTs into physiotherapy treatment of ME/CFS used this scale (1)
Multidimensional Fatigue Inventory (MFI)	A 20-item questionnaire with subscales: general fatigue, physical fatigue, mental fatigue, reduced motivation and reduced activity (29)	Found to have good internal consistency (Cronbach's alpha 0.84) in general population (29) Deemed not specific enough for ME/CFS, in that those with major depressive disorder would score similar to ME/CFS (15) The general and physical fatigue subscales had questionable or unacceptable internal consistency and ceiling effects (30)
Profile of Fatigue-Related Symptoms (PFRS)	A multidimensional measure with four scales: emotional distress, cognitive difficulty, fatigue and somatic symptoms (31)	Found to have high reliability (alpha 0.86–0.97) and high internal consistency in 'chronic fatigue syndrome' with scores correlating with severity of illness (31) Criticized for combining too many different fatigue states within the 'fatigue' subscale (15)

Cognitive dysfunction

While the measurement of cognitive function tends to be an area of speciality for occupational therapists or psychologists, a physiotherapist may still need to be aware of simple tools or measures to capture cognitive ability. For example, if a person reports cognitive symptoms a screening tool may be useful to determine whether a referral to a specialist is required.

Another situation where cognitive measures may be useful is when monitoring for signs of PEM. Some people with ME/CFS report cognitive dysfunction as a key symptom of their PEM, and therefore this may be an area that requires monitoring to determine the efficacy and safety of an intervention. In this case a simple numerical rating scale to rank the severity of their cognitive symptoms may be suitable to help track symptom behaviour.

More complex cognitive assessments may not be within the scope of practice or require additional training and certification so it is for each individual practitioner to determine whether they are capable of administering a test or should refer on for specialist input from other disciplines (Table 18.2).

More information on cognitive dysfunction in ME/CFS can be found in chapter 8.

Table 18.2 Measurements of cognitive function

Mini Mental State Examination (MMSE)	A 30-point screening tool to indicate potential cognitive impairment (32)	Not validated for use specifically for cognitive dysfunction with ME/CFS
		Good inter-observer reliability (kappa 0.95) in general population (33)
		Biased against people with poor education due to inclusion of language and mathematics questions (32)
Cognitive Failures Questionnaire	A patient reported measure that explores how often they make minor cognitive errors (34)	Not validated for use specifically for cognitive dysfunction with ME/CFS
		Test-retest reliability reported as 0.71 in general population (35)

Sleep dysfunction

Sleep dysfunction is a common symptom of ME/CFS and can have a significant impact on a person's function and quality of life. More information regarding sleep dysfunction can be found in chapter 9.

It is important to distinguish between sleep dysfunction and fatigue symptoms. The measures in Table 18.3 are designed to capture the quality of sleep and are not specific to ME/CFS, although they have been used as outcome measures in ME/CFS research.

Table 18.3 Subjective measurements of sleep dysfunction

Epworth Sleepiness Scale (ESS)	A self-administered questionnaire to measure levels of daytime sleepiness (36)	Not validated in people with ME/CFS Able to distinguish healthy subjects from people with obstructive sleep apnoea syndrome, narcolepsy and idiopathic hypersomnia (36) Good test-retest reliability (r = 0.82) and internal consistency (Cronbach's alpha 0.88) in general population (37)
Sleep Hygiene Index	A 13-item self-report measure to assess behaviours of sleep (38)	Not validated in people with ME/CFS Average internal consistency (alpha 0.66) and good test re-test reliability (0.71) in the general population (38)
The Pittsburgh Sleep Quality Index (PSQI)	A 24-item scale measuring sleep disturbances in 7 dimensions: subjective sleep quality, sleep latency, sleep duration, habitual sleep efficiency, sleep disturbances, use of sleep medication and daytime dysfunction (39)	Not validated in people with ME/CFS Good test re-test reliability (0.87) in people with insomnia (40) Score correlated with patient-reported sleep quality but not with an objective measure of sleep in the general population (41)

Autonomic function

Information regarding dysfunction of the autonomic nervous system, including orthostatic intolerance, can be found in chapter 12. Several subjective outcome measures have been developed to try to capture autonomic dysfunction and orthostatic intolerance symptoms (Table 18.4).

Table 18.4 Subjective measurements of autonomic dysfunction

Measure	Description	Comment
Autonomic Symptom Profile (ASP) and the Composite Autonomic Symptom Score (COMPASS)	A self-report questionnaire that assesses autonomic symptoms across 11 subscales, producing a 'COMPASS score' (42)	A COMPASS score has been reported as a valid diagnostic tool for autonomic dysfunction symptoms in people with ME/CFS (43) Only two of the individual domains had good reliability: orthostatic intolerance and erectile dysfunction (Cronbach's alpha 0.79 and 0.75) (44)
COMPASS 31	A more concise and simplified scoring system based on the ASP and COMPASS (44)	Not validated specifically for people with ME/CFS Improved reliability compared to COMPASS on all domains (Cronbach's alpha 0.40–0.70) (44)
Orthostatic Hypotension Questionnaire (OHQ)	Split into a six-item symptom assessment scale and a four-item daily activity scale (45)	Not validated specifically for ME/CFS Shows good validity and reliability (Cronbach's alpha >0.80) for measuring neurogenic orthostatic hypotension (45)

Objective measures of autonomic dysfunction

Objectively there are numerous methods of measuring autonomic dysfunction in the general population (46). There are two particular objective measures that a physiotherapist could use in clinical practice to provide information about the autonomic nervous system in relation to orthostatic intolerance.

Active stand test

The active stand test (47) involves measuring heart rate and blood pressure at set intervals:

- supine
- immediately upon standing
- after two, five and ten minutes' standing.

The active stand test has been shown to have comparable results to the head-up tilt-table test in people with orthostatic intolerance (48).

The NASA lean test

The NASA lean test has been used to identify orthostatic intolerance in people with ME/CFS (49).

- The person lies horizontally on a bed for 15 to 20 minutes to establish a resting baseline.
- Their blood pressure and heart rate are measured after this period, then repeated every minute until two consecutive readings are obtained – this provides information on the resting measures.
- The person then stands up and leans against a wall with just their shoulder blades resting.
- Heart rate and blood pressure measures are taken every minute over a ten-minute period in this upright position.

While the active stand test and NASA lean test are quite simple to carry out, an accurate interpretation of the results is key to maximize clinical benefit (47).

Orthostatic hypotension (OH) is seen as a sustained drop in blood pressure within three minutes of standing up, with a decrease of at least 20mm Hg in systolic or 10mm Hg in diastolic (50).

Postural orthostatic tachycardia syndrome (POTS) is characterized by an abnormal increase in heart rate when moving into a standing position, with diagnostic criteria in adults stipulating an increase of over 30 beats per minute or above 120 beats per minute within the first 10 minutes of standing, or an increase of over 40 beats per minute or above 130 beats per minute in children and adolescents (51).

These tests may be used as a screening tool for orthostatic intolerance and allow the physiotherapist to refer a person on for further investigation and treatment if results indicate an issue.

Heart rate variability

Heart rate variability (HRV) looks at the variability of the interval between consecutive heart beats (52) and has been shown to have good reliability (ICC 0.79–0.95) (53), although its validity has been questioned (54). Heart rate variability can be reflective of parasympathetic activity (53), which can allow for analysis of the function of the autonomic nervous system. This is discussed in more detail in chapter 12. A number of commercially available heart rate monitors can now measure HRV and it could provide an objective measure to determine the effect of any intervention aiming to affect the nervous system.

Respiratory measures

Breathlessness is a symptom included under the category of autonomic dysfunction on two of the diagnostic criteria for ME/CFS. If a person with ME/CFS lists breathlessness or breathing dysfunction as a priority symptom it may be beneficial to use an outcome measure to monitor this symptom.

While objective measures for respiratory function could be taken, such as oxygen saturation and respiratory rate, it may be beneficial to focus on symptoms related to breathing pattern disorders as part of an autonomic dysfunction manifestation (Table 18.5).

Table 18.5 Subjective measurements of respiratory function

Nijmegen Questionnaire	A commonly used brief questionnaire to screen for breathing pattern disorders (55)	Not validated for people with ME/CFS In relation to hyper-ventilation syndrome, the Nijmegen Questionnaire met criteria for content validity but not structural validity (56)
Brompton Breathing Pattern Tool (BPAT)	A simple screening tool to detect breathing pattern disorder	Not validated for people with ME/CFS Validated within asthma population only (57)
Self-Evaluation of Breathing Questionnaire (SEBQ)	A 25-item questionnaire to measure breathing related symptoms and their severity (58)	Not validated for people with ME/CFS Good test re-test reliability (Cronbach's alpha 0.89) and the SEBQ is considered to be a useful clinical screening tool for dysfunctional breathing (58)

Pain

There are a number of simple scales to measure pain subjectively, which are all valid and reliable for clinical practice (59) (Table 18.6). None of these scales have been validated for use specifically for people with ME/CFS.

Table 18.6 Subjective measurements of pain

Numerical Rating Scale (NRS)	This scale can be presented graphically or verbally, in which a scale up to 11, 21 or 101 points is presented and the person indicates their level of pain	The NRS has been found to have good sensitivity and produces data that can be analysed for audit purposes (59). A scale of either 11 or 21 has been found to be sufficient to show levels of pain severity in chronic pain (60)
Visual Analogue Scale (VAS)	A 10cm line, with 'no pain' at one end and 'worst imaginable pain' at the other. The person is asked to mark on the line where they would rate their pain, and the point at which they have marked is measured in millimetres, giving a possible score out of 100	The VAS has been found to be a satisfactory measure of chronic pain (59) (61) with good reliability in people with abdominal pain (ICC 0.99) (62)
Verbal Rating Scale (VRS)	The VRS involves a list of adjectives in relation to the severity of pain, ranging from 'no pain' to 'mild', 'moderate' and 'severe'	This scale is very simple but lacks sensitivity to change (59)

Physical function

Measuring the physical function of a person with ME/CFS can provide information as to the extent of their physical limitations, which may be of particular focus for a physiotherapist. However, the methods typically used to measure physical function may not be appropriate for people with ME/CFS due to the risks of causing PEM. A physiotherapist must therefore clinically reason whether any physical measurements are necessary and determine whether they will be tolerated.

Subjective measurements of physical function

Subjective information can be gathered to determine the current physical function of a person with ME/CFS. Information gained through the assessment of their current daily routine may be more than enough to identify their level of function. More information on assessment is in chapter 14. Subjective outcome measures for physical function include:

Short Form Health Survey (SF-36)

The physical function subscale of the SF-36 has been shown to have validity in discriminating between many diseases and health controls, and it has been used to show a clear distinction between various levels of severity of ME/CFS (2). Further information on the SF-36 is included later in this chapter.

Patient Reported Outcome Measurement Information System: Physical Function (PROMIS PF)

The PROMIS PF is an eight-item self-reported questionnaire that asks respondents to rate how easily they are able to manage general physical activities such as standing, washing and dressing, going for a 15-minute walk and taking part in vigorous exercise (63). The measure has good internal consistency in people with cancer (Cronbach's alpha 0.92–0.96) (64). The PROMIS PF has not been validated in people with ME/CFS.

Objective measurements of physical function

Objective measurements of physiological processes in response to physical function may be helpful for continuous monitoring during an intervention or as a means of establishing possible triggers of PEM (Table 18.7).

Table 18.7 Objective measurements of physiological function

Pulse oximeter	A device that fits on the end of the finger to measure oxygen saturation and heart rate (65)	Readings can be affected by skin colour, circulation, tobacco use and fingernail polish. Different manufacturers may have different levels of accuracy so blood oxygen results should be treated as an estimate (65)
		No significant difference has been found in heart rate measurement between a pulse oximeter and taking the radial pulse in the general population (66); however some inconsistencies have been found during intensive exercise with higher heart rates in healthy males (67)

Heart rate monitors	A wide range of monitors is commercially available, either worn on the wrist or with a chest strap	More discussion of heart rate monitoring is in chapter 16
Lactic acid monitors	Lactic acid can be measured by taking blood samples, but non-invasive monitors are now on the market, often aimed at athletes	Continuous lactic acid monitoring using an electrochemical biosensor can measure the intensity of an exercise and metabolic activity (68)
Cardiopulmonary Exercise Test (CPET)	CPET captures and analyses expired gas, heart rate and blood pressure as a participant works to a point of maximal physical exertion (69)	CPET has been used for people with ME/CFS in order to trigger and subsequently study PEM Sound reasoning should be in place before this test is considered as it is designed to cause PEM
Portable metabolic measurement system	A portable system designed to capture similar physiological data to the CPET: VO_2, VCO_2, ventilation capacity, respiratory rate	A reliable and valid method of measuring VO_2 (r = 0.86–0.94) (70) As this system is portable, it is feasible to use it with people with ME/CFS to capture physiological data in the home during normal daily activities (71)
Accelerometers	Accelerometers are movement sensors used to monitor and measure physical activity	Accelerometers have been used to measure disease severity in people with ME/CFS (72) Have been shown to have good test re-test reliability in people recovering from stroke (ICC 0.95–0.98) (73)

Other methods of measuring physical function through time and/or distance may be standard practice in typical physiotherapy assessments. Simple tests include the six-minute walk test, ten-metre walk test, timed up and go, and stair climb test (74). However, when considering the purpose of measuring physical function in relation to ME/CFS, the emphasis should be on how much physical function can be carried out without causing PEM, as opposed to how far or how fast a person can move. Given PEM can often be a delayed response, a person with ME/CFS may perform at one level during a physical function test such as the six-minute walk test, but then experience a deterioration in their symptoms a day later. The measurements taken during the test would therefore not reflect the true physical function of that person.

A physiotherapist should clinically reason whether a physical function test is appropriate during an assessment of someone with ME/CFS, considering the risks of physical exertion causing PEM and whether the tests would even successfully establish an accurate portrayal of the person's physical function.

Physical function could be measured by charting how many physical activities a person with ME/CFS can carry out within their daily routine. This would provide a more realistic measure of their physical function and allow for individualized monitoring over time.

Quality of life scales

ME/CFS has a profound effect on quality of life and function, so it can be appropriate to include a holistic measure to capture the impact on a person.

Short Form Health Survey (SF-36)

The most frequently used outcome measure in studies of physiotherapy interventions for people with ME/CFS was the Short Form Health Survey (SF-36) with 69% of randomized controlled trials using it as an outcome measure (1).

The SF-36 is a multi-item scale spanning eight areas (75):

1. physical functioning
2. role limitations – physical
3. bodily pain
4. general health
5. vitality
6. social functioning
7. role limitations – emotional
8. mental health.

The different subscales contribute in unequal proportions to produce two scores: a physical component summary and a mental component summary. All subscales have good reliability in the general population (Cronbach's alpha >0.75) apart from social functioning (76).

A review (77) of the use of the SF-36 in 172 studies found major discrepancies in how the outcome measure was used and scored, with some studies opting for single subscales and 75% failing to outline how the final score was calculated. Of the remaining 25% there were at least nine different ways of calculating the total score reported. The review summarized that the SF-36 measure has poor validity and

> **Oliver**: 'A physio assessment was really unhelpful when they asked me to do an exercise test even though I told them it would cause me PEM. They didn't listen to me.'

that it is important to take this into account if basing clinical decisions on interventions that have used an inaccurate recording of this outcome measure.

EuroQol EQ-5D-3L
This version of the EuroQol is split into two sections (78).

1. The EQ-5D descriptive system asks people to indicate their health status in relation to five dimensions: mobility, self-care, usual activities, pain/discomfort and anxiety/depression.
2. The EQ VAS (visual analogue scale) asks a person to rate their health on a vertical scale with the endpoints of 'best imaginable health' and 'worst imaginable health'.

EuroQol scores have been found to correlate strongly with scores from the SF-36 in people with ME/CFS and it is a quick tool to determine health status; however there were issues in determining appropriate severity of disability (79).

Hospital Anxiety and Depression Scale (HADS)
The Hospital Anxiety and Depression Scale (HADS) was designed to detect states of anxiety or depression in a hospital medical outpatient clinic (80), but is also valid in community settings (81). The HADS has been found to be a reliable measure of psychological distress for people diagnosed with ME/CFS using the Fukuda Criteria (which do not include PEM) (82), and it is often utilized in ME/CFS research. For example in a review of studies on physiotherapy interventions for ME/CFS the HADS was used as an outcome measure in 44% of papers (1).

The scale is a self-assessment and therefore only valid as a screening tool (81) and there may be an inflation of scores if the questionnaire is administered virtually (82). As it is only a screening tool, a clinical diagnosis in relation to anxiety or depression must be made by a relevant health professional who is also familiar with ME/CFS. This is especially important given there is an overlap in symptoms between depression and ME/CFS that can lead to misdiagnosis. For example one paper found 68% of 31 people with ME/CFS had been misdiagnosed with a psychiatric disorder (83), which could lead to inappropriate treatments (84).

SUMMARY

▸ There are a wide range of outcome measures and screening tools that may be applicable when working with a person with ME/CFS.

▸ A physiotherapist must use their clinical reasoning skills to determine which measures are the most reliable and valid in relation to the individual they are working with, and the purpose of the physiotherapy intervention.

▸ Choosing a suitable measurement of the symptoms of PEM is necessary regardless of the reason for physiotherapy, so that symptoms can be monitored for signs of deterioration, stability or improvement.

▸ Understanding the limitations of many outcome measures will help to critically appraise the evidence base.

References

1. Wormgoor, M.E.A. & Rodenburg, S.C. (2021) 'The evidence base for physiotherapy in myalgic encephalomyelitis/chronic fatigue syndrome when considering post-exertional malaise: a systematic review and narrative synthesis.' *Journal of Translational Medicine 19* (1).
2. van Campen, C.M.C., Rowe, P.C. & Visser, F.C. (2020) 'Validation of the severity of myalgic encephalomyelitis/chronic fatigue syndrome by other measures than history: activity bracelet, cardiopulmonary exercise testing and a validated activity questionnaire: SF-36.' *Healthcare 8.*
3. Stokes, M. (2004) *Physical Management in Neurological Rehabilitation.* London: Elsevier Health Sciences.
4. Lachin, J.M. (2004) 'The role of measurement reliability in clinical trials.' *Clinical Trials 1* (6).

5. Bean, J.F., Olveczky, D.D., Kiely, D.K., LaRose, S.I. & Jette, A.M. (2011) 'Performance-based versus patient-reported physical function: what are the underlying predictors?' *Physical Therapy 19* (12).
6. Weldring, T. & Smith, S.M. (2013) 'Patient-reported outcomes (PROs) and patient-reported outcome measures (PROMs).' *Health Service Insights 4* (6).
7. Greenhalgh, J. (2009) 'The applications of PROs in clinical practice: what are they, do they work, and why?' *Quality of Life Research 18* (1).
8. Haywood, K.L., Staniszewska, S. & Chapman, S. (2012) 'Quality and acceptability of patient-reported outcome measures used in chronic fatigue syndrome/myalgic encephalomyelitis (CFS/ME): a systematic review.' *Quality of Life Research 21* (1).
9. Jason, L.A. & Sunnquist, M. (2018) 'The development of the DePaul Symptom Questionnaire: original, expanded, brief, and pediatric versions.' *Frontiers in Pediatrics 6* (6).
10. Jason, L.A., So, S., Brown, A.A., Sunnquist, M. & Evans, M. (2015) 'Test-retest reliability of the DePaul Symptom Questionnaire.' *Fatigue 3* (1).
11. Conroy, K., Bhatia, S., Islam, M. & Jason, L.A. (2021) 'Homebound versus bedridden status among those with myalgic encephalomyelitis/chronic fatigue syndrome.' *Healthcare 9* (106).
12. Bedree, H., Sunnquist, M. & Jason, L.A. (2019) 'The DePaul Symptom Questionnaire-2: a validation study.' *Fatigue 7* (3).
13. Bell, D.S. (1994) *CFIDS Disability Scale.* OI Resource. Accessed on 6/12/2022 at www.oiresource.com/cfsscale.htm.
14. Stouten, B. (2005) 'Identification of ambiguities in the 1994 chronic fatigue syndrome research case definition and recommendations for resolution.' *BMC Health Services Research 13* (5).
15. Jason, L.A., Evans, M., Brown, M., Porter, N., *et al.* (2011) 'Fatigue scales and chronic fatigue syndrome: issues of sensitivity and specificity.' *Disability Studies Quarterly* 31 (1).
16. Krupp, L.B., LaRocca, N.G., Muir-Nash, J. & Steinberg, A.D. (1989) 'The fatigue severity scale: application to patients with multiple sclerosis and systemic lupus erythematosus.' *Archives of Neurology 46* (10).
17. Krupp, L.B., LaRocca, N.G., Muir-Nash, J. & Steinberg A.D. (1989) 'The fatigue severity scale. Application to patients with multiple sclerosis and systemic lupus erythematosus.' *Archives of Neurology 46* (10).
18. Yang, M., Keller, S. & Lin, J.S. (2019) 'Psychometric properties of the PROMIS® Fatigue Short Form 7a among adults with myalgic encephalomyelitis/chronic fatigue syndrome.' *Quality of Life Research 28* (12).
19. Ameringer, S., Elswick, R.K., Jr., Menzies, V., Robins, J.L., *et al.* (2016) 'Psychometric Evaluation of the patient-reported outcomes measurement information system fatigue-short form across diverse populations.' *Nursing Research 65* (4).
20. Fisk, J.D., Ritvo, P.G., Ross, L., Haase, D.A., Marrie, T.J. & Schlech, W.F. (1994) 'Measuring the functional impact of fatigue: initial validation of the fatigue impact scale.' *Clinical Infectious Diseases 18* (1).
21. Mathiowetz, V. (2003) 'Test–retest reliability and convergent validity of the fatigue impact scale for persons with multiple sclerosis.' *American Journal of Occupational Therapy 57* (4).
22. Jackson, C. (2015) 'The Chalder Fatigue Scale (CFQ 11).' *Occupational Medicine 65* (1).
23. Jason, L., Ropacki, M.T., Nicole, B., Santoro, N.B., Richman, J.A., *et al.* (1997) 'A screening instrument for chronic fatigue syndrome.' *Journal of Chronic Fatigue Syndrome 3* (1).
24. Friedberg, F. & Jason, L.A. (2002) 'Selecting a fatigue rating scale.' *CFS Research Review 35* (7).
25. Lewis, I., Pairman, J., Spickett, G. & Newton, J.L. (2013) 'Clinical characteristics of a novel subgroup of chronic fatigue syndrome patients with postural orthostatic tachycardia syndrome.' *Journal of Internal Medicine 273* (5).

26. Goudsmit, E.M., Stouten, B. & Howes, S. (2008) 'Fatigue in myalgic encephalomy-elitis.' *Bulletin of IACFS/ME 16* (3).
27. Chalder, T., Berelowitz, G., Pawlikowska, T., Watts, L., *et al.* (1993) 'Development of a fatigue scale.' *Journal of Psychosomatic Research 37* (2).
28. Worm-Smeitink, M., Gielissen, M., Bloot, L., van Laarhoven, H.W.M., *et al.* (2017) 'The assessment of fatigue: psychometric qualities and norms for the checklist individual strength.' *Journal of Psychosomatic Research 98.*
29. Smets, E.M., Garssen, B., Bonke, B. & De Haes, J.C. (1995) 'The Multidimensional Fatigue Inventory (MFI) psychometric qualities of an instrument to assess fatigue.' *Journal of Psychosomatic Research 39* (3).
30. Murdock, K.W., Wang, X.S., Shi, Q., Cleeland, C.S., Fagundes, C.P. & Vernon, S.D. (2017) 'The utility of patient-reported outcome measures among patients with myalgic encephalomyelitis/chronic fatigue syndrome.' *Quality of Life Research 26* (4).
31. Ray, C., Weir, W., Phillips, S. & Cullen, S. (1992) 'Development of a measure of symptoms in chronic fatigue syndrome: the profile of fatigue-related symptoms (pfrs).' *Psychology & Health 7* (1).
32. Oxford Medical Education (2022) 'Mini Mental State Examination.' Accessed on 6/12/2022 at https://oxfordmedicaleducation.com/geriatrics/mini-mental-state-examination-mmse.
33. O'Connor, D.W., Pollitt, P.A., Hyde, J.B., Fellows, J.L., *et al.* (1989) 'The reliability and validity of the Mini-Mental State in a British community survey.' *Journal of Psychiatric Research 23* (1).
34. Broadbent, D.E., Cooper, P.F., FitzGerald, P. & Parkes, K.R. (1982) 'The Cognitive Failures Questionnaire (CFQ) and its correlates.' *British Journal of Clinical Psychology 21.*
35. Bridger, R.S., Johnsen, S.Å. & Brasher, K. (2013) 'Psychometric properties of the Cognitive Failures Questionnaire.' *Ergonomics 56* (10).
36. Johns, M.W. (1991) 'A new method for measuring daytime sleepiness: the Epworth Sleepiness Scale.' *Sleep 14* (6).
37. Johns, M.W. (1992) 'Reliability and factor analysis of the Epworth Sleepiness Scale.' *Sleep 15* (4).
38. Mastin, D.F., Bryson, J. & Corwyn, R. (2006) 'Assessment of sleep hygiene using the Sleep Hygiene Index.' *Journal of Behavioural Medicine 29.*
39. Buysse, D.J., Reynolds, C.F., III, Monk, T.H., Berman, S.R. & Kupfer, D.J. (1989) 'The Pittsburgh Sleep Quality Index: a new instrument for psychiatric practice and research.' *Psychiatry Research 28* (2).
40. Backhaus, J., Junghanns, K., Broocks, A., Riemann, D. & Hohagen, F. (2002) 'Test-retest reliability and validity of the Pittsburgh Sleep Quality Index in primary insomnia.' *Journal of Psychosomatic Research 53* (3).
41. Grandner, M.A., Kripke, D.F., Yoon, I.Y. & Youngstedt, S.D. (2006) 'Criterion validity of the Pittsburgh Sleep Quality Index: investigation in a non-clinical sample.' *Sleep and Biological Rhythms 4* (2).
42. Suarez, G.A., Opfer-Gehrking, T.L., Offord, K.P., Atkinson, E.J., O'Brien, P.C. & Low, P.A. (1999) 'The Autonomic Symptom Profile: a new instrument to assess autonomic symptoms.' *Neurology 52* (3).
43. Newton, J.L., Okonkwo, O., Sutcliffe, K., Seth, A., Shin, J. & Jones, D.E.J. (n.d.) 'Symptoms of autonomic dysfunction in chronic fatigue syndrome.' *QJM: An International Journal of Medicine 100* (8).
44. Sletten, D.M., Suarez, G.A., Low, P.A., Mandrekar, J.& Singer, W. (2012) 'COMPASS 31: a refined and abbreviated composite autonomic symptom score.' *Mayo Clinic Proceedings 87* (12).
45. Kaufmann, H., Malamut, R., Norcliffe-Kaufmann, L., Rosa, K. & Freeman, R. (2012) 'The Orthostatic Hypotension Questionnaire (OHQ): validation of a novel symptom assessment scale.' *Clinical Autonomic Research 22* (2).

46. Low, P.A., Tomalia, V.A. & Park, K.J. (2013) 'Autonomic function tests: some clinical applications.' *Journal of Clinical Neurology 9* (1).
47. Finucane, C., van Wijnen, V.K. & Fan, C.W. (2019) 'A practical guide to active stand testing and analysis using continuous beat-to-beat non-invasive blood pressure monitoring.' *Clinical Autonomic Research 29*.
48. Kirbiš, M., Grad, A., Meglič, B. & Bajrović, F.F. (2013) 'Comparison of active standing test, head-up tilt test and 24-h ambulatory heart rate and blood pressure monitoring in diagnosing postural tachycardia.' *Functional Neurology 28* (1).
49. Lee, J., Vernon, S.D. & Jeys, P. (2020) 'Hemodynamics during the 10-minute NASA Lean Test: evidence of circulatory decompensation in a subset of ME/CFS patients.' *Journal of Translational Medicine 18* (314).
50. Freeman, R., Wieling, W., Axelrod, F.B., Benditt, D.G., *et al.* (2011) 'Consensus statement on the definition of orthostatic hypotension, neurally mediated syncope and the postural tachycardia syndrome.' *Clinical Autonomic Research 21* (2).
51. Fedorowski, A. (2019) 'Postural orthostatic tachycardia syndrome: clinical presentation, aetiology and management.' *Journal of Internal Medicine 285* (4).
52. Tracy, L.M., Ioannou, L., Baker, K.S., Gibson, S.J., Georgiou-Karistianis, N. & Giummarra, M. (2016) 'Meta-analytic evidence for decreased heart rate variability in chronic pain implicating parasympathetic nervous system dysregulation.' *Pain 157* (1).
53. Bertsch, K., Hagemann, D., Naumann, E., Schächinger, H. & Schulz, A. (2012) 'Stability of heart rate variability indices reflecting parasympathetic activity.' *Psychophysiology 49* (5).
54. Thomas, B.L., Claassen, N., Becker, P. & Viljoen, M. (2019) 'Validity of commonly used heart rate variability markers of autonomic nervous system function.' *Neuropsychobiology 78* (1).
55. Dixhoorn, J.V. & Folgering, H. (2015) 'The Nijmegen Questionnaire and dysfunctional breathing.' *ERJ Open Research 1* (1).
56. Li Ogilvie, V., Kayes, N. & Kersten, P. (2019) 'The Nijmegen Questionnaire: a valid measure for hyperventilation.' *New Zealand Journal of Physiotherapy 47* (3).
57. Todd, S., Walsted, E.S., Grillo, L., Livingston, R., Menzies-Gow, A. & Hull, J.H. (2018) 'Novel assessment tool to detect breathing pattern disorder in patients with refractory asthma.' *Respirology 23* (3).
58. Mitchell, A.J., Bacon, C.J. & Moran, R.W. (2016) 'Reliability and determinants of Self-Evaluation of Breathing Questionnaire (SEBQ) score: a symptoms-based measure of dysfunctional breathing.' *Applied Psychophysiology and Biofeedback 41* (1).
59. Williamson, A. & Hoggart, B. (2005) 'Pain: a review of three commonly used pain rating scales.' *Journal of Clinical Nursing 14*.
60. Jensen, M.P., Turner, J.A. & Romano, J.M. (1994) 'What is the maximum number of levels needed in pain intensity measurement?' *Pain 58* (3).
61. Joyce, C.R.B., Zutshi, D.W. & Hrubes, V. (1975) 'Comparison of fixed interval and visual analogue scales for rating chronic pain.' *European Journal of Clinical Pharmacology 8*.
62. Gallagher, E.J., Bijur, P.E., Latimer, C. & Silver, W. (2002) 'Reliability and validity of a visual analog scale for acute abdominal pain in the ED.' *American Journal of Emergency Medicine 20* (4).
63. Shirley Ryan AbilityLab (2018) 'PROMIS – physical function.' Accessed on 6/12/2022 at www.sralab.org/rehabilitation-measures/promis-physical-function.
64. Jensen, R.E., Potosky, A.L., Reeve, B.B., Hahn, E., *et al.* (2015) 'Validation of the PROMIS physical function measures in a diverse US population-based cohort of cancer patients.' *Quality of Life Research 24* (10).
65. US Food and Drug Administration (2021) 'Pulse oximeter accuracy and limitations: FDA safety communication.' US Food and Drug Administration. Accessed on 12/01/23 at www.fda.gov/medical-devices/safety-communications/pulse-oximeter-accuracy-and-limitations-fda-safety-communication.

66. Losa-Iglesias, M.E., Becerro-de-Bengoa-Vallejo, R. & Becerro-de-Bengoa-Losa, K.R. (2016) 'Reliability and concurrent validity of a peripheral pulse oximeter and health-app system for the quantification of heart rate in healthy adults.' *Health Informatics Journal 22* (2).
67. Iyriboz, Y., Powers, S., Morrow, J., Ayers, D. & Landry, G. (1991) 'Accuracy of pulse oximeters in estimating heart rate at rest and during exercise.' *British Journal of Sports Medicine 25* (3).
68. Enomoto, K., Shimizu, R. & Kudo, H. (2018) 'Real-time skin lactic acid monitoring system for assessment of training intensity.' *Electronics and Communications in Japan 101.*
69. Albouaini, K., Egred, M., Alahmar, A. & Wright, D.J. (2007) 'Cardiopulmonary exercise testing and its application.' *Postgraduate Medical Journal 83* (985).
70. Melanson, E.L., Freedson, P.S., Hendelman, D. & Debold, E. (1996) 'Reliability and validity of a portable metabolic measurement system.' *Canadian Journal of Applied Physiology 21* (2).
71. Clague-Baker, N., Dawes, H., Tyson, S., Bull, M., Leslie K. & Hilliard, N. (2021) 'Feasibility of investigating oxygen consumption (VO2), heart rate, blood pressure, lactic acid levels and activity levels of people with myalgic encephalomyelitis during normal daily activities.' Physios for ME. Accessed on 7/12/2022 at www.physiosforme.com/feasabilitymeasuressummary.
72. Palombo, T., Campos, A., Vernon, S.D. & Roundy, S. (2020) 'Accurate and objective determination of myalgic encephalomyelitis/chronic fatigue syndrome disease severity with a wearable sensor.' *Journal of Translational Medicine 18* (1).
73. Lee, J.Y., Kwon, S., Kim, W.S., Hahn, S.J., Park, J. & Paik, N.J. (2018) 'Feasibility, reliability, and validity of using accelerometers to measure physical activities of patients with stroke during inpatient rehabilitation.' *PLOS ONE 13* (12).
74. Bennell, K., Dobson, F. & Hinman, R. (2011) 'Measures of physical performance assessments: Self-Paced Walk Test (SPWT), Stair Climb Test (SCT), Six-Minute Walk Test (6MWT), Chair Stand Test (CST), Timed Up & Go (TUG), Sock Test, Lift and Carry Test (LCT), and Car Task.' *Arthritis Care & Research 53* (Suppl. 11).
75. Ware, J.E. & Sherbourne, C.D. (1992) 'The MOS 36-item Short-Form Health Survey (SF-36): I. conceptual framework and item selection.' *Medical Care 30* (6).
76. Brazier, J.E., Harper, R., Jones, N.M., O'Cathain, A., *et al.* (1992) 'Validating the SF-36 health survey questionnaire: new outcome measure for primary care.' *British Medical Journal 305* (6846).
77. Lins, L. & Carvalho, F.M. (2016) 'SF-36 total score as a single measure of health-related quality of life: scoping review.' *SAGE Open Med 4.*
78. EuroQol Group (1990) 'EuroQol – a new facility for the measurement of health-related quality of life.' *Health Policy 16* (3).
79. Myers, C. & Wilks, D. (1999) 'Comparison of Euroqol EQ-5D and SF-36 in patients with chronic fatigue syndrome.' *Quality of Life Research 8.*
80. Zigmond, A.S. & Snaith, R.P. (1983) 'The Hospital Anxiety and Depression Scale.' *Acta Psychiatrica Scandinavica 67.*
81. Zigmond, A.S. & Snaith, R.P. (1983) 'The Hospital Anxiety and Depression Scale.' *Acta Psychiatrica Scandinavica 67.*
82. McCue, P., Buchanan, T. & Martin, C.R. (2006) 'Screening for psychological distress using internet administration of the Hospital Anxiety and Depression Scale (HADS) in individuals with chronic fatigue syndrome.' *British Journal of Clinical Psychology 45.*
83. Deale, A. & Wessely, S. (2000) 'Diagnosis of psychiatric disorder in clinical evaluation of chronic fatigue syndrome.' *Journal of the Royal Society of Medicine 93* (6).
84. Shepherd, C. & Chaudhuri, A. (2019) *ME/CFS/PVFS: An Exploration of the Key Clinical Issues.* Gawcott: The ME Association.

CASE STUDIES

CASE STUDY: KIM

Age	56
Present condition and reason for seeking physiotherapy	Increase in severity of ME/CFS symptoms following COVID-19 infection Previously moderate ME/CFS, currently severe ME/CFS Seeking physio for support and advice to help her get back to pre-COVID-19 baseline
History of present condition	ME/CFS symptoms for over thirty years Progressed from mild to moderate ME/CFS after further viral illness seven years ago Recent COVID-19 infection and subsequent flare in ME/CFS symptoms has led to severe presentation and new orthostatic intolerance symptoms
Past medical history and co-morbidities	Thirty+ years ago: post viral fatigue syndrome Seven years ago: viral illness followed by ME/CFS diagnosis Five years ago: diagnosed mild sleep apnoea Now under investigation for POTS/orthostatic intolerance
Past experience of physiotherapy	Attended fatigue clinic after original ME/CFS diagnosis. Given cognitive behavioural therapy, which was not helpful, and advised to incrementally increase her walking speed, which made her deteriorate. Kim self-discharged from the fatigue clinic as she felt it was not a safe service Seen several private physiotherapists in the past: • one had no experience with ME/CFS and gave exercises that were unmanageable • one had personal understanding of fatigue and gave advice on core strength and safe exercise, which was helpful
Medication	B12 patches Vitamin drink
Hydration and nutrition	Stays well hydrated, which helps to manage symptoms
Social history	Supportive husband Unable to work, some voluntary work when able
Home environment	Block at end of bed to slightly elevate head Wheelchair for outdoor mobility Shower stool
Activities of daily living	Manages most ADLs with pacing Unable to stand for long periods Husband does most cooking and cleaning Able to self-care at the moment

Daily routine	8–9am: breakfast
	9–9.30am: sits to do teeth and hair
	Coffee break
	1 hour: admin/voluntary work from home
	Lunch prep
	1pm–3pm: 'down time' including body scan meditation, breathing exercises
	3–4pm: dinner prep
	5pm: dinner and rest
	8pm: shower/bath
	9.30pm: bed

Subjective symptoms

Post exertional malaise (PEM)	Triggers: physical, cognitive and social exertion, heat, cold, infection
	PEM causes severe sleep dysfunction (awake 2–5am) and significant cognitive dysfunction
	Rest eases PEM
Fatigue	Physical, cognitive and emotional fatigue – at worst dependent for basic needs
Cognitive dysfunction	Difficulty with processing, concentrating, word finding
Sleep dysfunction	Difficulty sleeping and unrefreshing sleep during PEM
Pain	No pain
Neurological impairments	Sound hypersensitivity
Autonomic dysfunction	Elevated heart rate on standing, currently being investigated for POTS; exacerbated by heat
Neuroendocrine manifestations	Intolerant to heat
Immune dysfunction	Viral flares, very frequent cold symptoms, takes a long time to get over them and they set her back
Any other reported symptoms?	N/A
Which symptoms are the patient's current priority?	All, but feels new orthostatic intolerance symptoms are exacerbating all other symptoms and limiting progress

Objective assessment

Observation	Cognitive decline noted after 20 minutes of assessment
Muscle, joint and skin integrity	Beighton score – 5/9 suggesting generalized hypermobility
Muscle strength	Not formally assessed
Neurological testing	Not assessed
Neurodynamic testing	Not assessed
Movement analysis	Normal – observed throughout the assessment, no indication for specific functional assessment
Orthostatic intolerance	NASA lean test: increase of 30bpm on standing
Dysfunctional breathing	Not assessed
Exercise tolerance	Not appropriate due to PEM caused by physical exertion
Any other objective assessment	Looked at heart rate data that Kim had collected Observable spikes in heart rate throughout the day Analysis of her heart rate variability data showed her sympathetic system was dominant 90–95% of the time including during sleep Step-count data: managing 3000–4000 steps per day

Management plan

Symptom to address	Management strategy
PEM (causing cognitive dysfunction and physical fatigue)	Energy management: increase structured rests during the day
Orthostatic intolerance	Provide supporting letters to consultants/GP and report results of NASA lean test Advice on hydration
Viral flares	Refer for medical review
Heat intolerance	Provide supporting letter for funding of air conditioning unit for use over summer months
Autonomic nervous system dysfunction	Explore self-treatment with transcutaneous vagus nerve stimulation

Outcome

Kim had lived with ME/CFS for so long that she already had a good grasp of energy management strategies; however adding further rest periods to her routine helped to stabilize her symptom flare. Kim was also encouraged to use her heart rate variability data for pacing, by checking it each morning and planning her activities for the day according to whether she had higher levels of dysfunction.

Kim was willing to try self-treatment with transcutaneous vagus nerve stimulation, and this appeared to have a positive impact with Kim reporting that her sleep quality had improved as well as her digestive health.

Provision of an air-conditioning unit provided significant relief to Kim in respect of her heat intolerance, which reduced her triggers of PEM.

After further appointments and investigations with medical consultants Kim was formally diagnosed with postural orthostatic tachycardia syndrome and prescribed medication. She was also given antivirals. This treatment improved her symptoms further and once Kim had an established period of symptom stability she began to slowly and carefully increase the amount of activity aiming towards her previous baseline, while continuing to ensure she paced and incorporated adequate rest periods throughout the day.

Kim is now mostly back at her pre-COVID-19 baseline of moderate ME/CFS, with her new orthostatic intolerance managed medically. Kim can manage three to four hours of activity per day, including gentle walking. She can tolerate standing again, allowing her to do light tasks in the kitchen. While she is still significantly impacted by her ME/CFS, her quality of life has improved now that her post-COVID-19 symptom flare has subsided.

CASE STUDY: OLIVER

Age	14
Present condition and reason for seeking physiotherapy	Moderate ME/CFS Would like help with reducing PEM, leg pain and migraines
History of present condition	Post viral onset after illness aged 12 Took six weeks to recover but never got back to full fitness, then had major relapse after playing football Since then has been off school, as every time he tried to go in he had significant increase in symptoms Has seen little improvement since onset
Past medical history and co-morbidities	Severe nut allergy requiring EpiPen Hayfever
Past experience of physiotherapy	Only for sporting injuries
Medication	Nil at initial assessment
Hydration and nutrition	Drinks constant amount of water during day Diet fairly limited – typical meal is pasta and cheese
Social history	Unable to go into school Studying online: maximum two hours per day, fifty minutes at a time Listens to music Used to be very sporty (football, cycling) but now unable Social contact limited to immediate family (used to have wide group of friends)
Home environment	Lives with family, parents provide support
Activities of daily living	When first ill aged 12 spent most of time in bed or chair in bedroom, went downstairs once a day Can now leave room more often and able to sit at desk for lessons for about fifty minutes' duration at a time Able to wash, dress and shower (although needs to rest after shower and does nothing else that day) Needs help with laundry and food prep other than simple sandwiches

Daily routine	Takes a long time to get up and going
	Online school during week and homework
	Reads, listens to music, watches TV at weekend
	Eats lunch
	Long wind-down before bed
	Sleep

Subjective symptoms

Post exertional malaise	Minimal exertion is enough to trigger PEM
	On a good week can manage 45 minutes of cognitive effort for schooling 2–3 times a week, and an occasional trip outside the house for a very short walk or short drive
Fatigue	Describes as simply 'massive fatigue'
Cognitive dysfunction	Reports brain fog; word finding difficulty
	Takes significantly longer to work through tasks
	Describes as 'like wading through treacle in the brain'
Sleep dysfunction	Sleep reversal – often still awake at 1:30/2am
	Unrefreshing sleep – wakes up in the morning not feeling as if has slept well
	Sometimes falls asleep in the middle of the day if really tired
Pain	Myalgia reported in leg muscles especially after physical exertion
	Migraines
Neurological impairments	Bright light when studying can lead to migraines; may suggest hypersensitivity to light
Autonomic dysfunction	None diagnosed
Neuroendocrine manifestations	N/A
Immune dysfunction	Repeated colds and viruses every couple of weeks
Any other reported symptoms?	N/A
Which symptoms are their current priority?	PEM, migraines, leg pain

Objective assessment

Observation	After 10 minutes of discussion there was noticeable cognitive fatigue. Most of discussion took place with Oliver lying down or sitting with feet up (preferred position)
	Poor sitting posture – head poked forward, thoracic slump. Particularly noticeable in chairs with poor lumbar support, including existing workstation arrangements
Muscle, joint and skin integrity	Noticeable, significant range of movement at hip, knee, elbows and fingers/thumbs, suggesting hypermobility
	Fingers and thumbs reported to be particularly susceptible to subluxation with low force, such as contact against chair or bedclothes
Muscle strength	Reports decreased muscle strength since developing ME/CFS but not appropriate to objectively test all muscle groups due to low threshold of exertion before onset of PEM
	Can sit to stand, manage stairs, lift books
Neurological testing	Not assessed
Movement analysis	No movement disorders noted
Orthostatic intolerance	No abnormal response during sit to stand
Dysfunctional breathing	Good diaphragmatic breathing observed at rest
Exercise tolerance	Formal exercise tests not appropriate due to potential for PEM
Any other objective assessment	CFIDS scale: 20

Management plan

Symptom to address	Management strategy
PEM	Energy management Activity diary to identify pattern in onset of PEM Planning/pacing activities: • chunking of schoolwork to allow rest breaks between lessons • scheduling to avoid early starts as late morning/early afternoon identified as best time for activity • activities planned in small amounts spread through day rather than single high intensity activity • scheduling activities throughout the week to spread out major demands If PEM stabilizes, consider adding in activity as appropriate/tolerated
Posture/migraines	Postural exercises to improve head position when in sitting Assess workstation ergonomics and advise re positioning for school work Advice re environment (lighting) Refer for Disability Support Assessment
Myalgia	Gentle massage Advice on lower limb stretching Energy management to avoid triggering PEM, as myalgia was a main symptom of PEM Try magnesium spray
Finger and thumb subluxations	Strapping, ice and rest when injury occurs Advice on dictation software and/or a scribe for lessons when injuries occur
Medical review	Referred for review of medications

Outcome

The activity diary highlighted that Oliver's PEM would have a delay of two to three days after an activity. This information helped with further planning and pacing.

Following initial assessment Oliver had regular monthly appointments to check in on progress and see whether there was a need to amend his routine. As education was his priority, an additional school lesson was added when Oliver managed six weeks without an episode of PEM. He was provided with a laptop, split keyboard and software to support studying by reducing cognitive demands.

After a medical review Oliver was put on antivirals and B12 injections, which further helped to stabilize symptoms and improve his cognitive function. Magnesium spray also helped to manage his myalgia.

Once Oliver had experienced a six-month period of stability, with no instances of PEM and a consistent ability to complete his workload, he began to explore the addition of physical activity and targeted exercise to address his posture and hypermobility. He began isometric exercises using simple resistance equipment for chest, back, legs and core, starting with three repetitions of each exercise and a gap of three days in between sessions in order to rule out PEM.

Once it was established that Oliver could manage this without triggering PEM, walking was also added to his routine, with a very short, low intensity walk of less than five minutes, which was also spaced out by three days to monitor for PEM. The length of time spent walking was increased after each six-week period of stability.

Strength work and walking routines were reduced during any symptom flares, if Oliver felt generally unwell, or if there were other demands on his energy such as exams, hospital appointments or social events.

After the age of 16 his physiotherapy input reduced to an 'SOS' approach, where Oliver could contact the physiotherapist as and when he needed advice. More intensive input was required when he started studying for another set of exams aged 18 and experienced an exacerbation of symptoms, and he received physiotherapy support fortnightly until he had stabilized, which then reduced back to monthly and then resumed the 'SOS' approach. Oliver most often sought assistance for strapping after digit subluxations.

Now aged 22, Oliver's frequency of PEM has reduced so significantly that he rarely experiences an episode. This has also reduced the myalgia in his lower limbs and frequency of migraines, and improved his sleep patterns. He still uses energy management strategies to manage his symptoms with a daily routine that he adapts depending on how he is feeling, and he can still only engage in minimal social activities. He has reduced the doses of his antivirals and B12 injections to a maintenance level.

Oliver is now studying at university and he can attend classes every day for two to three hours and attends them in person two to three times per week. He walks 25 minutes each way to university, and on days he isn't in class he walks for 30 minutes as part of his exercise routine. His strengthening routine now involves dynamic exercises using dumbbells and resistance bands, and he works at eight to ten repetitions of each exercise, three times per week. His posture has significantly improved.

He has lived independently since starting further education and has planned and cooked his meals, cleaned, and done his washing with minimal assistance from his parents.

His CFIDS (Chronic Fatigue and Immune Dysfunction Syndrome) score is now 75 (previously 20).

CASE STUDY: MO

Age	37
Present condition and reason for seeking physiotherapy	Referred by respiratory physio as not following 'normal' rehab trajectory following infection with COVID-19 Suffering with crippling fatigue, extreme brain fog and significant pain Unable to function normally
History of present condition	Post viral onset after COVID-19 infection 18 months ago Never got back to full fitness after covid infection but was making steady progress with walking and starting couch to 5k programme Eight months later, during a national lockdown, he had to combine home schooling and working from home while continuing with his exercise programme. This resulted in a major relapse with significant increase in symptoms and he has been struggling ever since
Past medical history and co-morbidities	Nil of note. Previously fit and healthy, working full time, active family life and enjoyed playing team sports
Past experience of physiotherapy	Nil
Medication	Pain relief 3 × per day. Reports minimal benefits
Hydration and nutrition	Often forgets to drink enough during the day as finds it hard to remember everything Often doesn't eat much as too busy working
Social history	Lives with wife and three children of primary school age Wife often works away so manages all school drop-offs and pick-ups. No close family support Used to be very sporty and enjoyed fitness activities but not able to get back to those since initial infection Used to enjoy walks with family at weekends, but not been able to since initial infection
Home environment	Lives in a house with bathroom upstairs No aids or adaptations
Activities of daily living	Responsible for all cooking and food preparation for children and wife Drives for school run Drives to shops for food Able to wash, dress and shower independently. Recently needed wife to assist in shower as feels like he is about to collapse when washing his hair Responsible for all household chores

Daily routine	Wake up early as takes long time to prepare school packed lunches
	Does school run
	Works from home on computer
	Cleans and tidies house. Has to vacuum every day due to cat with long hair
	School run in afternoon
	Cooks evening meal and cleans up afterwards
	Sleep
	Describes himself as 'always on the go'

Subjective symptoms

Post exertional malaise	Symptoms are constant at present
Fatigue	Fatigue is overwhelming but he will push through
	Sometimes needs to have a nap early afternoon
Cognitive dysfunction	Reports brain fog, word finding difficulty and sometimes can't remember what activity he had started doing
Sleep dysfunction	Unrefreshing sleep – wakes up in the morning not feeling as if has slept well
	Sometimes falls asleep in the middle of the day if really tired
Pain	Describes pain in whole body. Pain killers can take edge off the pain but rarely take it all away
Neurological impairments	Some severe headaches when very tired
Autonomic dysfunction	Reported dizziness and light-headedness
	Finds it easier to work if legs are elevated
Neuroendocrine manifestations	N/A
Immune dysfunction	None reported
Any other reported symptoms?	Hair loss on crown
Which symptoms are their current priority?	Fatigue and brain fog

Objective assessment

Observation	During initial phone call to arrange appointment there was significant word finding trouble and difficulty in constructing sentences after first five minutes Initial assessment was via phone call. After 15 minutes there was word finding trouble and some slurring of speech, so arranged follow-on call the next week
Muscle, joint and skin integrity	Virtual appointments so N/A
Muscle strength	Subjectively reports can sit to stand, manage stairs, lift shopping but feels fatigued constantly
Neurological testing	Virtual appointments so N/A
Movement analysis	Virtual appointments so N/A
Orthostatic intolerance	Virtual appointments so N/A
Dysfunctional breathing	Virtual appointments so N/A Had previously been seen by respiratory consultant and nothing abnormal detected
Exercise tolerance	Virtual appointments so N/A Exercise tests not appropriate due to level of symptoms reported
Any other objective assessment	None

Management plan

Symptom to address	Management strategy
PEM	Activity diary to identify a 'typical' day and a 'typical' week Recommend a two-week period of rest to stabilize symptoms by reducing all non-essential activities and getting help from others (e.g. children to pack their own lunches the night before school to reduce morning workload) Keep a symptom and activity diary during rest period Refer for equipment assessment with occupational therapy
Medical review	Referred to general practitioner for review of pain relief

Outcome

Following initial assessment a video-call was scheduled one week later. Mo reported he could barely remember the details of the first assessment and had been in bed for three days following the call as he had felt so unwell. The discussion of which activities he could remove for his period of rest was repeated and this was written up for him to refer back to. Mo was reviewed fortnightly via video call.

Mo was able to moderately reduce his activity levels and saw an associated minor reduction in his symptoms. During the next appointment, activities that he had to add back in were reviewed to see if they could be modified to reduce the exertional load. Examples include:

- batch cooking to reduce meal prep workload
- children to continue assisting with packing their own lunches
- using online shopping for weekly food shop.

Mo was encouraged to set alarms as reminders to take a break from work and to hydrate. His workstation was adjusted to allow him to raise his feet.

Occupational therapists provided Mo with a shower stool and perching stool to reduce the time spent in standing. His general practitioner changed his medication which helped to address his pain symptoms.

With the new equipment and energy management strategies, Mo began to experience some improvements in his symptoms, only rarely needing to rest in bed during the day. However, Mo continued to report dizziness and light-headedness, even on days his other symptoms were improved. He was therefore referred for an assessment for orthostatic intolerance. An active stand test showed he was borderline for postural orthostatic tachycardia syndrome and he was started on medication to reduce his heart rate, which provided some improvement to these symptoms.

Mo was very keen to increase his activity levels and decided to take a weekend walk with his family. He enjoyed this so much that they ended up walking for an hour, and the following day his symptoms were exacerbated so severely that he was unable to work and needed most of the week to stabilize. The setback was upsetting and Mo felt he would never be able to do normal things with his children again. With support and reassurance, Mo resumed his energy management techniques to re-establish stability in his symptoms. A walking frame with a seat component or a wheelchair were suggested alternatives to allow him to engage in walking activities with his family.

Mo was understandably struggling with the emotional impact of such significant changes to his life, and his general practitioner therefore referred him for psychological support.

Mo continues to use energy management techniques but has regular episodes of PEM due to a tendency to overdo activity when his symptoms are stable. He has reduced his working days down to three times per week, which means he can manage to keep on top of basic household tasks. Mo understands he would probably be able to reduce his episodes of PEM even further by cutting down on more activity, but his family commitments mean this is not possible.

Mo will need ongoing periodic input to help him deal with any future relapses.

CASE STUDY: ANA

Age	53
Present condition and reason for seeking physiotherapy	Severe/very severe ME/CFS Significant relapse three months ago following chest infection and asthma flare, which required a course of steroids. Ana does not tolerate steroids and this led to her being 100% bedbound and needing 24/7 care She is now improving and seeking physio to get back to her pre-relapse baseline, which involved: • mobile short distances around house • daily care/support with meal prep, laundry, heavier housework duties, e.g. vacuuming, bed making • friends and mother supporting with admin and other household duties; 80–90% bedbound/sofabound • able to go out once every two to four weeks with assistance from friend/carer
History of present condition	21-year history of severe/very severe ME/CFS Initial onset from viral infection leading to post viral fatigue syndrome and severe asthma. This developed into severe ME/CFS and Ana was completely bedbound for the first year, needing a brace to support her back and neck Experienced some recovery after first year but still severely affected and has had a number of significant relapses over the years, needing 24/7 care. Worst relapses last up to 18 months
Past medical history and co-morbidities	Fibromyalgia, autoimmune thyroiditis, thalassaemia trait, GERD, atypical asthma (likely MCAS related, not diagnosed), POTS, chronic migraine
Past experience of physiotherapy	Varied and mostly poor experience of physiotherapy to date Inpatient rehabilitation programme Physiotherapy stretches in morning followed by 40-minute exercise programme in afternoon. One day of this programme caused Ana to relapse so severely that she had to be discharged from the programme. The relapse resulted in Ana being fully bedbound requiring continuous care at home for nine months Outpatient rehabilitation programmes: tried twice, both times resulted in severe relapses. The programmes involved circuit training in a bright gym with loud music, and encouragement to push to complete all the exercises

	Community physiotherapy input following relapses: • Home visits were more helpful, but some physiotherapists used graded exercise therapy approaches that pushed beyond limitations, set unrealistic timeframes or used rigid incremental increases in activity Private physiotherapy input: • Acupuncture and gentle bed-based exercises. The acupuncture provided some pain relief, but sessions were clinic based and the symptom exacerbation from attending these appointments was over-riding any benefits
Medication	Levothyroxine, paracetamol, HRT, Oramorph PRN, ondansetron, omeprazole, Fostair, Seretide, Spiriva Respimat, senna, Ventolin and saline nebulizers
Hydration and nutrition	Lost weight due to relapse, now able to drink and eat in small quantities. Dietician has been involved
Social history	24-hour care at home Minimal family support Unable to work Unable to socialize Very poor quality of life
Home environment	Hoist, slide sheets, commode, shower stool, toilet frame, rollator frame, electric profiling bed
Activities of daily living	Currently requires assistance of two for all activities of daily living Baseline is assistance of one person
Daily routine	Currently 80–90% bedbound; all care and meals delivered by carer

Subjective symptoms

Post exertional malaise	Describes as being in a state of continuous PEM Triggers can be cognitive, sensory, physical and orthostatic
Fatigue	Severe, fluctuating, sleeping during daytime
Cognitive dysfunction	Severe Now improving as coming out of relapse, but unable to talk for more than five minutes
Sleep dysfunction	Very poor and dysregulated sleep due to chronic pain History of insomnia Currently in bed 80–90% of the time, resting and sleeping as body needs

Pain	Severe pain in whole body, constant; can reach 9/10 on numerical rating scale during relapse; 'normal' is 7/10
Neurological impairments	Painful to touch, especially lower limbs Extremely sensitive to light, noise and smell Social contact can cause pain Neurogenic bladder dysfunction
Autonomic dysfunction	Urinary dysfunction, bowel (constipation and diarrhoea) Postural orthostatic tachycardia syndrome; changes to blood pressure and heart rate. Can faint even when sitting up in bed for short periods Temperature dysregulation
Immune dysfunction	Allergies increase during relapse Sensitive to medications, chemicals and some foods Viral symptoms – severe flu-like symptoms that fluctuate
Any other reported symptoms?	Asthma flare (initial infection post viral asthma)
Which symptoms are the patient's current priority?	To return to baseline pre-chest infection

Objective assessment

Observation	Frail due to weight loss
Muscle, joint and skin integrity	Soreness from mattress in several places but skin intact Restricted active range of movement for shoulder Difficult to fully assess due to severe limitations
Hypermobility	Global hypermobility
Muscle strength	Generalized muscle weakness Inappropriate to repeat testing due to symptom severity
Neurological testing	Not appropriate to assess due to symptom severity
Neurodynamic testing	Not appropriate to assess due to symptom severity
Movement analysis	Slow movement Requires assistance of one to move Immediate exacerbation of symptoms on movement

Orthostatic intolerance	Not appropriate to conduct standing tests Orthostatic intolerance symptoms reported subjectively and evident on sitting/standing – became tachycardic, very faint and sweaty
Autonomic dysfunction	Heart rate and blood pressure extremely variable
Dysfunctional breathing	Increased respiratory rate
Exercise tolerance	Very poor, managed two minutes sitting on edge of bed before symptoms triggered No further testing appropriate

Management plan

Symptom to address	Management strategy
Managing emergence from relapse in respect of PEM, fatigue, and orthostatic intolerance	All sessions home-based or virtual Moving and handling training with care team on use of slide sheet and hoist Aim to gradually increase functional movement practice as able, e.g. rolling, lie to sit, sit to lie and gradually increasing sitting on edge of bed, sit to stand and walking with rollator frame Taught carers how to assist with these movements but educated on importance of only doing this when she is able and not to let her over-exert Educated (along with care team) on importance of rest
Asthma/chest infection prevention	Improve fluid intake Arrange regular input from respiratory nurse Regular repositioning in bed including sitting out of bed for short periods as able Deep breathing exercises
Weight loss	Refer to dietician

Outcome

Ana was very motivated to improve and do as much as she could, but it was so easy to trigger PEM that much of her physiotherapy input was initially around prompting her to prioritize rest and take her time. Progress was very much determined by the severity of her symptoms, and therefore it was important to work within her limits rather than try to follow any strict timed goals.

After four months Ana had regained the ability to walk around her house for short periods. A dietician prescribed drink supplements to help with her weight loss, although these were difficult to tolerate due to their richness.

It took another four months for Ana to return to her baseline prior to her chest infection. Each relapse has a negative impact on her overall health, which makes recovery prolonged.

Ana continues to have severe ME/CFS. She is housebound and has to spend long periods in bed. She still uses a walking frame and toilet frame, but she no longer requires continuous care support or the hoist. It is likely Ana will need ongoing periodic physiotherapy support to help her manage future relapses.

CASE STUDY: FAITH

Age	42
Present condition and reason for seeking physiotherapy	Moderate to severe ME/CFS Looking for any further advice on how to pace more efficiently Interested in using a heart rate monitor but finding it difficult to understand the method and equipment
History of present condition	Ten-year history of ME/CFS following viral infection
Past medical history and co-morbidities	Fatty liver – under control Food intolerances, multiple chemical sensitivities and dysautonomia
Past experience of physiotherapy	Following initial diagnosis was referred to occupational therapy department. Given information and advice regarding pacing Graded exercise therapy was suggested, but she had already experienced negative effects of exercise and seen research advising caution against it, so she refused Further pacing advice provided by a specialist ME/CFS service Support from specialist ME/CFS physiotherapist to minimize back pain from lying down most of the time due to ME/CFS
Medication	Nil
Hydration and nutrition	Drinks three strong coffees a day Reasonable diet – lots of food intolerances from ME/CFS impacting diet and leading to mainly meals prepared from scratch
Social history	Runs local charity group Unable to work Meets with friends regularly to play card games Meet up online to socialize with a friend once a week Spends time with family
Home environment	Lives with husband, child and dog Shower seat and hand rails in bathroom Wheelchair, walking stick and portable seat for mobilizing
Activities of daily living	Showering is exhausting and sometimes requires assistance from others Spends most of the day lying down, able to take part in small amounts of activity as long as rests before and after Can take a long time to recover if overdoes it

Daily routine	Wake up, feed dog Get (or help get) child ready for school and walk dog Rest for one hour Catch up on emails/social media/charity work Manages two × 30–45 min activities (one physical like housework, one cognitive like reading or charity work) Walk the dog Lunch One to two further periods of activity with rests Make dinner for family Rest Evening activities – TV, talking with family, sometimes further charity work. Once a week goes out, but needs more rest on that day

Subjective symptoms

Post exertional malaise	Physical and cognitive exertion are triggers. Managing OK with current energy management routine but still triggered especially with extra events such as hospital appointments
Fatigue	Always present and restricts activities but manageable with good pacing
Cognitive dysfunction	Always present, worse if tired/fatigued Can mix up basic words and forget conversations part way through
Sleep dysfunction	Always wake up feeling unrefreshed
Pain	Mild back pain
Neurological impairments	Hypersensitive to sound
Autonomic dysfunction	None identified
Neuroendocrine manifestations	N/A
Immune dysfunction	Seem to get ill often and can last a long time
Any other reported symptoms?	N/A
Which symptoms are their current priority?	PEM

Objective assessment

Formal objective assessment was not carried out. Implementation of heart rate monitor will form basis of objective measures to further assessment and develop management strategy.

Management plan

Symptom to address	Management strategy
PEM	Explore how heart rate monitoring can assist with energy management

Outcome

The first step was to help Faith to find a heart rate monitor. She had already looked at what was available on the market but she found the vast array of devices available overwhelming, especially with her cognitive dysfunction. The device was chosen based on price and platform familiarity.

Faith wore the monitor for three days to first establish her typical resting heart rate, then she trialled a two-week period with the limit set to 15 beats above her resting heart rate. After two weeks of using the heart rate monitor Faith discovered:

- she was setting the alert off almost constantly
- brushing her teeth was an activity that had a surprising effect on her heart rate
- many activities that would trigger the alert were hard to avoid, such as walking the dog or taking her child to school.

Based on these findings and on joint discussion, the following was decided:

- the alert limit would be raised
- Faith would use an electric toothbrush rather than a manual brush to reduce the workload of this task
- Faith would add in an additional rest prior to walking the dog or doing the school run.

With these modifications, Faith continued to trial the heart rate monitor and began to find it provided her with many benefits. An electric toothbrush reduced the physical exertion of her morning routine and resting prior to walking the dog resulted in a reduction in raised heart rate during the walks.

During physical tasks such as housework or walking, she now had a quick way of observing when she was starting to over-exert and began to take quick rests throughout the duration of a task, or experiment with modifications to the task in order to reduce their overall physical demands. However, cognitive exertion did not always set off the alert, so she had to pace cognitive tasks irrespective of her heart rate.

Faith found that the heart rate monitor was also helpful when talking to her family about what activities she was able to take part in each day, providing her with objective information to show them rather than having to explain how she was feeling. This allowed the family to plan activities together that met Faith's needs.

Faith remarked that she wished she had used heart rate monitoring at the beginning of her journey with ME/CFS as it made learning how to pace much quicker and easier. Certain experiences whose physical toll had taken her years to understand or discover, for example choosing what temperature to set the shower water, were almost instantly shown with the heart rate monitor.

Faith feels she has experienced fewer PEM episodes and less fatigue since implementing the heart rate monitor. The device has reduced the effort she has to put in to pacing and given her more confidence to try new experiences because she has an instant method of assessing how they are affecting her.

Appendix: Common Medications

This list is for reference only.

Any medication or supplement should be introduced under guidance of a trained medical practitioner.

Medications	Symptom treated
Pain relief	
• Analgesics/NSAIDs	Pain
– Paracetamol	
– Aspirin	
– Ibuprofen	
– Naproxen	
• Opioids	Pain
– Codeine	
– Dihydrocodeine	
– Tramadol	
– Low Dose Naltrexone (LDN) (1)	Pain, brain fog, sleep
• Local anaesthetics	
Benzodiazepines:	Sleep and brain fog
– Diazepam	
– Clonazepam	
– Lorazepam	
– Zopiclone	
Cardiovascular system	
• HCN channel blockers (for heart failure)	
– Ivabradine (2)	POTS
• Low BP	Low BP
– Midodrine	Autonomic dysfunction
• Beta blocker (for high HR)	POTS
– Bisoprolol	
– Propranolol	

cont.

Medications	Symptom treated
Gastrointestinal system	
• Antacid	
– Lansoprazole	
– Omeprazole	
• Laxatives	
– Laxido	
• Antiflatulent	
– Simethicone	
• Antispasmodics	IBS pain relief
– Mebeverine hydrochloride	
Kidneys	
• Antidiuretic	Low BP
– Desmopressin	
– Fludrocortisone	
Endocrine	
• Thyroid	
– Levothyroxine (3)	
• Diabetes	
– Metformin	
• Steroid	
– Fludrocortisone	POTS
Nervous system	
• Antiemetic	
– Ondansetron	Central fatigue and nausea
– Metoclopramide	
• ANS dysfunction	Low BP and POTS
– Midodrine	
• Antidepressant	
– Fluoxil	
– Fluoxetine	
– SSRI	
– Amitriptyline	Pain relief and sleep
– Duloxetine	Pain relief
– Doxepin	Sleep
• Anticonvulsants	Pain relief
– Gabapentin	
• Parasympathometic	
– Mestinon/pyridostigmine (4)	POTS and fatigue
• Stimulants	Brain fog
– Amphetamine	
– Methylphenidate	

• Muscle relaxants	
– Cyclobenzaprine	Sleep
– Carisoprodol	
Immune system	
• Ampligen (rintatolimod) (5)	
• Immunoglobulins	
Obstetrics and gynaecology	
• Estrogen	
• Progesterone	
Antiviral	
• Paxlovid	
• Acyclovir	
• Amantadine	Central fatigue
Allergies/antihistamine	MCAS
• Phenylephrine	
• Hydrocortisol (6)	
• Cinnarizine	
• Loratadine	
• Fexofenadine	
• Sodium cromoglicate	
• Ketotifen	
• Diphenhydramine	Sleep
• Promethazine	Sleep
Vitamins	
• B12 inj./patches/oral/sublingual (7)	
• B complex (8)	
• Multivitamins	
• Vit D	Muscle pain
• Vit C	
• Folic acid	
Minerals	
• Magnesium (9)	Muscle pain
• Zinc (10) (11)	
• Iron	Fatigue
• Calcium	
Supplements	
• Ubiquinol (reduced CoQ10) (12)	Brain fog and sleep
• Carnitine (13)	Fatigue
• D ribose	
• Omega 3 (14)	
• Melatonin (10)	Sleep disturbances

cont.

Medications	Symptom treated
Other	
• Amino acids – L-lysine	
• Electrolytes	
• Probiotics (15)	
• Antioxidants	
• Glutathione (16)	
• Cannabis	Sleep
• IV Saline (17)	POTS
• Phospholipids (18)	
• Creatine (19)	Post viral fatigue syndrome

References

1. Bolton, M.J., Chapman, B.P. & Van Marwijk, H. (2020) 'Low-dose naltrexone as a treatment for chronic fatigue syndrome.' *BMJ Case Report 13*.
2. Tahir, F., Bin Arif, T., Majid, Z., Ahmed, J. & Khalid, M. (2020) 'Ivabradine in postural orthostatic tachycardia syndrome: a review of the literature.' *Cureus 12*.
3. Ruiz-Núñez, B., Tarasse, R., Vogelaar, E.F., Janneke Dijck-Brouwer, D.A. & Muskiet F.A.J. (2018) 'Higher prevalence of "low T3 syndrome" in patients with chronic fatigue syndrome: a case-control study.' *Frontiers in Endocrinology (Lausanne) 20*.
4. Kawamura, Y., Kihara, M., Nishimoto, K. & Taki, M. (2003) 'Efficacy of a half dose of oral pyridostigmine in the treatment of chronic fatigue syndrome: three case reports.' *Pathophysiology 9*.
5. Strayer, D.R., Carter, W.A., Stouch, B.C., Stevens, S.R., *et al.* (2012) 'A double-blind, placebo-controlled, randomized, clinical trial of the TLR-3 agonist rintatolimod in severe cases of chronic fatigue syndrome.' *PLOS ONE 7*.
6. Cleare, A.J., Heap, E., Malhi, G.S., Wessely, S., O'Keane, V. & Miell, J. (1999) 'Low-dose hydrocortisone in chronic fatigue syndrome: a randomised crossover trial.' *Lancet 353*.
7. van Campen, C.L.M., Riepma, K. & Visser, F.C. (2019) 'Open trial of vitamin B12 nasal drops in adults with myalgic encephalomyelitis/chronic fatigue syndrome: comparison of responders and non-responders.' *Frontiers in Pharmacology 10*.
8. Heap, L.C., Peters, T.J. & Wessely, S. (1999) 'Vitamin B status in patients with chronic fatigue syndrome.' *Journal of the Royal Society of Medicine 92*.
9. Cox, I.M., Campbell, M.J. & Dowson, D. (1991) 'Red blood cell magnesium and chronic fatigue syndrome.' *Lancet 337*.
10. Castro-Marrero, J., Zaragozá, M.C., López-Vílchez, I., Galmés, J.L., *et al.* (2021) 'Effect of melatonin plus zinc supplementation on fatigue perception in myalgic encephalomyelitis/chronic fatigue syndrome: a randomized, double-blind, placebo-controlled trial.' *Antioxidants (Basel) 10*.
11. Maes, M., Mihaylova, I. & De Ruyter, M. (2006) 'Lower serum zinc in chronic fatigue syndrome (CFS): relationships to immune dysfunctions and relevance for the oxidative stress status in CFS.' *Journal of Affective Disorders 90*.
12. Fukuda, S., Nojima, J., Kajimoto, O., Yamaguti, K. *et al.* (2016) 'Ubiquinol-10 supplementation improves autonomic nervous function and cognitive function in chronic fatigue syndrome'. *Biofactors 42*.
13. Reuter, S.E. & Evans, A.M. (2011) 'Long-chain acylcarnitine deficiency in patients with chronic fatigue syndrome: potential involvement of altered carnitine palmitoyltransferase-I activity.' *Journal of Internal Medicine 270*.

14. Castro-Marrero, J., Zaragozá, M.C., Domingo, J.C., Martinez-Martinez, A., Alegre, J. & von Schacky, C. (2018) 'Low omega-3 index and polyunsaturated fatty acid status in patients with chronic fatigue syndrome/myalgic encephalomyelitis.' *Prostaglandins Leukot Essent Fatty Acids 139.*

15. Roman, P., Carrillo-Trabalón, F., Sánchez-Labraca, N., Cañadas, F., Estévez, A.F. & Cardona, D. (2018) 'Are probiotic treatments useful on fibromyalgia syndrome or chronic fatigue syndrome patients? A systematic review.' *Beneficial Microbes 9.*

16. Godlewska, B.R., Williams, S., Emir, U.E., Chen, C., *et al.* (2022) 'Neurochemical abnormalities in chronic fatigue syndrome: a pilot magnetic resonance spectroscopy study at 7 Tesla.' *Psychopharmacology (Berl) 239.*

17. Ruzieh, M., Baugh, A., Dasa, O., Parker, R.L., *et al.* (2017) 'Effects of intermittent intravenous saline infusions in patients with medication-refractory postural tachycardia syndrome.' *Journal of Interventional Cardiac Electrophysiology 48.*

18. Nicolson, G.L. (2014) 'Mitochondrial dysfunction and chronic disease: treatment with natural supplements.' *Integrated Medicine (Encinitas) 13.*

19. Ostojic, S.M. (2021) 'Diagnostic and pharmacological potency of creatine in post-viral fatigue syndrome.' *Nutrients 13.*

Subject Index

Author Index

Note markers are indicated with the letter 'n'.